#1402-1338 W. Broadway
Vanc. BC
V6H 1H2.
604-738-7710

The Clinical Applications for the Er,Cr:YSGG Laser System

An Atlas by Dr. William H. Chen

Library of Congress Control Number: 2008939504
ISBN: 978-09822073-0-7

Table of Contents

Preface

No significant new modality has been introduced in the field of dentistry since the use of the belt-driven hand piece gave way to the use of the air-turbine hand piece. The technique of air-abrasion was introduced in the fifties and again in the nineties, and yet it could not overtake the popularity of the air-turbine hand piece. The use of lasers in dentistry has the potential to provide groundbreaking changes in the field of dentistry. Especially during the last decade, the Er,Cr:YSGG (erbium, chromium, yttrium, scandium, gallium and garnet) laser system has developed into a very versatile modality. Its applicability to a variety of tissues (i.e., tooth, gingival, mucogingival, tongue, lip and bone tissues), and the fact that Er,Cr:YSGG procedures provide more comfort to patients during and after the completion of procedures attracts clinicians to the use of the laser system. It seems we have another significant change in dentistry at hand.

I have been fortunate to use all three models of the Er,Cr:YSGG laser – from the Millennium® system in 1999 to the newest version, the Waterlase MD™ laser system. Beyond the "wow" factor of laser dentistry, beyond the hype, is a simple fact: lasers hurt less. They cause less post-operative discomfort. They don't sound like drills. Anything that takes patients' minds off the sounds and feelings they associate with pain is a benefit to our profession and to the public in general. Even though links between oral health and systemic health are well-known, the average American patient would rather be anywhere other than at the dentist's office. And we all understand why – those necessary twin evils of the bur and the needle keep half of our potential patient base away.

By using the Er,Cr:YSGG, many procedures can be performed without using injection anesthesia and without causing pain and distress to the patient. These procedures include all classes of cavity preparations, gingivectomies, crown lengthening procedures, biopsies, frenectomies, laser-assisted periodontal therapy, uncovering implant healing caps, deciduous tooth pulpotomies, extraction of loose deciduous teeth, and very selective cases of laser-assisted root canal therapy. The phenomenon of how the laser works without causing significant pain to the patient has still not been thoroughly explained. However, effort is under way to investigate the science on this subject. Some explanations are discussed in the chapter on Laser Analgesia. The hypothesis involves starting the procedure with a form of low level laser therapy ("LLLT"), which is utilized to pre-condition the tissue before ablation takes place. LLLT has the capabilities of causing pain reduction, anti-inflammatory action and better and faster healing. In the chapter on Laser Analgesia, the enzymatic, chemical and physical effect on laser analgesia is discussed.

It is true that the dental laser is not yet a complete replacement for the dental drill, and will not always replace injectable anesthetic. On the other hand, I have found it possible to avoid using the high-speed drill or injectable anesthetic altogether in almost all cases; there remain a handful of procedures where the old technology is entirely appropriate. Beyond that, and with applicable training, the laser enables a practicing dentist to safely perform many procedures – operative, periodontal, endodontic, or oral surgical – that they may otherwise have referred out to another dentist. In writing this book, I hope to provide you with suggested techniques for achieving success with your laser system. Congratulations, and I hope your purchase was as life-changing for you as it was for me.

To my staff and associates, I offer gratitude for their hard work, patience and support, especially the many hours of video taping, photographing and organizing laser procedures. Without their contribution of time and effort in this project, the book could not have been written. I wish to thank the following individuals:

Bethann Autery, for her computer work in editing and organizing countless clinical cases for the book.

Melissa Meyer, my chief dental nurse, for her dedication and hard work in helping me with the recording and organizing the laser procedures.

Crissy French, Amanda Rall, Kristina Wolfe and Melissa Pryor for their team work with Melissa Meyer.

Linda Knobeloch and Tina Autery, for their teamwork of managing and coordinating schedules for our documentation of the clinical cases.

Joni Blus and Sarah Fultz, my dental hygienists, for their contribution in patient education and selection for our documentation.

Dr Angelina Fu, for her contribution in some of the art work.

Dr. Charles Lockhart, for helping me at my practice for a duration of time to allow me being out my practice to teach, train and educate colleagues on laser dentistry and for being my best friend and colleague who has been encouraging me to finish this book.

My gratitude also goes to **Ioana Rizoiu**, VP of Biolase® Research and Development, **Dmitri Boutoussov**, VP of Biolase Engineering for recruiting me to be involved with clinical laser research. I am very appreciative of their support, encouragement and advice on the clinical applications of the Er,Cr:YSGG.

Most importantly, I want to mention that my authoring of this book could not have been possible without the support, love, patience and understanding of my wife, Alison, and daughters Audrey and Bianca.

Introduction

I have a deep and abiding passion for the use of lasers in dentistry, and see a very bright future for lasers in dentistry and surgery. As a clinical trainer for the Er,Cr:YSGG laser system since 2000, I have taught laser dentistry to clinicians all over the world, and have conducted numerous studies at my dental office and in conjunction with other dentists showing the benefits of the system.

Pain Management and the Four Warmups

One well-known concept which I have successfully turned into a technique over the past several years is 'Low Level Laser Therapy' and the inducement of an analgesic effect using Er,Cr:YSGG laser on the tooth by utilization of subablative levels of laser energy. Beyond LLLT, understanding patients' pain tolerance has resulted in the development of different techniques in patient management during the laser procedure to attain a higher percentage of success in delivering comfortable laser dentistry. In general, I divide patients into five categories of pain tolerance:

1. Patients who are most tolerant to pain
3. Patients who are moderately tolerant to pain
5. Patients who are least tolerant to pain
Categories 2 and 4 fall between categories 1, 3 and 5

Different techniques should be considered for different category of patients, and will be discussed at greater le ngth in the chapter on Laser Analgesia. Ultimately, the technique that is selected is based on recognizing a given individual patient's tolerance to pain. Consideration should be given to the fact that lower laser sound to start the procedure could serve the purpose of "warming up" the least tolerant patient to painless dentistry. The low sound and low power setting is more patient friendly.

In my courses and training programs, I have talked about the Four Warm-Ups in my philosophy of gentle laser dentistry. The Four Warm-Ups are as follows:

1. The Patient Warm-Up:
 Using low power and low sound laser to start a procedure, it is more likely that the patient will not complain about any discomfort. The comfortable start will give the patient the confidence that the procedure will be pain-free. The use of the LLLT could precondition the tissue, providing an analgesic effect, before a higher power is used to ablate the tissue.

2. The ToothWarm-Up:
 When lower power is applied to the tissue, not much ablation can be witnessed. However, the tissue is affected by this low power of laser energy. There is a softening effect on the tissue. Increase the level of power in gradual increments. The composition of teeth and gingival may differ from patient to patient. Some may have softer teeth than others. The gradual increase in power will allow the operator to use

the least amount of laser energy to ablate the most tenacious enamel. Once the power setting has reached the stage where it can ablate the enamel, one can stop selecting higher power settings – reducing and minimizing pain or discomfort to the patient, and consequently giving the patient a positive attitude towards laser dentistry.

3. The Doctor Warm-Up:

Starting at a lower power setting allows the doctor focus on aiming the laser energy at the target tissue. In the non-contact mode of laser energy, this is a beneficial approach. Minimally invasive dentistry is heavily promoted among laser users. The low power start gives the operator a chance to not make the mistake in cutting more tissues than one has planned.

4. The Laser Warm-Up:

Using low power to start the procedure will allow time for the laser energy to be transmitted in full efficiency when the power adjustment has reached the ablation rate.

These "Four Warm-ups" are rationales for choosing lower power to start a procedure. In addition, during a patient's first experience with laser dentistry, I prefer to start on a cavity of a smaller lesion rather than a deeper lesion, as there is less chance of giving the patient a negative experience with the treatment of the shallower cavity preparation. A positive experience will give the patient a sense of confidence. This is huge in creating the mind-set in the patient that laser dentistry can be painless. I believe that confidence builds success.

Time Management

Keeping track of time can be an art if you do not want to engage in using a stop watch. You could count "by heart". My usual counting is about 2 counts to a second. In other words, the time that takes me to count from 1 to 60 is about 30 seconds. However, the rate of counting may differ on a given day. If you are happy and excited, there is a tendency to count a little faster. Calibrating yourself in counting at the beginning of the day will give you a good guideline in the accuracy of counting "by heart". A perfectly acceptable alternative is to have your assistant keep track of time, but please note that techniques described in this text often involve using a particular setting for a duration of time, and frequent changes to settings in between.

One may argue that it takes too long to change settings several times. As I estimate it, since most procedures do not require injection, by using the laser we actually reduce the duration of each patient's appointment by a minimum of 7-15 minutes. For example, if a procedure would ordinarily require the use of topical anesthesia gel, it would take approximately 15 minutes to give an injection and wait for the local anesthesia to take effect. The time saved here more than makes up for the time used to perform the laser procedure. Any setting changes and the use of lower power to apply the "Four Warm-ups", which typically only takes a few minutes, can be administered without much stress. Furthermore, each time the setting is changed, the patient has a chance to relax and avoid straining the facial muscles.

Words I often use to describe laser dentistry are "no shot" and "no pain", which conveniently rhyme with "no stress" and "no strain". I have noticed over the past nine years of utilizing Er,Cr:YSGG lasers daily in my practice, that my philosophy about comfort laser dentistry usually results in shorter appointments with no post-operative dysfunction such as numbness in the lip, face or tongue from injectable anesthetic, and a lesser chance for sore muscles to develop from keeping the patient's mouth open too long during the appointment.

The intent of this book is not to replace any training exercise. Correct use of the Er,Cr:YSGG laser system does require that you advance along a fairly steep learning curve, since use of the laser can seem counter-intuitive when compared to use of the dental drill. There is much in this book for a novice laser user, but I also strongly emphasize extensive training alongside it.

This textbook will show, in some detail, my techniques for using the Er,Cr:YSGG laser system and avoiding the high-speed drill and the needle. These techniques have been gathered and refined through experience over the years and have served me well; I trust they will do the same for you.

EXPLANATION OF LASER SETTINGS AND TERMS

End-firing: Typically, the Er,Cr:YSGG laser system cuts away from the distal end of the fiber optic tip in the handpiece – compared to the drill, which is held laterally against tissue to achieve cutting (side-cutting). This is the first and most important distinction between lasers and high speed drill.

Focused mode: For hard tissue applications, because the Er,Cr:YSGG laser system wavelength is highly absorbed in water, and water is used as an integral part of the cutting process, the Er,Cr:YSGG laser system has a limited range of cutting. Optimal cutting is best achieved with a 1-2mm distance between the distal end of the fiber optic tip and the tissue being ablated. This distance is generally referred to as 'focused mode'.

Defocused mode: If the distance between the distal end of the fiber optic tip and the tissue increased beyond 2mm, a decrease in cutting speed will be observed. Typically, the laser will not ablate tissue when the distance between tip and tissue is above 5mm, and except where otherwise specified, 'defocused mode' generally means that distance between 2-5mm.

Watts A unit of power; the expression of energy over time. The Er,Cr:YSGG laser system has a maximum power output of 300 millijoules per pulse; if you fired one pulse, that would be expressed as 0.3 Watts; ten pulses would be expressed as 3 Watts, twenty pulses as 6 Watts, and so on. Throughout this book, 'Watts' shall be abbreviated to 'W'.

Hertz (Hz): The rate of fire of laser pulses per second. The older model Er,Cr:YSGG laser systems have a fixed Hertz setting of 20 pulses per second. The Hertz rate in the new models can be varied from 10-50 pulses per second, in 5 Hz increments. Throughout this book, "Hertz" shall be abbreviated to "Hz".

Air/Water The Er,Cr:YSGG laser system allows for user control of the air and water outputs. In practice, the actual quantity of air and water may vary between units (different models of the same device can have different air/water output ratios, for instance). Relative % is used to control output through the main display.

H / S Mode A feature of the Waterlase MD Er,Cr:YSGG system allows the user to switch between H (Hard Tissue) and S (Soft Tissue) modes. S mode is useful for several soft tissue applications and the differences between the two are explained later in this chapter. Please note that unless S mode is specifically stated for a given set of parameters, all parameters described herein use H mode on the Waterlase MD.

Er,Cr:YSGG Laser System

An Introduction to Er,Cr;YSGG Laser Systems

The first Er,Cr:YSGG system developed for dental purposes in the United States was the original Elmer model produced by Biolase® Technology. Originally cleared for soft tissue indications in August 1995, hard tissue indications – including cavity preparations – came in October 1998. Since that time, Biolase has increased the laser's capabilities to perform periodontal procedures (July 2001 and January 2004), endodontic procedures (January 2002 and February 2003) and bone ablation (February 2002). To date, Biolase Technology has obtained the only hard tissue clearance for Er,Cr:YSGG laser systems.

Several different models – three of them significantly different – have been developed over the years. The first model produced and sold in the United States was the Millennium®. The second model was the 'Millennium II', which came to be known as the Waterlase® Millennium and finally the Waterlase. Both models employed essentially the same concept and design; the second benefited from advances in laser technology and was considerably lighter and more user-friendly.

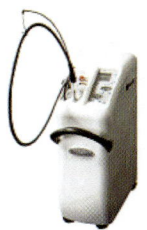

Series two, also known as the Millennium II, Waterlase Millennium, or simply, Waterlase.

The third series, the Waterlase MD™, incorporates the same conceptual design but with significantly enhanced functionality. Throughout this text, "Other Er,Cr:YSGG systems" refer to the first and second models of Er,Cr:YSGG models produced by Biolase Technology. Because of enhancements to the air/water spray, trunk fiber and handpiece, the Waterlase MD typically requires different settings to accomplish the same tasks.

Waterlase MD

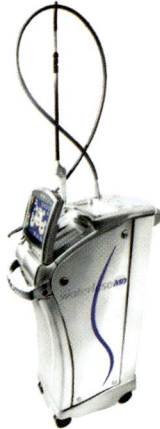

*Series three, the
Waterlase MD.*

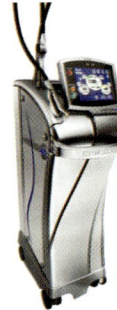

Er,Cr:YSGG Laser Technology

Laser Specifications

One common feature of all the Er,Cr:YSGG laser systems referred to are the laser parameters. The systems all operate at a wavelength of 2.78 microns, have a pulse width of 140 microseconds, and laser energy fires 20 times per second (20 Hz).

Functionality

The Waterlase MD has additional functionality settings that allow the pulse width to be increased (in the "S" mode) to about 700 microseconds, and modify the number of times the laser may fire per second (from 10 – 50 times per second, or 10-50Hz).

Although the shorter pulse width ("H" mode in the Waterlase MD) works for both hard and soft tissue applications, the S mode should only be used on soft tissue, never on or near hard tissue structures. The longer pulse width in the S mode allows for deposition of energy over a longer period of time, and consequently results in more heat being generated at the target tissue site. While ideal for hemostasis and ablation of soft tissue, this can cause charring and burning in bone or tooth tissue if the laser is improperly used.

The variability in Hz in the Waterlase MD allows greater amounts of power to be used than in earlier systems. Up to 8 Watts of power can be used with the Waterlase MD, compared to 6 Watts for the others. However, higher power is not the only benefit of a higher pulse rate. For soft tissue applications, higher pulse rates are useful for accuracy and cleanliness of incisions. For desensitization of teeth – as will be described later – the higher pulse rates result in lower power density, optimal for Low Level Laser Therapy.

Accessories

In all models, the laser energy is delivered from the Er,Cr:YSGG crystal through a trunk fiber approximately 2 meters long. The long, gray tube also contains the air and water lines that deliver the atomized air/water spray through the handpiece. The trunk fiber is extremely fragile and care should always be taken in its handling; avoid excessive twisting or bending, as well as contact against hard surfaces. Properly handled, your trunk fiber will not degrade or burn out, but is fragile and easy to damage.

All models are accompanied by two types of handpieces. The first and second models have a standard-issue 90-degree handpiece which directs laser energy from the trunk fiber through the fiber tips that connect, in turn, to it. An internal mirror reflects and refocuses light from the trunk fiber into the rear of the fiber tip. With the Waterlase MD, the standard-issue handpiece is a contra-angle 70-degree handpiece; it utilizes a slightly different mirror design but the essential concept remains the same. All models also have a straight handpiece which eliminates the head, the angulation of the tip, and the internal mirror. The straight handpiece is primarily useful for oral surgical applications.

Additionally, Biolase Technology has recently developed a new handpiece design for the Waterlase MD. Incorporating a more efficient mirror design, the new handpiece promises greater cutting efficiency and a lower risk of burning out tips. Specific settings for this new design will be addressed in a separate chapter towards the end of the book.

User Controls

The user controls for the Er,Cr:YSGG laser systems have expanded and improved with the changes to the models over the years – from a relatively crude LED display on the original Millennium, to the touch-screen available for the Waterlase MD. All of the controls have common elements:

Power Setting

The power setting may be increased or decreased in 0.25 Watt increments by simply pressing the + or – button. The maximum power output is 300mJ per pulse; on the first two Er,Cr:YSGG models, which had a pulse rate of 20Hz, that equated to 6 Watts. On the Waterlase MD, the maximum power output is set at 8 Watts; the highest power output based on mJ/pulse is 7.5W and 25 Hz.

Air/Water Settings

Both air and water rates are expressed as a % on the screen. A 0% water setting means no water will exit the handpiece on firing the laser. A 100% water setting means as much water as possible will exit the handpiece. When combined with the air setting, an air/water spray is formed.

The %'s do not represent an actual volume, and may in fact differ between units. Because both the air and water are competing for space in exiting the narrow exit apertures from the handpiece, each setting should be considered relative to the other. In fact, the largest volume of water will not be achieved by a 100% Air / 100% Water setting.

Preset Settings

Each model allows for preset settings – predetermined combinations of Power, Air and Water settings (and, with the Waterlase MD, Rep Rate and Pulse Width). The first two models only have the capability for 4 presets each, while the Waterlase MD allows for up to 16 presets.

Rep Rate/Hz (Waterlase MD only)

The first two Er,Cr:YSGG models utilize a standard 20Hz. The Waterlase MD allows the user to modify the pulse rate from 10 – 50 Hz in 5 Hz increments. As you will see throughout this text, I have found certain pulse rates to have certain applications.

Pulse Width (Waterlase MD only)

The Waterlase MD allows the ability to change between a short ("H", for hard tissue) and long ("S", for soft tissue) mode. The short pulse, 140 microseconds in length, is the same pulse width used in all previous models and is ideally suited for any type of ablation of hard or soft tissues. The long pulse, 700 microseconds in length, is ideal for certain soft tissue applications but should not be used for any hard tissue ablation at all.

Er,Cr:YSGG Fiber Tips

Before introducing the fiber tips that are available with the Er,Cr:YSGG laser system, I want to review some important background information concerning the understanding of power density.

Power density means the amount of actual energy that is absorbed into any given target tissue that lies within the laser's area of effect.

Power density is affected, therefore, by the following five factors:

1) Starting power

   For any given pulse repetition rate (Hz), the <u>higher</u> the power, the <u>higher</u> the power density will be.

2) Pulse repetition rate (Hz)

For any given power setting, the <u>higher</u> the number of pulses per second, the <u>lower</u> the power density will be.

3) Diameter of the tip

The <u>wider</u> the tip diameter, the <u>lower</u> the power density.

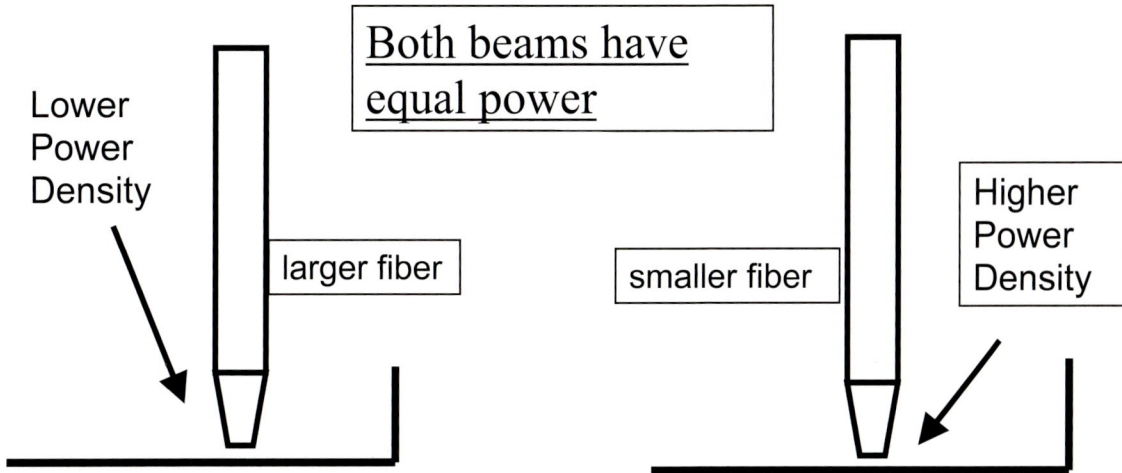

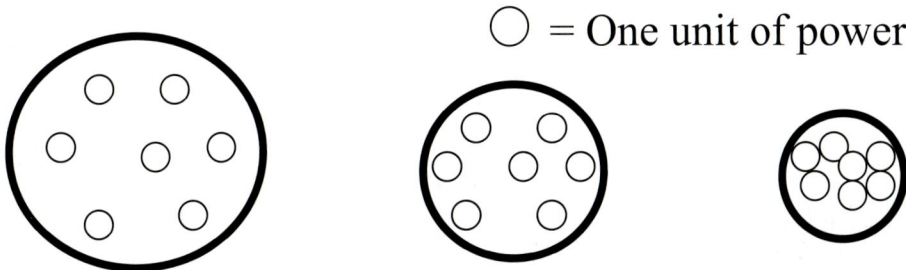

Lower Power Density

Both beams have equal power

larger fiber

smaller fiber

Higher Power Density

◯ = One unit of power

The smaller the diameter of the fiber, the more power per square centimeter.

4) Distance to tissue

Because there is some divergence of the laser beam from the fiber tip, then the <u>further</u> the distance between the tip and the tissue is, the <u>lower</u> the power density and the larger the beam size interacting with the tissue will be.

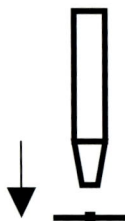

1. Focused – Shorter distance to tissue, higher power density

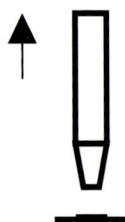

2. Defocused – Longer distance to tissue, lower power density

5) <u>Interference between the tip and tissue</u>

The Er,Cr:YSGG laser is typically used with an air/water spray. Because the laser energy is highly absorbed in water, the <u>higher</u> the levels of water spray, the more laser energy will be absorbed prior to contacting the tissue, and the <u>lower</u> the power density of laser energy interacting with the tissue.

While the exact numbers related to power density are almost impossible to quantify given all the factors listed above, they can be generally known and understood, and all settings suggested in this Atlas have been developed with these five factors in mind.

You should also consider the following when utilizing your Er,Cr:YSGG laser:
1. The laser fiber tip delivers energy mostly linearly past the end of the tip. While there may be some divergence, there is no sideways firing from standard operative tips.
2. The tip should be aimed perpendicular (90 degrees) to the target tissue for analgesia, but angled towards tissue for faster cutting.
3. Unless otherwise suggested or recommended, the tip should be moved slowly around target tissue. Faster movements will generally result in slower ablation rate, which may in specific circumstances be desirable.
4. For most effective cutting, the tip should be placed approximately 1-2mm from the target tissue in a "focused" mode.
5. When the tip is moved further away from the target tissue (2-5mm), less energy will be applied to the target (see information above on power density).
6. Beyond 5mm, no ablation should be observed.

Description of Tips for the Waterlase MD

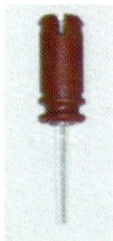

G- and MG-series tips are 750μm tips that taper to a 600μm diameter at the exit and are considered the 'work horses' for most hard and soft tissue procedures. The hotspot of these two fiber tips lie in the center of the beam. These tips are ideal for Class I – V cavity preparations, caries removal, etching of the enamel, root canal access opening, pocket reduction, gingivoplasty, operculectomy, frenectomy and excision of soft tissue lesions.

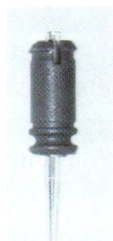

MG4 fiber tip

The MT-4 is a 750μm diameter tip that tapers to 400μm at the exit. This fiber tip can be used in incision for a flap, in breaking tenacious enamel in posterior teeth, crown troughing, retrofill preparation/apicoectomy, complete excavation of pits and fissures for placement of sealants and removal of incipient caries, as well as any refined procedure that requires more precision and smaller diameter of ablation.

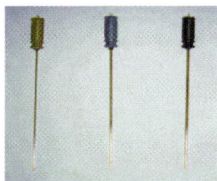

MT-4 fiber tip

Z- and MZ-series fiber tips (Z2, Z3 and Z4: 200, 300 and 400μm diameter tips respectively) are mainly used in laser endodontics and periodontics, as well as extraction of loose teeth without anesthesia and crown lengthening. The hot spot for any of these tips is somewhat centered, but the radiation is mostly evenly distributed over the beam.

MZ-2, MZ-3 and MZ-4 tips

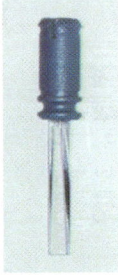

MC-3 fiber tip

C3 is a rectangular-shaped ("chisel") tip 300µm thick by 1200µm wide. This tip can be used for crown and veneer preparations, soft tissue surgery such as frenectomy, gingivectomy and operculectomy, and hard tissue preparations such as osteoplasty and torus removal. At the chisel end, the hot spot is in the center but radiates out to the periphery. At the bevel of the flat side, the energy is lower but is distributed more evenly along the flat side with a side-firing effect.

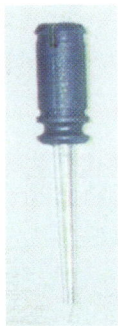

MC-6 Fiber Tip

C6 is a 1200µm tip that tapers down to a 600µm diameter end; can be used for the same applications as the MG4/MG6 tips. The hot spot is in the periphery of the diameter, which makes this tip very attractive for soft tissue applications.

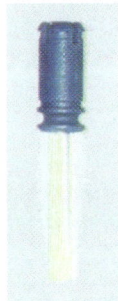

MC-12 Fiber Tip

C12 is a 1200µm diameter cylindrical tip that can be used to apply laser energy to a large surgical site. Particularly effective for aphthous ulcer therapy and desensitizing teeth. What little hot spot there is, lies within the very center of the beam but most laser energy is well distributed across the entire beam.

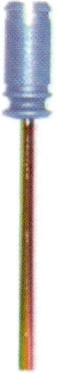

Z6 is a 600μm diameter tip made of quartz. The tip can be used in bony crown lengthening and all soft tissue applications that are suitable for an MG4 or MG6. Like the C12, the hot spot is in the center but most laser energy is well distributed over the entire beam.

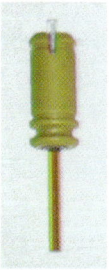

MZ6 fiber tip

Z5 is a 500μm diameter tip made of quartz. The tip is designed for optimal general usage, but has a shorter useful life than other tips. Like the C12, the hot spot is in the center but most laser energy is well distributed over the entire beam.

MZ-5 Fiber tip

Laser Analgesia

Introduction

A few studies have been done with different wavelengths (diode, Nd:YAG) to show the effectiveness of pain attenuation through low level laser therapy ("LLLT"). In vivo laboratory studies were performed on rats to study the use of a diode laser and the effect of LLLT irradiation of the trigeminal caudal neurons by tooth pulp stimulation. The evoked potential was recorded by electrodes inserted in the trigeminal subnucleus candalis and tooth pulp stimuli. The conclusion of this study was that LLLT could suppress the excitation of unmyelinated C-fiber afferents of the pulp.

Another experiment was performed on conscious rabbits to study somatosensory evoked potential by electro-acupuncture and low power laser stimulation. The results in the study showed decrease in mean peak amplitude in the evoked potential when electro-acupuncture was applied. This showed pain attenuation following stimulation. The study was repeated by substituting low power laser diode irradiation to achieve a LLLT effect. A similar result from the recordings of the evoked potential to show pain attenuation by the low laser irradiation is obtained. In the conclusion, the author hypothesized that pain is primarily a perceptual experience that is characterized by motivational-emotional arousal and cognitive judgments, and that it had been demonstrated that LLLT caused the release of beta-endorphins from the mid-brain neurons, activating serotonergic descending fibers which through a relay of influence inhibits ascending pain messages. It had been suggested that LLLT irradiation activates similar descending pain inhibitory pathways.

There are few studies conducted with the Er,Cr:YSGG laser system that specifically address reduced pain through LLLT. However, the fact remains that numerous Er,Cr:YSGG laser system practitioners, myself included, have been successful in performing a variety of hard and soft procedures without the application of local analgesia, and do not cause pain and discomfort to the patients. These include all classes of cavity preparation, soft tissue procedures, some veneer and crown preparations, pedodontic, endodontic, periodontic and even some oral surgery. These are evidence-based experiences that have not been formally studied and are not yet published. It leads us to believe there is laser analgesia in the use of the Er,Cr:YSGG laser system.

Professor Andreas Moritz's "Oral Laser Application" (Quintessence Book 2006), cited "the use of LLLT to achieve an analgesic effect in the dental pulp prior to restorative procedures", stating that the clinical use of "pre-emptive laser analgesia" is becoming more widespread now as a clinical technique with Er:YAG and Er,Cr:YSGG lasers. When operated at pulse rates between 15 and 20 Hz, the pulse energies below the ablation threshold of tooth structure, the low level laser energy penetrates into the tooth, and is directed along hydroxyapatite crystals (which function like waveguides) towards the elevated pulp. Here, the pulses of energy coincide with the natural by a resonance frequency of Type C and other nerve fibers in the dental pulp. The action of this type of LLLT is to cause a reduction in the action of Na-K pump in the cell membrane, resulting in a loss of impulse conduction, and this is an analgesic effect.

In my experience with laser systems, I have determined techniques to treat even very sensitive patients. The following sections describe each technique and when they should be applied.

Technique 1: For Patients with Low Tolerance (Apprehensive Adult Patients)

Class I and Class II Preparation

Low laser power is used to start the preparation. The sound of laser energy applied to the molar is less irritating when the energy is lower. After the low-level laser has been used to precondition the pulp, gradual higher power is used to ablate the enamel. Once ablation has reached the dentin, the laser power is reduced to ablate dentin. Even lower laser power is used to finish cleaning and etching the cavity. This technique is described as the "Turtle Technique".

For the Er,Cr:YSGG laser system Waterlase MD, the recommended settings are:

2.00W, 30 Hz, 60% Water, 80% Air, 30 seconds

3.00W, 30 Hz, 60% Water, 80% Air, 30 seconds

4.50W, 30 Hz, 60% Water, 80% Air, 30 seconds

6.00W, 30 Hz, 60% Water, 80% Air, 30 seconds

7.50W, 30 Hz, 60% Water, 80% Air, until enamel ablation is complete

3.00W, 30 Hz, 60% Water, 80% Air, for caries removal

2.00W, 30 Hz, 60% Water, 80% Air, to finish

For the Er,Cr:YSGG laser system (model: Millennium Waterlase, Millennium 2, Waterlase), the recommended settings are:

1.25W, 15% Water, 15% Air, 30 seconds

2.00W, 30% Water, 30% Air, 30 seconds

4.00W, 60% Water, 65% Air, 30 seconds

5.50-6.00W, 75% Water, 90% Air until enamel ablation is complete

2.00W, 30% Water, 30% Air until caries removal is finished

If it were expressed in graph form, the overall power delivered to the patient over time might look as follows:

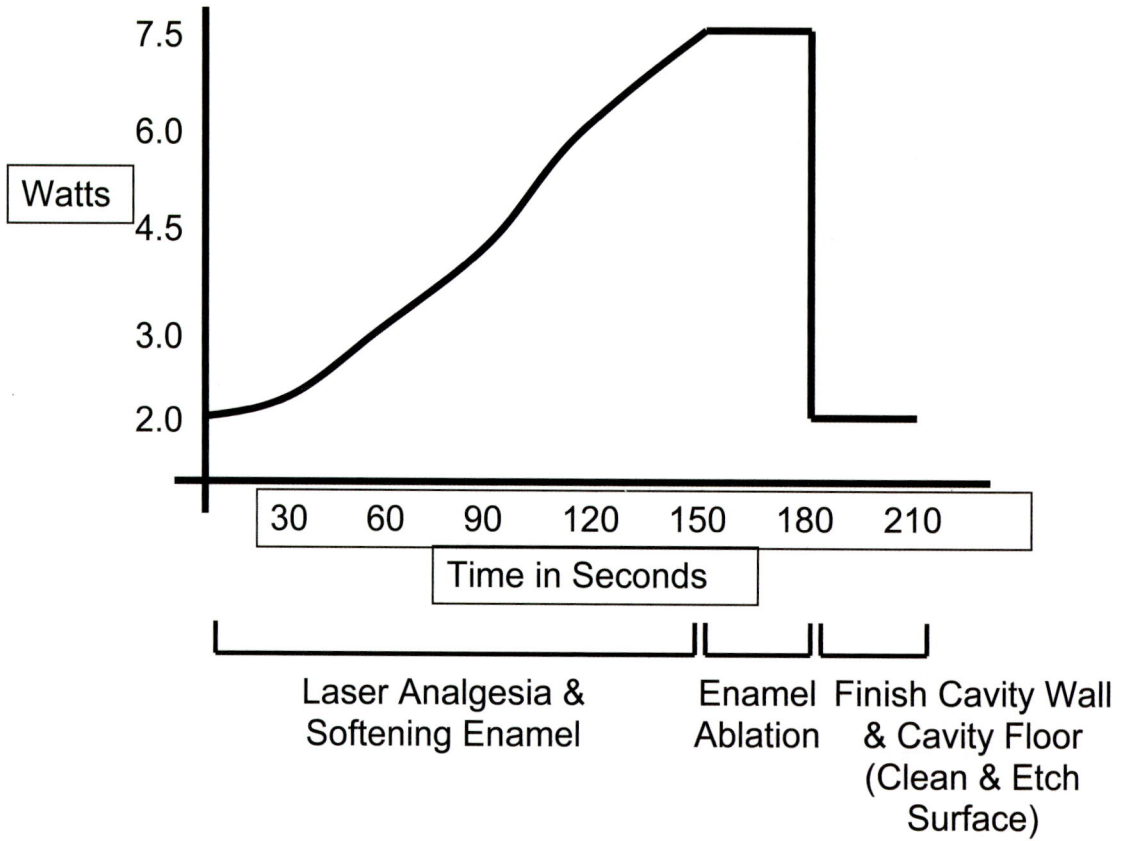

Laser Analgesia & Softening Enamel

Enamel Ablation

Finish Cavity Wall & Cavity Floor (Clean & Etch Surface)

Case 1: For patient with Low Tolerance (Apprehensive Adult Patient , Permanent Molar, Class I)

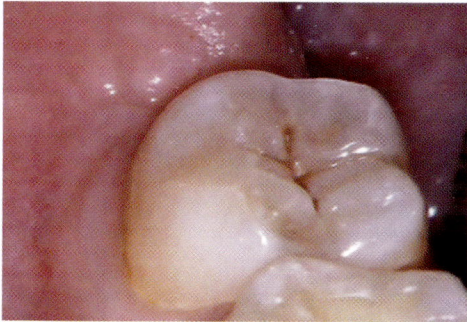

Fig. 1: Pre-op. An occlusal caries is noted in mandibular right 2nd molar.

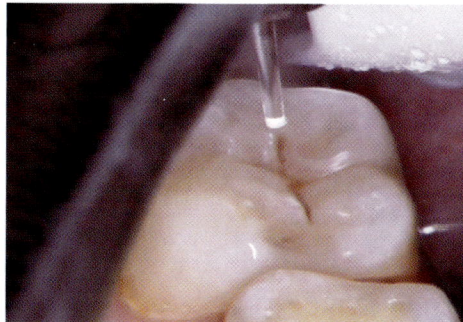

Fig. 2: A MG-6 tip is focused at 1-2mm aiming at the fossa. The setting is 2.00W, 60% Water, 80% Air, 30 Hz.

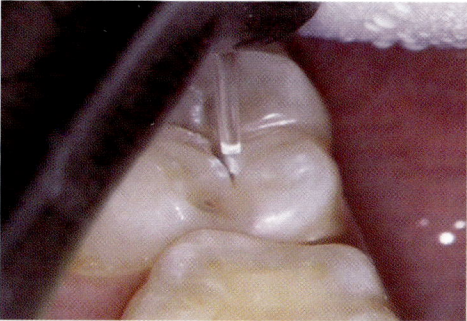

Fig. 3: The setting is 3.00W, 60% Water, 80% Air, 30 Hz.

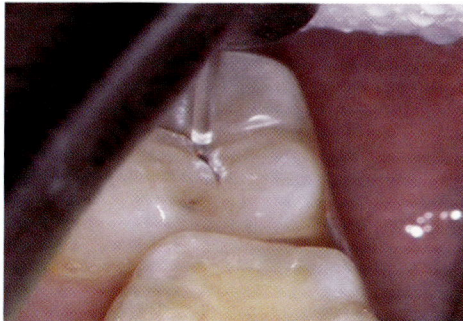

Fig. 4: The setting is 4.50W, 60% Water, 80% Air, 30 Hz.

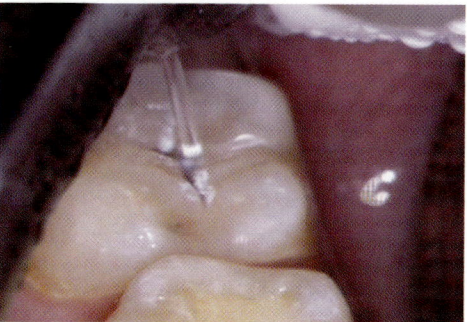

Fig. 5: The setting is 6.00W, 60% Water, 80% Air, 30 Hz. The tip is focused and angled to aim at extending the border of the preparation on one side.

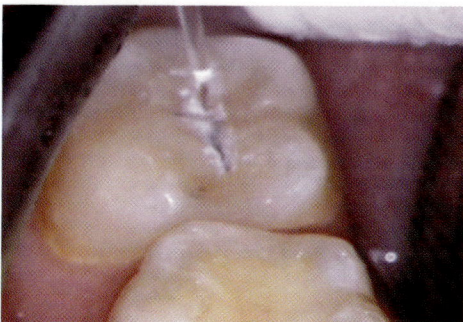

Fig. 6: The setting is 7.50W, 60% Water, 80% Air, 30 Hz. The tip is focused and angled to aim at extending the other border of the preparation.

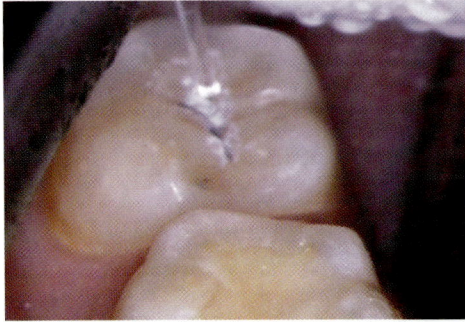

Fig. 7: The tip is focused and aimed to ablate the pulpal floor.

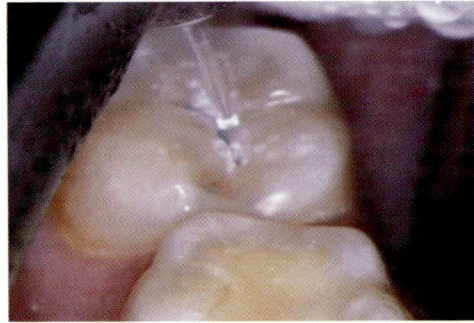

Fig. 8: The tip is focused and angled at tubules exposed under the margin of the prep.

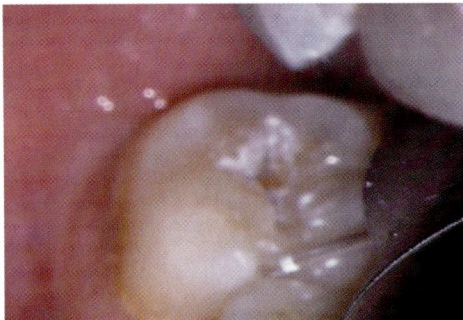

Fig. 9: With sides of tubules exposed, caries removal and dentin preparation is performed more rapidly.

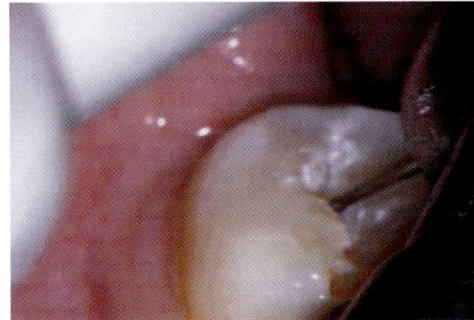

Fig. 10: A slow speed round bur is used to remove and check caries.

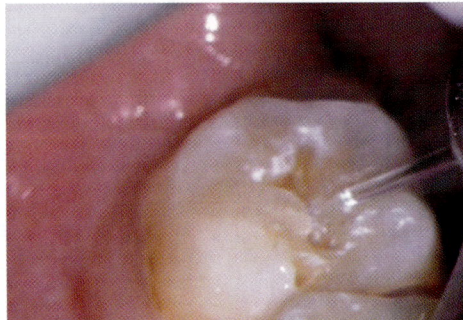

Fig. 11: The setting is 2.00W, 60% Water, 80% Air, 30 Hz. Laser energy is used to remove smear, debris, and finish the preparation.

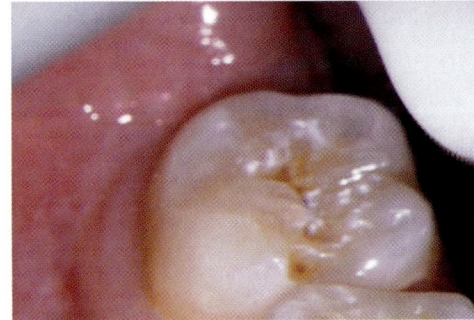

Fig. 12: The Class I preparation is complete.

Technique 2: For Patients with Low Tolerance (Apprehensive Adult and Pedo Patients)

Bicuspid and Deciduous Molar Preparation

The approach here is similar to the one used in Technique One. The difference is that a lower maximum laser power is needed to ablate enamel. This technique is also described as the "Turtle Technique".

For the Er,Cr:YSGG laser system Waterlase MD, the recommended settings are:

> 2.00W, 30 Hz, 60% Water, 80% Air, 30 seconds

> 3.00W, 30 Hz, 60% Water, 80% Air, 30 seconds

> 4.50W, 30 Hz, 60% Water, 80% Air until enamel ablation is complete

> 2.00W, 30 Hz, 60% Water, 80% Air to finish

For the Er,Cr:YSGG laser system (model: Millennium Waterlase, Millennium 2, Waterlase), the recommended settings are:

> 1.25W, 15% Water, 15% Air, 30 seconds

> 2.00W, 30% Water, 30% Air, 30 seconds

> 4.00W, 60% Water, 65% Air until enamel ablation is complete

> 2.00W, 30% Water, 30% Air to finish

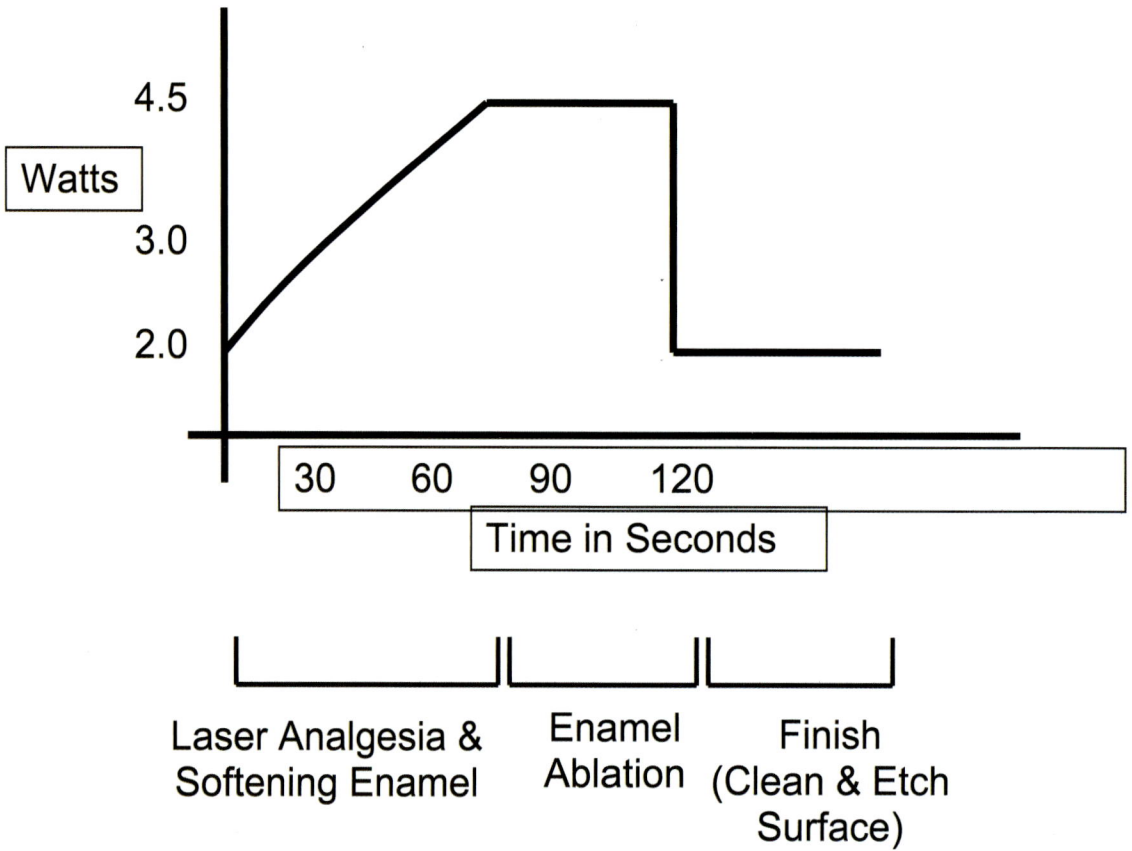

Watts

4.5

3.0

2.0

30   60   90   120

Time in Seconds

Laser Analgesia &   Enamel   Finish
Softening Enamel   Ablation   (Clean & Etch
                                        Surface)

Case 1: For patient with Low Tolerance (Permanent Bicuspid, Class I)

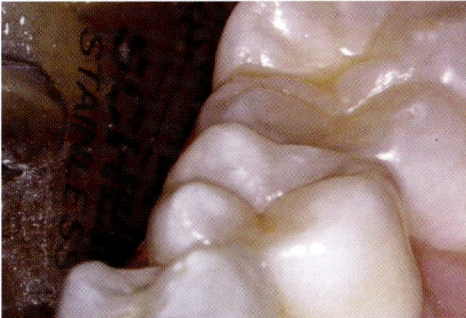

Fig. 1: Pre-op. An occlusal caries is noted at left mandibular 1st premolar.

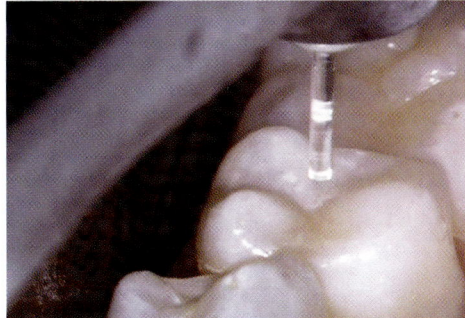

Fig. 2: A MG-6 tip is focused and aimed at the fossa. The setting is 2.00W, 60% Water, 80% Air, 30 Hz.

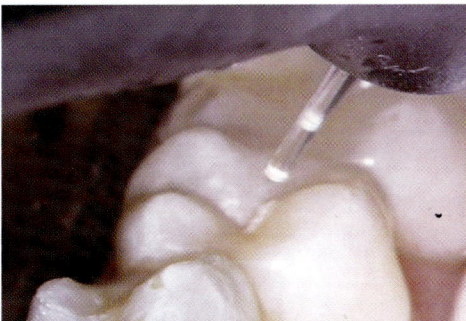

Fig. 3: The tip is focused and angled aiming at the border of caries on one side. The setting is 4.50W, 60% Water, 80% Air, 30 Hz.

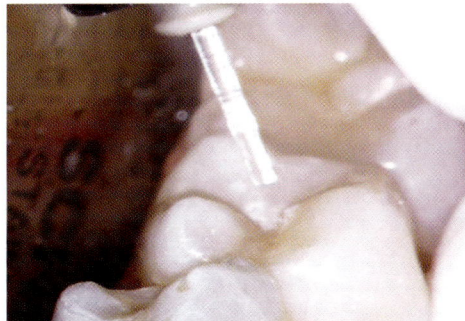

Fig. 4: The tip is focused and angled, aiming at the other border of caries. The setting is 4.50W, 60% Water, 80% Air, 30 Hz.

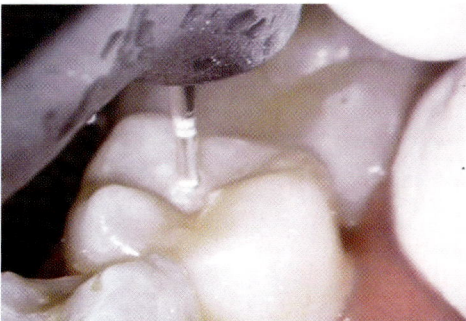

Fig. 5: The tip is focused and aimed at ablating the pulp floor. The setting is 4.50W, 60% Water, 80% Air, 30 Hz.

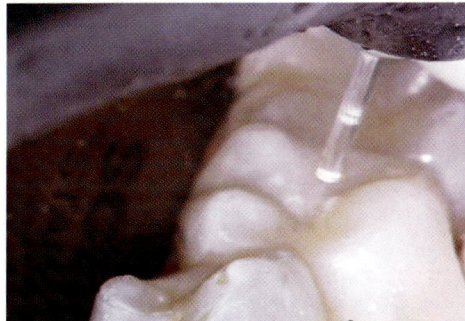

Fig. 6: The setting is 2.00W, 60% Water, 80% Air, 30 Hz. Preparation is being completed.

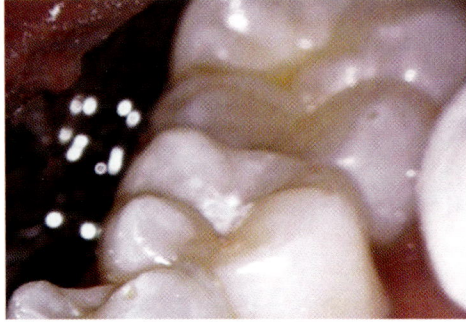
Fig. 7: Post-op. Preparation is complete.

Technique 3: For Patients with Low Tolerance (Apprehensive Adult and Pedo Patients)

Anterior Teeth

Lower laser power is used to start. The power is raised 0.25W at a time until efficient enamel ablation is complete. This technique is described as the "Turtle Technique".

For the Er,Cr:YSGG laser system Waterlase MD, the recommended settings are:
>1.50W, 30 Hz, 60% Water, 80% Air, 30 seconds
>Increase the laser power at 0.25-0.50W increments at a time until enamel ablation is complete
>1.75-2.50W, 30 Hz is the highest power setting
>1.50-2.00W, 30 Hz, 60% Water, 80% Air to finish

For the Er,Cr:YSGG laser system (model: Millennium Waterlase, Millennium 2, Waterlase), the recommended settings are:
>1.25W, 15% Water, 15% Air, 30 seconds
>Increase the laser power at 0.25-0.50W increments at a time until enamel ablation is complete
>1.50-2.25W is the highest power setting
>1.50-2.00W, 15% Water, 15% Air to finish

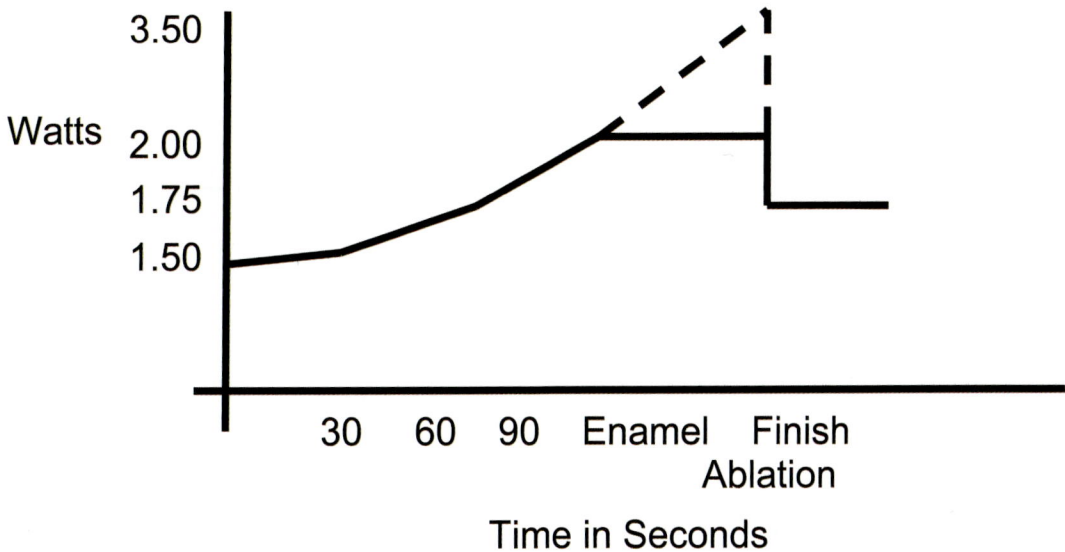

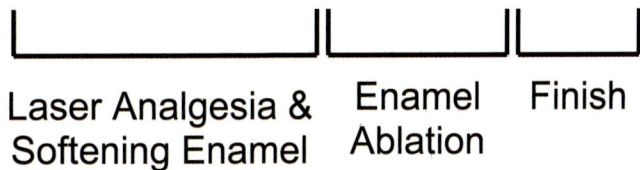

Case 1: For patient with Low Tolerance (Permanent Cuspid, Class V)

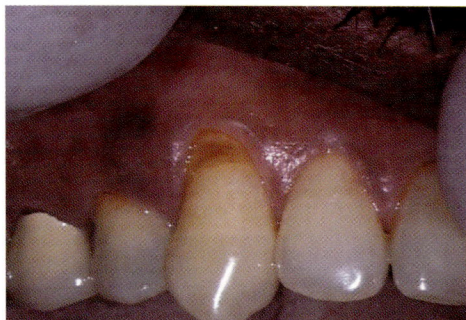

Fig. 1: Pre-op. A Class V lesion is present in maxillary right cuspid labial surface.

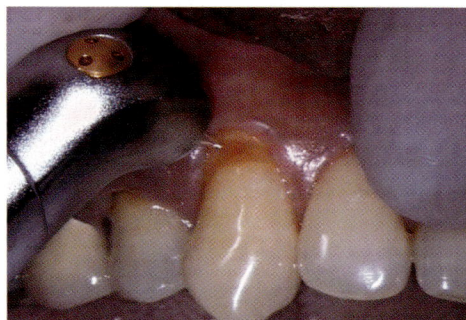

Fig. 2: A MG-6 tip is focused and aimed at the caries. The setting is 0.25W, 0% Water, 0% Air, 50 Hz.

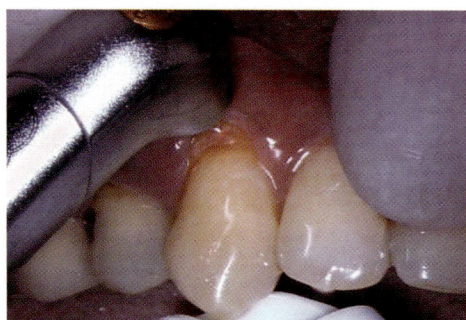

Fig. 3: After 30 seconds, the power is raised 0.25W to 1.75W.

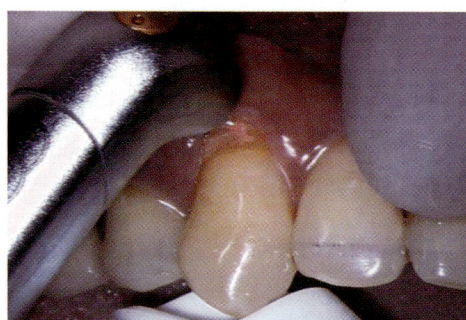

Fig. 4: After another 30 seconds, the power setting is raised another 0.25W to 2.00W.

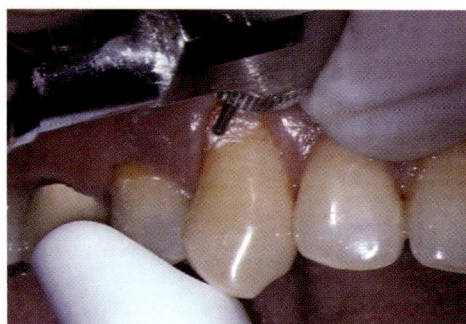

Fig. 5: A slow speed round bur is used to remove and check caries.

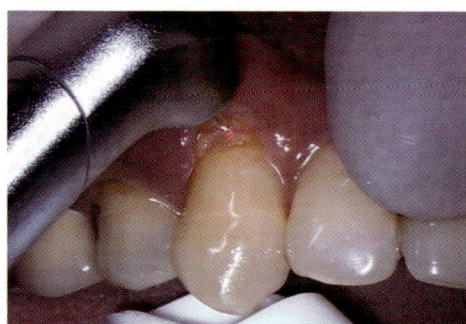

Fig. 6: The preparation is finished with laser. The setting is 1.75W, 60% Water, 80% Air, 30 Hz.

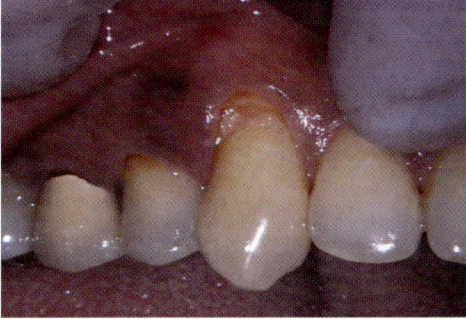

Fig. 7: Post-op. Composite restoration is placed.

Technique 4: For Patients with Higher Tolerance (Non-Apprehensive Adult Patients, Laser Familiar Adult and Pedo Patients)

Bicuspid, Molar and Deciduous Molar

Low laser power is used to pre-condition the pulp. This is followed by high laser energy to ablate enamel. To finish, low laser power is used. This technique is described as the "Modified Rabbit Technique".

For the Er,Cr:YSGG laser system Waterlase MD, the recommended settings are:

> 2.00W, 30 Hz, 60% Water, 80% Air, 60 seconds
>
> 2.00W, 30 Hz, 60% Water, 80% Air, 45 seconds
>
> 3.00W, 15 Hz, 60% Water, 80% Air, enamel ablation
>
> In case of tenacious enamel, increase power setting to
> 3.50-4.50W, 15 Hz, 60% Water, 80% Air to complete enamel ablation
>
> 2.00W, 30 Hz, 60% Water, 80% Air to finish

For the Er,Cr:YSGG laser system (model: Millennium Waterlase, Millennium 2, Waterlase), the recommended settings are:

> 1.25W, 15% Water, 15% Air, 60 seconds
>
> 1.25W, 15% Water, 15% Air, 60 seconds
>
> 5.00W, 75% Water, 90% Air, enamel ablation
>
> In case of tenacious enamel, increase power setting to
> 5.50-6.00W, 75% Water, 90% Air to complete enamel ablation
>
> 2.00W, 30% Water, 30% Air to finish

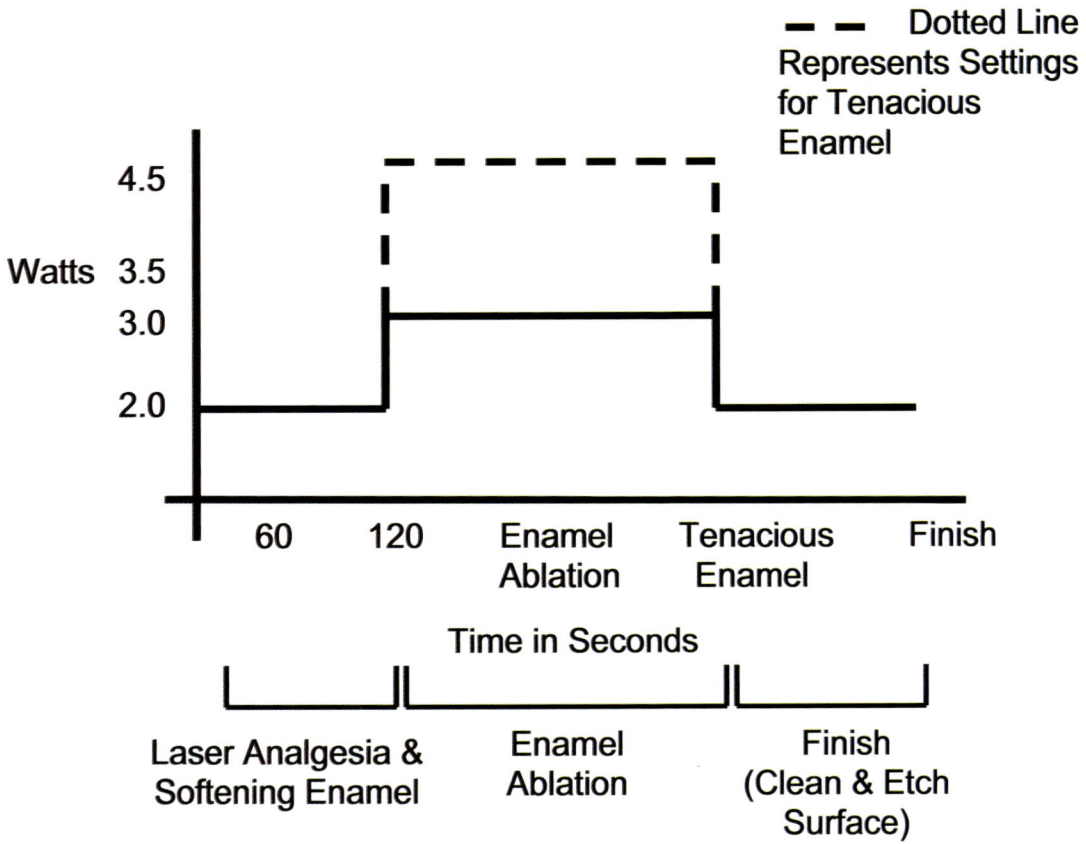

Case 1: For patient with Higher Tolerance (Permanent Bicuspid, Class I)

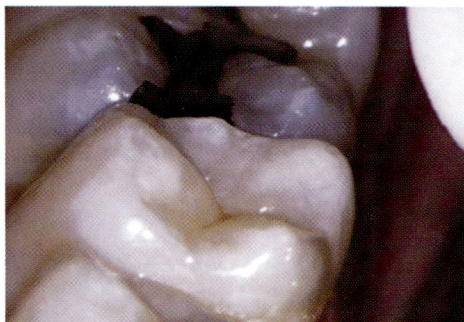

Fig. 1: Pre-op. An occlusal caries is noted in mandibular 2nd premolar.

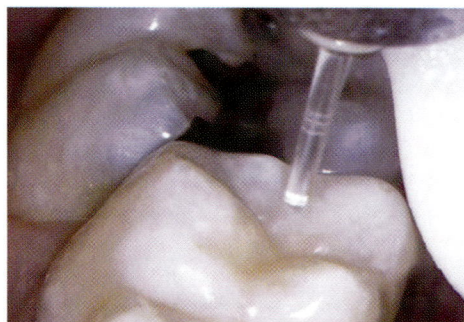

Fig. 2: A MG-6 tip is focused and aimed at the fossa. The setting is 2.00W, 60% Water, 80% Air, 30 Hz.

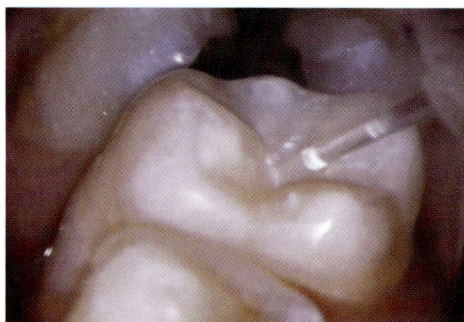

Fig. 3: The tip is focused and angled aiming at extending the border on one side. The setting is 3.00W, 60% Water, 80% Air, 15 Hz.

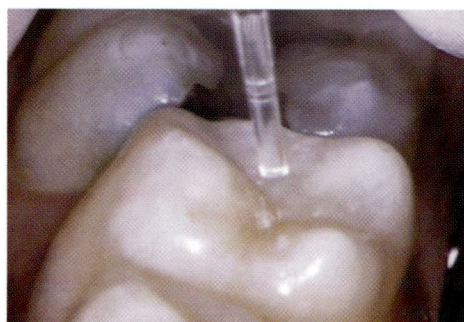

Fig. 4: The tip is focused and angled aiming at extending the border on the other side.

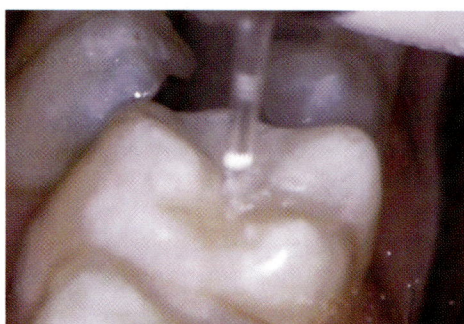

Fig. 5: The tip is focused and aimed at deepening the preparation.

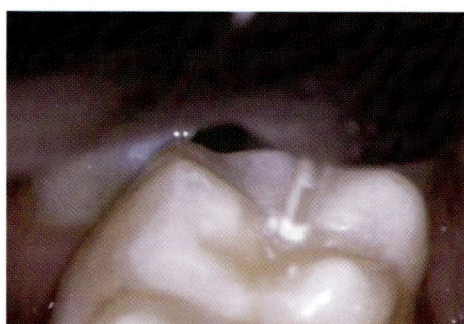

Fig. 6: The preparation is completed by using the setting of 2.00W, 60% Water, 80% Air, 30 Hz.

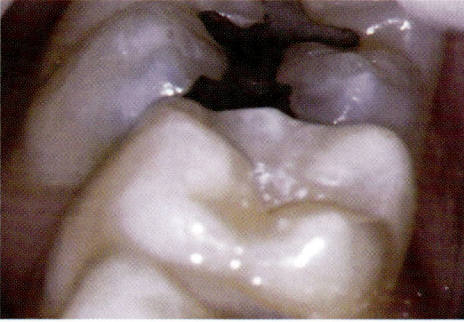

Fig. 7: Post-op. The preparation is complete.

Technique 5: For Patients with Higher Tolerance (Less Apprehensive Adult Patients, Laser Familiar in Adult and Pedo Patients)

Bicuspids, Molars and Deciduous Molars

A different low laser power is used to precondition the pulp. This is followed by a high laser power to ablate enamel. To finish the prep, lower power is used.

For the Er,Cr:YSGG laser system Waterlase MD, the recommended settings are:
  0.25W, 50 Hz, 0% Water, 0% Air, 120 seconds
  2.00-4.50W, 15 Hz, enamel ablation
  2.00W, 30 Hz, 60% Water, 80% Air to finish

For the Er,Cr:YSGG laser system (model: Millennium Waterlase, Millennium 2, Waterlase), the recommended settings are:
  0.25W, 7% Water, 7% Air, 3-5 minutes.
  2.00-6.00W, enamel ablation
  1.50-2.00W to finish

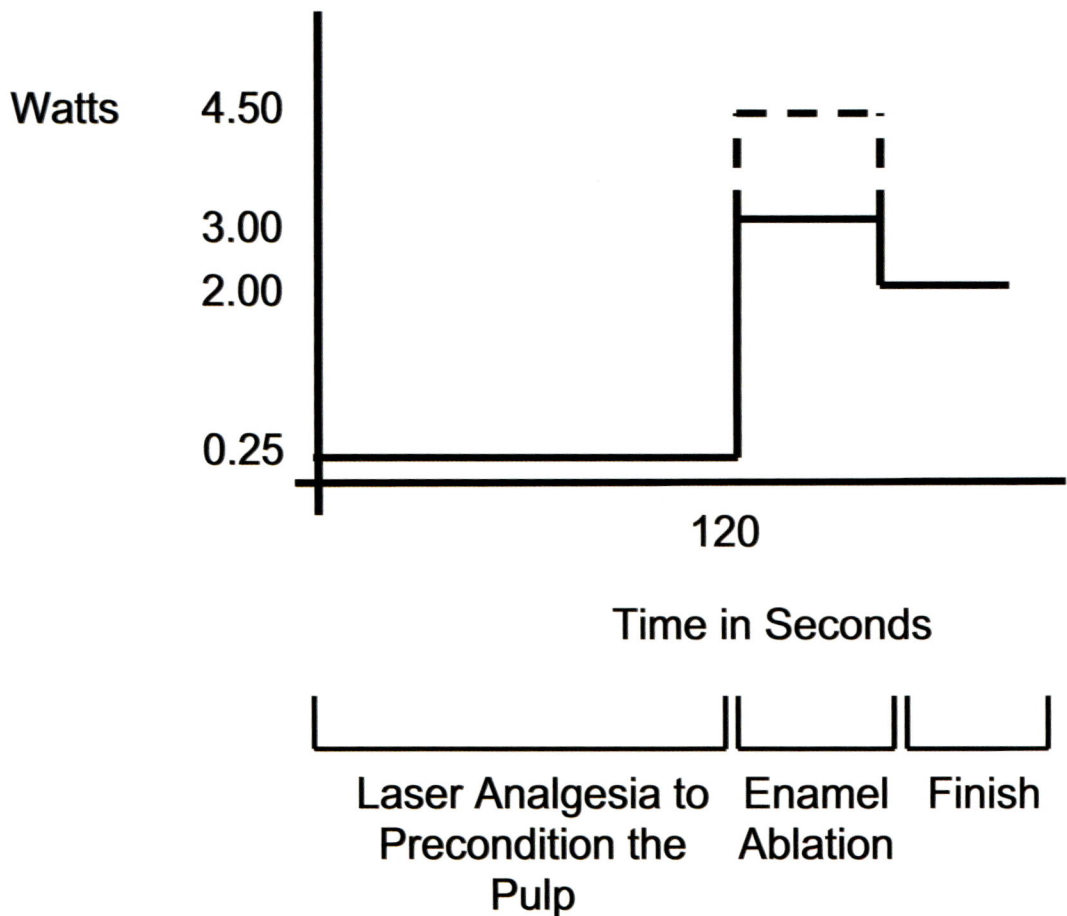

Watts 4.50 3.00 2.00 0.25

120

Time in Seconds

Laser Analgesia to Precondition the Pulp   Enamel Ablation   Finish

Case 1: For patient with Higher Tolerance , Permanent Cuspid, Class V

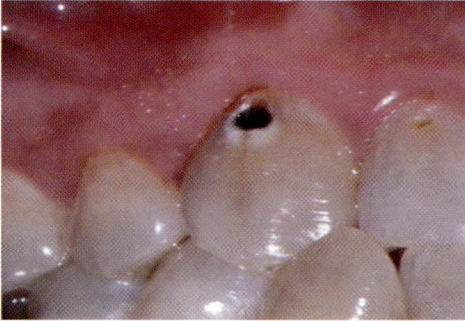

Fig. 1: Pre-op. A Class V lesion is present in maxillary right cuspid labial surface.

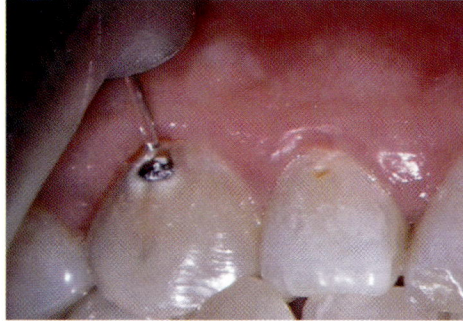

Fig. 2: A MG-6 tip is focused and aimed at the caries. The setting is 0.25W, 0% Water, 0% Air, 50 Hz.

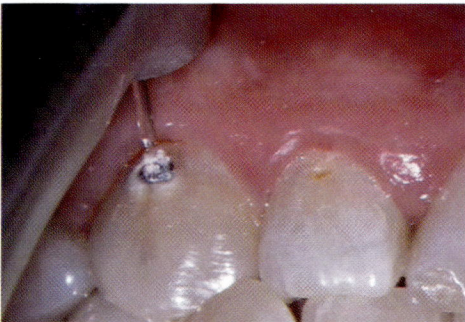

Fig. 3: Two minutes is spent with the setting to pre-condition the pulp.

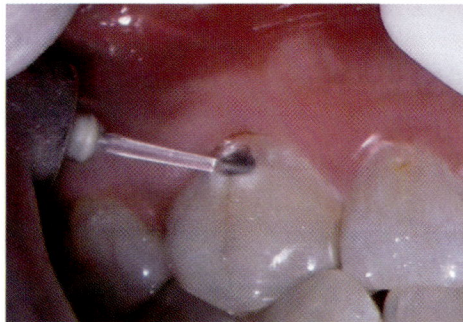

Fig. 4: The tip is focused and angled, aiming at ablating the sides of the exposed caries. The setting is 2.00W, 60% Water, 80% Air, 15 Hz.

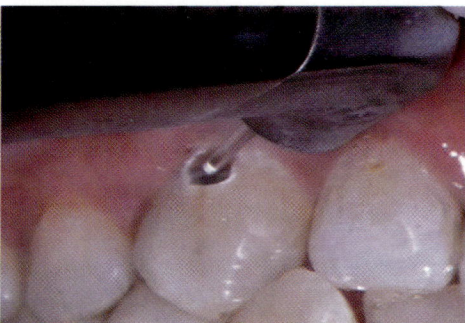

Fig. 5: The tip is focused and angled, aiming at ablating the sides of the other border.

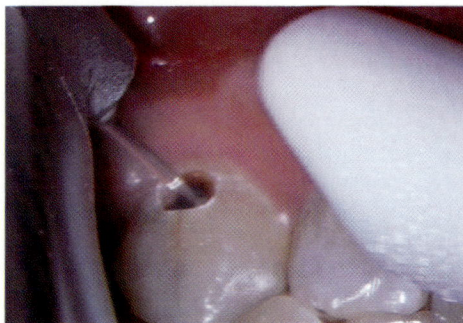

Fig. 6: The tip is focused and aimed at removing decay.

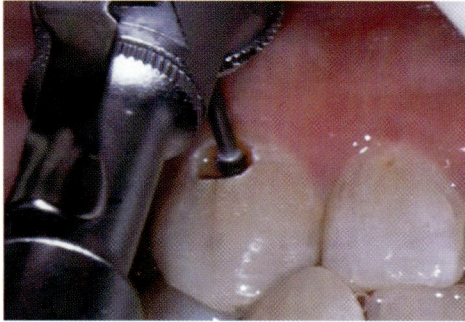

Fig. 7: A slow speed round bur is used to remove and check caries.

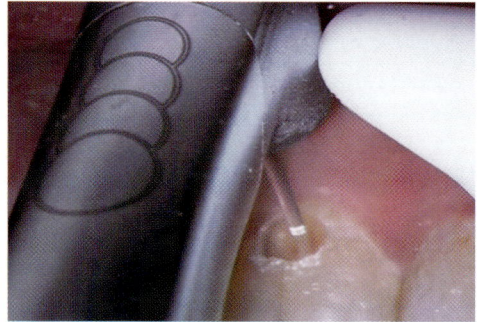

Fig. 8: The preparation is finished with lower laser power. The setting is 2.00W, 60% Water, 80% Air, 30 Hz.

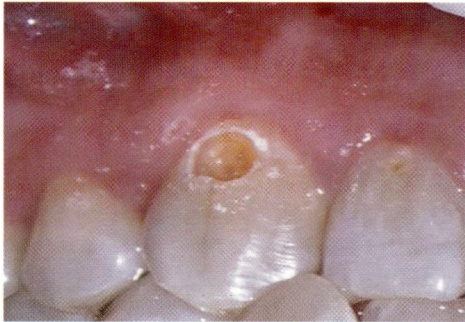

Fig. 9: The Class V prep is complete.

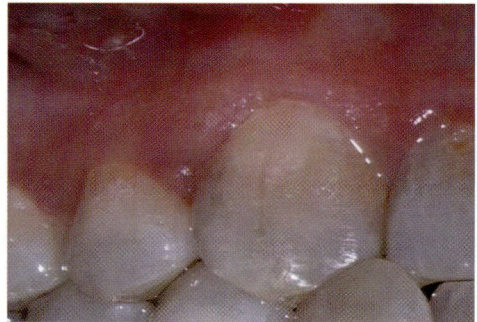

Fig. 10: Post-op. Composite restoration is placed.

Case 2: For patient with higher tolerance, Permanent Bicuspid, Class I

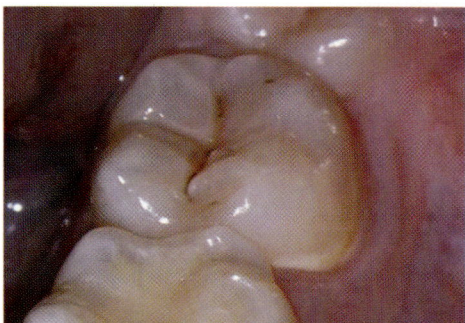

Fig. 1: Pre-op. An occlusal caries is present in mandibular left 2nd molar.

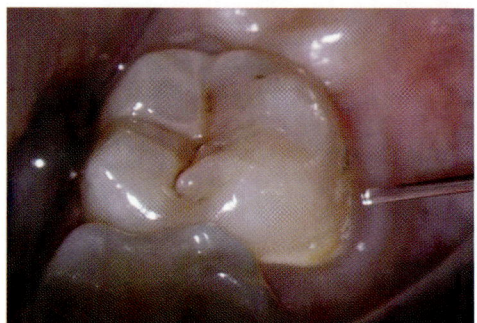

Fig. 2: A MG-6 tip is focused at 1-2mm aiming at the cervical area of the buccal surface. The setting is 0.25W, 0% Water, 0% Air, 50 Hz.

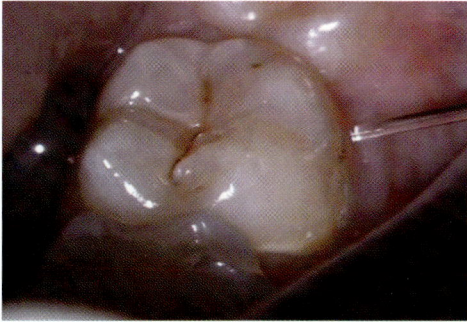

Fig. 3: The tip is moved in the shape of the pulp.

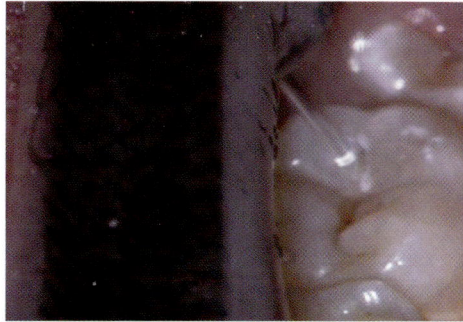

Fig. 4: The tip is focused and angled to aim at the border of the caries. The setting is 4.50W, 60% Water, 80% Air, 15 Hz.

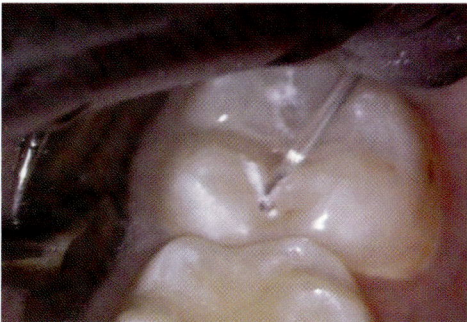

Fig. 5: The tip is focused and angled to ablate and extend the border of the other side.

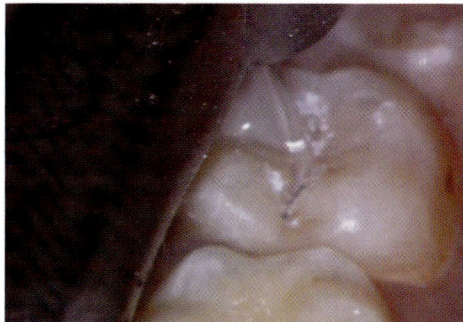

Fig. 6: The tip is focused and aimed to deepen the prep.

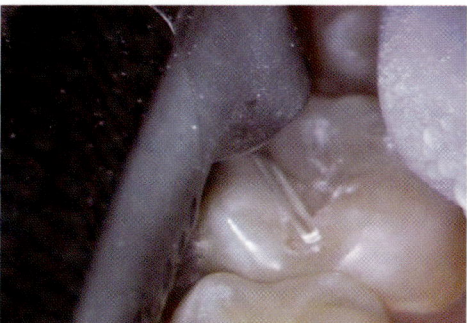

Fig. 7: The tip is focused and angled aiming at ablating the sides of tubules beneath the border of the prep.

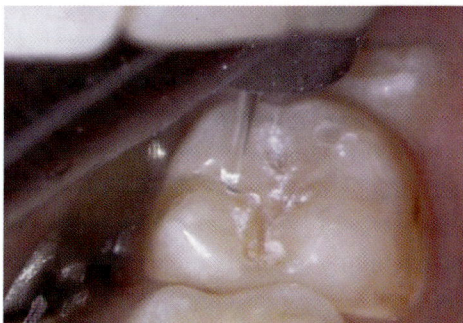

Fig. 8: To finish the prep, the setting is changed to 2.00W, 60% Water, 80% Air, 30 Hz.

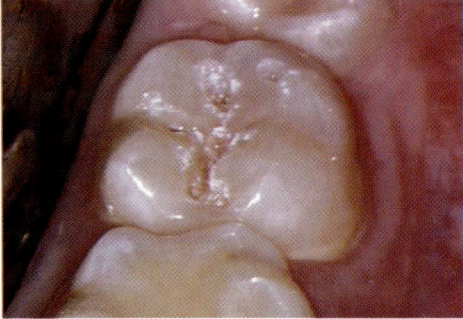

Fig. 9: Post-op. The preparation is complete.

Technique 6: Customizing Individual Preferred Power Settings

Use a low or very low power setting to precondition the pulp before using the individual preferred high-power setting. This technique is described as the "Modified Rabbit Technique".

Customizing Technique 1:

For the Er,Cr:YSGG laser system Waterlase MD, the recommended settings are:
>2.00W, 30 Hz, 60% Water, 80% Air, 60 seconds
>2.00W, 30 Hz, 60% Water, 80% Air, 60 seconds
>Individual practitioner's favorite high-power setting, enamel ablation
>2.00W, 30 Hz, 60% Water, 80% Air to finish

For the Er,Cr:YSGG laser system (model: Millennium Waterlase, Millennium 2, Waterlase), the recommended settings are:
>1.25W, 15% Water, 15% Air, 60 seconds
>1.25W, 15% Water, 15% Air, 60 seconds
>Individual practitioner's favorite high-power setting, enamel ablation.
>2.00W, 30% Water, 30% Air to finish

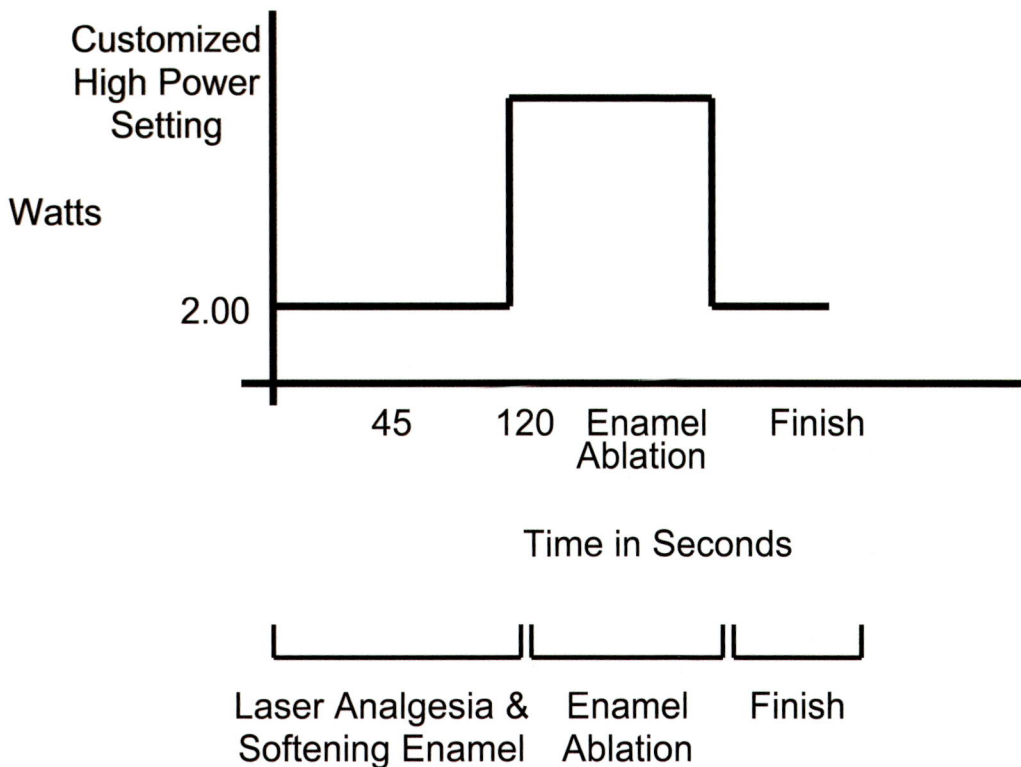

Customizing Technique 2:

For the Er,Cr:YSGG laser system Waterlase MD, the recommended settings are:
 0.25W, 50 Hz, 0% Water, 0% Air, 120 seconds
 Individual practitioner's favorite high-power settings for enamel ablation, but my preferred settings are:
 2.00W, 30 Hz, 60% Water, 80% Air to finish

For the Er,Cr:YSGG laser system (model: Millennium Waterlase, Millennium 2, Waterlase), the recommended settings are:
 0.25W, 7% Water, 7% Air, 200 seconds
 Individual practitioner's favorite high-power settings for enamel ablation, but my preferred settings are:
 2.00W, 30% Water, 30% Air to finish

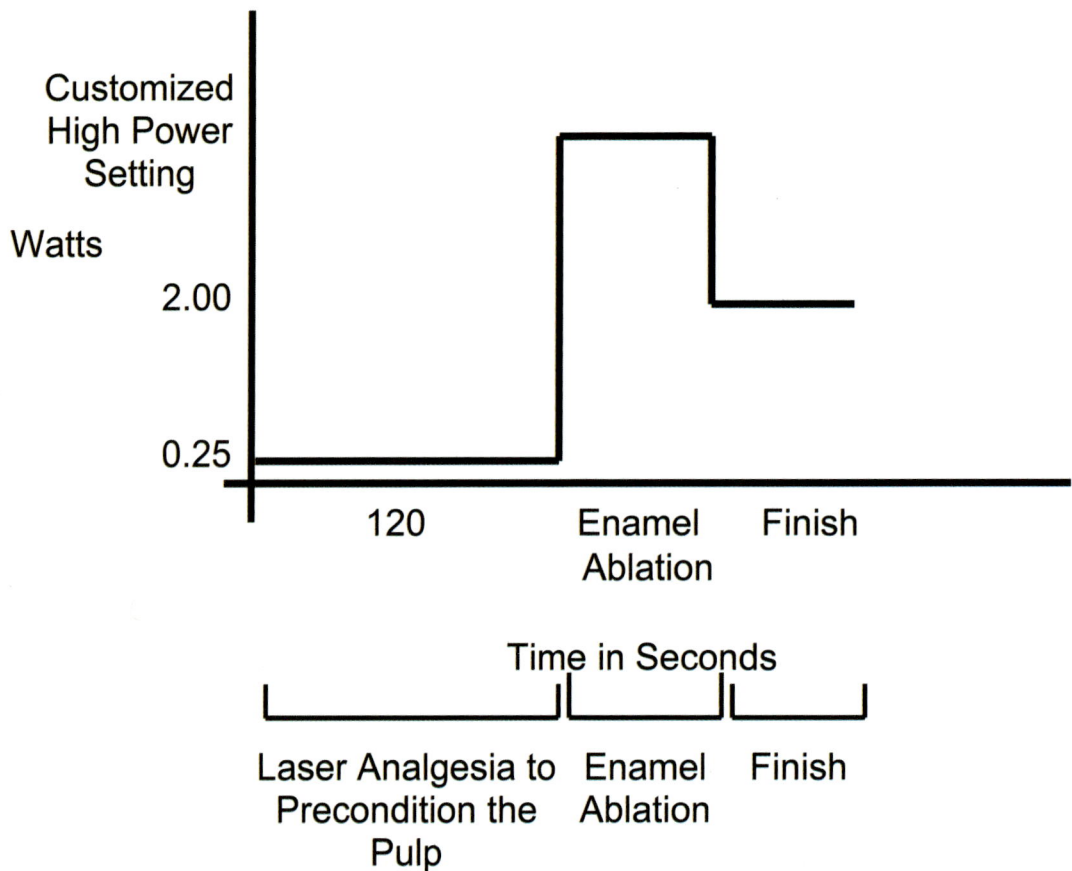

Technique 7: Amalgam Removal

A very low laser power is used to precondition the pulp. This is followed by a high-speed drilling by a one-quarter or one-half round new carbide bur channeling the old amalgam restoration. This is aimed to fragment the old amalgam restoration before being removed. Laser power is then used to clean the cavity and finish the preparation.

For the Er,Cr:YSGG laser system Waterlase MD, the recommended settings are:
MC-12 tip, 0.50W, 50 Hz, 0% Water, 0% Air, 120 seconds. The tip is aimed at the cervical portion of the tooth. The tip should be defocused 1-2mm and should be moving and aiming at the tooth in the direction and around the approximate shape of the pulp.

High-speed drill (¼ or ½ round bur) to fragment the amalgam restoration and remove the old amalgam.

A favorite high-power setting can be used to remove the recurrent decay:
2.00-4.00W, 30 Hz, 60% Water, 80% Air

2.00W, 30 Hz, 60% Water, 80% Air to finish.

For the Er,Cr:YSGG laser system (model: Millennium Waterlase, Millennium 2, Waterlase), the recommended settings are:
0.25W, 7% Water, 7% Air, 120 seconds; or
0.25W, 15% Water, 15% Air, 45 seconds per site.
High-speed drill (¼ or ½ round bur) to fragment the amalgam restoration, and remove the old amalgam.
2.00-3.00W, 30% Water, 30% Air to remove recurrent decay.
2.00W, 30% Water, 30% Air to finish.

Case 1: Laser-assisted Amalgam Removal, Permanent Bicuspid, Class I

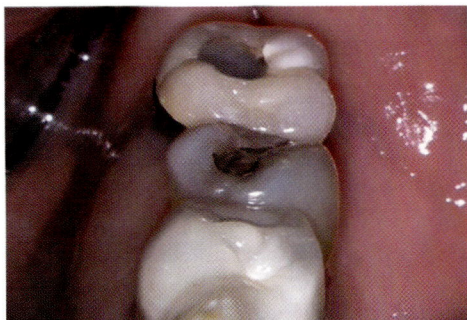

Fig. 1: Pre-op. Recurrent decay is present in the mandibular right 2nd premolar.

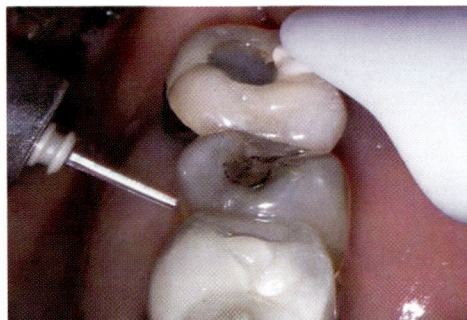

Fig. 2: A MG-6 tip is focused at 1-2mm aiming at the buccal surface cervical area. The setting is 0.25W, 0% Water, 0% Air, 50 Hz.

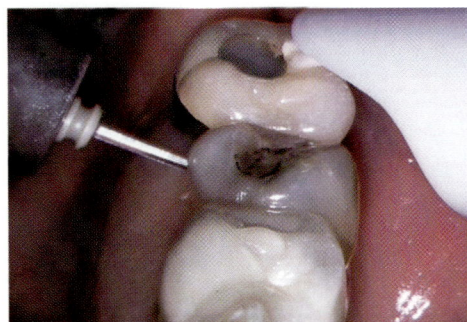

Fig. 3: The pre-conditioning continues on to a total of 120 seconds.

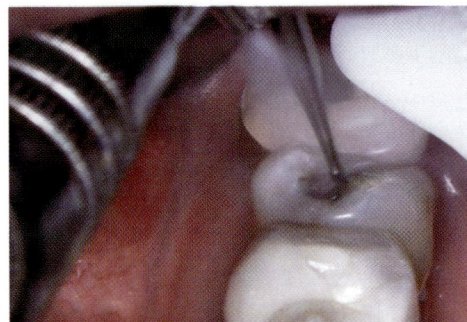

Fig. 4: A ¼ round high-speed bur is used to channel the amalgam and fragmentize the old restoration.

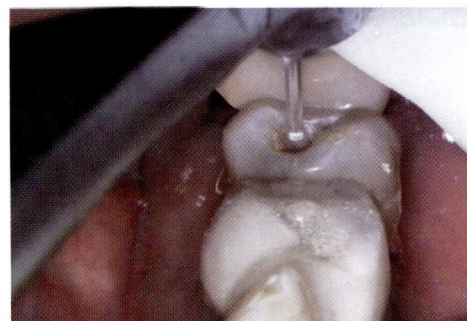

Fig. 5: The tip is focused and aimed at clean pulpal floor. The setting is 2.00W, 60% Water, 80% Air, 30 Hz.

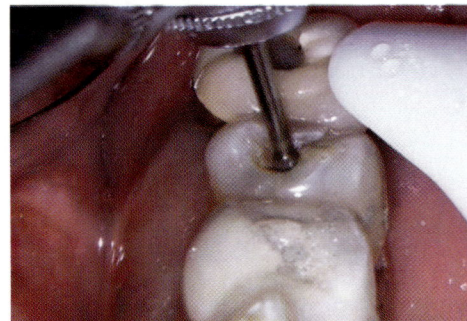

Fig. 6: A slow speed round bur is used to remove shavings of amalgam left on the internal wall and caries.

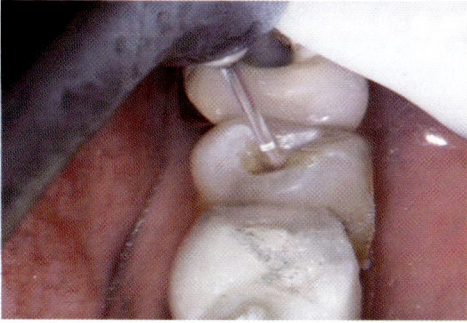

Fig. 7: The tip is focused to debride, clean, and finish the preparation.

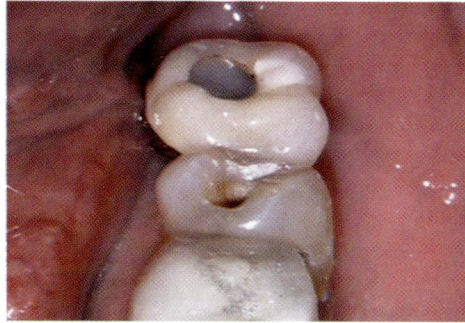

Fig. 8: The preparation is complete.

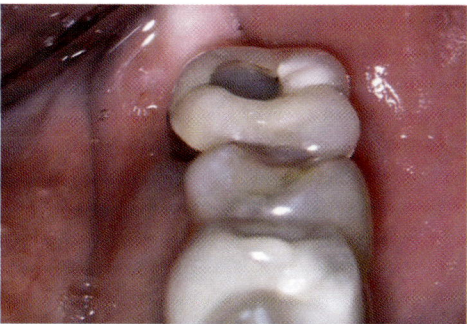

Fig. 9: Post-op. Composite restoration is placed.

Operative Dentistry

I apply principles of minimally invasive dentistry in laser cavity preparations whenever possible. The goal is to produce a final restoration that provides the best aesthetic result, by removing the minimum amount of tooth structure while eliminating diseased tissue and restoring the tooth with a conservative approach in design and with the least amount of discomfort to the patient.

In order to carry out micro-dentistry, proper and accurate detection of caries at its earliest stage is essential. This typically involves the use of good quality X-ray, physical assessment, and the utilization of caries detection systems. Early caries can be detected more accurately to allow micro-dentistry to be performed on them. Because of its end-firing nature, the Er,Cr:YSGG laser system is an ideal tool for preparation of minimally invasive procedures.

From discussions with my peers and my own experience, I have identified two commonly used laser cavity preparation techniques, which could appropriately be named the "Rabbit" and "Turtle" Techniques.

The Rabbit Technique

In the Rabbit Technique, a high power setting is used all throughout the procedure. To start, the fiber tip is defocused at 6-10mm from the target tissue. The intent of the defocused mode is to apply lower levels of laser energy to the pulp and induce laser analgesia. After a period of time, the fiber tip is focused to 1-2mm to ablate enamel. Once in dentin, the fiber tip is defocused again to reduce the power reaching the surface, to finish the cavity preparation. While I have found some efficacy in use of the Rabbit Technique, my personal experience is that – like in the fable – it will finish last; I tend to encounter increased patient sensitivity, which results in a longer treatment time, and less patient satisfaction.

The Turtle Technique

In the Turtle Technique, the laser fiber tip is focused at 1-2mm from the target tissue all through the procedure. To start the procedure, low power settings are used to apply laser analgesia to the pulp. The power setting is increased gradually until enamel ablation is complete. To finish the procedure, the power setting is normally reduced to lower power to debride and condition the surface before placement of the restoration.

The Modified Turtle Technique

There is a fairly simple modification to the Turtle Technique, especially appropriate for tenacious enamel, or for dentists who are still not quite confident enough to use the laser for the entire procedure. Once laser analgesia is achieved, a high-speed handpiece with a ¼ round bur can be used to remove enamel and outline the cavity preparation. To finish the procedure, lower power laser setting is used to debride and condition the surface before placement of the restoration.

In all the techniques listed above, the laser may be used solely, without requiring the use of any other ablating/cutting tools such as the high-speed or low-speed drill. I have used the laser without turning to the drill in many procedures; however, especially with large preparations, a drill will considerably speed up the procedure time. The need for improved speed led me to the Modified Turtle Technique. If the techniques have been properly observed, the patient will have greatly reduced sensitivity; you can still use the high-speed or slow-speed drills to assist in removal of gross caries without requiring the use of injectable anesthetic.

I use the Modified Turtle Technique for any patients who have large caries, or underlying caries that the laser could not reach without removal of more surrounding healthy tissue. It is my belief that research and development of dental lasers will lead to a point where they can match the drill for speed, without losing any of the benefits that the laser offers.

Class I Cavity Preparation – Turtle Technique

Laser Parameters, Set 1: Pre-Conditioning

Waterlase MD laser system settings: MG-6 tip, 2.00W, 60% Water, 80% Air, 30 Hz
Other Er,Cr:YSGG laser system settings: G-6 tip, 1.25W, 15% Air, 15% Water

Keeping the fiber tip in focused mode at all times (1–2mm), direct the fiber tip perpendicular towards the fissure, down the long axis of the tooth. When ablating, the motion used is semi-circular and back-and-forth, but primarily aiming at the area where the lesion is located. Move slowly along the length of the lesion. Fire the laser at starting settings for 30 seconds.

Laser Parameters, Set 2: Continuation of Pre-Conditioning and Enamel Ablation

Waterlase MD laser system settings: 3.00W, 60% Water, 80% Air, 30 Hz
Other Er,Cr:YSGG laser system settings: 2.00W, 30% Water, 30% Air

Continue to direct the fiber tip in focused mode towards the fissure and down the long axis of the tooth for a further 30 seconds. At this stage, not much ablation will be noticed.

Laser Parameters, Set 3: Continued Enamel Ablation

Waterlase MD laser system settings: 4.50W, 60% Water, 80% Air, 30 Hz
Other Er,Cr:YSGG laser system settings: 4.00W, 60% Water, 65% Air

Note: More noticeable ablation of the enamel should take place at this power setting. In my experience, more than 80% of bicuspid and deciduous molar enamel ablations can occur with 4.00W.

After ablation of the fissure groove has started to take place, aim the fiber tip within the boundary of the fissure so that it is directed at one side of the fissure wall. This will assist in establishing a small opening of approximately 0.5mm. The angle of the fiber tip is approximately 45 degrees to the plane perpendicular to the long axis of the tooth. Repeat the same motion onto the opposite side of the fissure wall to further widen the cavity. The effect of this is to widen the fissure allowing fiber tip access to the lesion.

After the initial opening of the lesion has been established, deepen the cavity preparation through enamel, aiming the tip perpendicular to the target surface. If the lesion is still wider than the opening you have prepared, continue to widen and deepen the prep until access to the lesion is established.

Laser Parameters, Set 4 (Optional): Continued Enamel Ablation

Waterlase MD laser system settings: 6.00W, 60% Water, 80% Air, 30 Hz
Alternatively: 7.50W, 75% Water, 90% Air, 30 Hz

Other Er,Cr:YSGG laser system settings: 5.00W, 75% Water, 90% Air
  Alternative: 6.00W, 75% Water, 90% Air

> After 30 seconds with Laser Parameter, Set 3, and if the enamel ablation is not complete, or not proceeding to your satisfaction, then the settings may be increased. The more tenacious the enamel, the higher the power setting that should be used. Advance through the opening and aim at the sides of tubules. Remove the enamel above the lesion and establish the cavity outline. The intent is to perform a conservative occlusal preparation with pits and fissures cleaned out.

Laser Parameters, Set 5: Dentin Ablation

Waterlase MD laser system settings: 3.50W, 60% Water, 80% Air, 30 Hz
Other Er,Cr:YSGG laser system settings: 2.50-3.50W, 60% Water, 65% Air

> Once the preparation reaches the dentin, the power setting is lowered; any ablation in dentin using the laser should take place in a slightly defocused mode, about 2.5-4mm away from the target. To ensure all soft caries are removed, use a slow-speed round bur (#2 or #4) to check and/or remove gross soft caries. The cavity should have a sound dentin floor and walls that do not have caries.

Laser Parameters, Set 6: Complete Preparation

Waterlase MD laser system settings: 2.00W, 60% Water, 80% Air, 30 Hz
Other Er,Cr:YSGG laser system settings: 2.00W, 30% Water, 30% Air

> To finish the cavity preparation, lower the power settings further. Move the tip over the cavity surface in focused mode to remove any smear layer or debris. Dry the surface with an air syringe to visualize the completeness of the preparation and etching, and to check if there is any sclerotic dentin left. Any remaining sclerotic dentin should be removed using the above settings.

Class I Turtle Technique – Supplementary Drawings

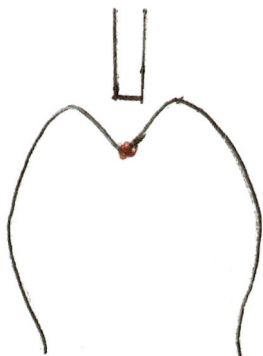

Fig. 1: The tip is focused at 1-2mm and is perpendicular to the fossa (pre-conditioning).

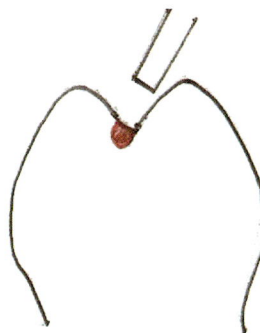

Fig. 2: The tip is angled and aimed at one border of the caries to ablate.

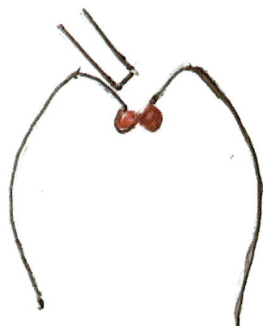

Fig. 3: The tip is angled and aimed at the opposite border of the caries to ablate.

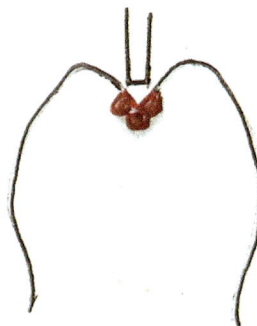

Fig. 4: The tip is perpendicular and aimed at the pulpal floor to ablate.

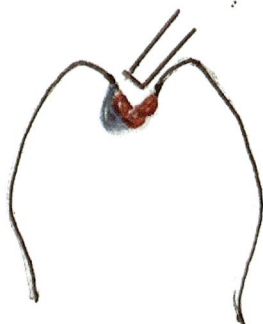

Fig. 5: The tip is angled and at open tubules beneath the margin to ablate.

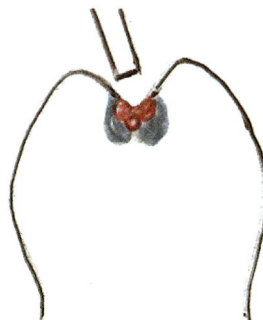

Fig. 6: The tip is angled and aimed at the open tubules beneath the margin at the opposite side to ablate.

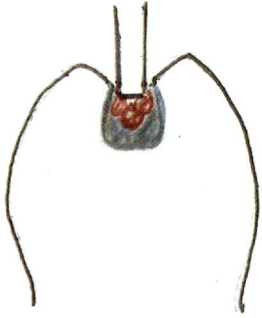

Fig. 7: The tip is perpendicular and aimed at the pulp floor to ablate.

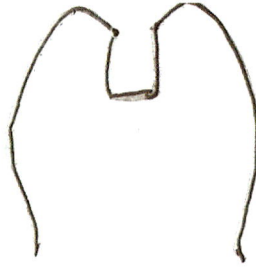

Fig. 8: The finished preparation.

Class I Cavity Preparation – Rabbit Technique

Laser Parameters, Set 1: Pre-Conditioning

Waterlase MD laser system settings: MG-6 tip, 3.00-4.50W, 60% Water, 80% Air, 15Hz
Other Er,Cr:YSGG laser system settings: G-6 tip, 5.50–6.00W, 75% Water, 90% Air

Defocus the fiber tip to 6-10mm from the tooth surface, aiming laser energy towards the fissure. Spend 90 seconds going back and forth over the fissure, keeping the defocused distance as constant as possible.

Laser Parameters, Set 2: Enamel / Dentin Ablation

Retain the same settings as in Set 1.

After 90 seconds, focus the tip within the fissure to start ablation of enamel. After the fissure groove has been established, aim the fiber tip towards one side of the groove wall to widen it, and then repeat for the other side of the groove wall. After a small opening of at least 0.75mm has been established, continue the preparation through enamel with the fiber tip aimed as perpendicular as possible to the target surface. Advance the ablation through the opening to remove the enamel above the lesion, and prepare a conservative cavity preparation with pits and fissures.

Once the preparation reaches the dentin, slightly defocus the fiber tip to about 3-5mm to reduce the laser energy applied to the dentin and caries. (Note: If the fiber tip stays focused, it may cause discomfort for the patient.) For large lesions, a slow-speed round bur may be used to remove decay and soft dentin. It also serves the purpose of caries check. The cavity should have a sound dentin floor and walls that do not have caries.

To finish the cavity preparation, use the laser, again in defocused mode of about 4-5mm, to etch the cavity surface. Dry the surface with an air syringe to visualize the completeness of the preparation and etching, and to check if there is any sclerotic dentin left. Any remaining sclerotic dentin should be removed using the above settings.

Class I Rabbit Technique – Supplementary Drawings

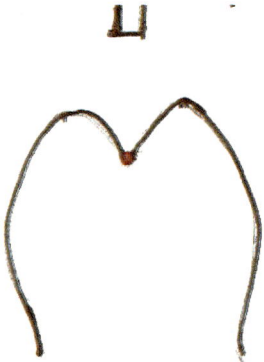

Fig. 1: The tip is defocused 6-10mm and is perpendicular to the fossa (pre-conditioning).

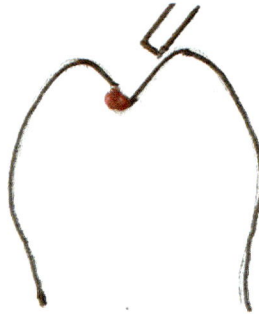

Fig. 2: The tip is angled and aimed at one border of the caries to ablate.

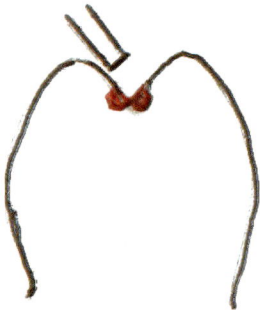

Fig. 3: The tip is angled and aimed at the opposite border of the caries to ablate.

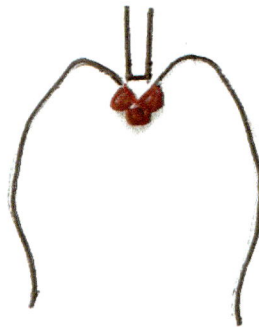

Fig. 4: The tip is perpendicular and aimed at the pulpal floor to ablate.

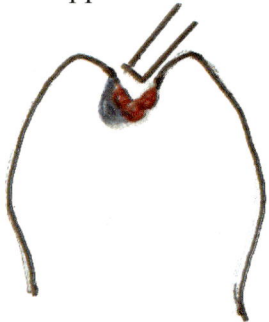

Fig. 5: The tip is angled and at open tubules beneath the margin to ablate.

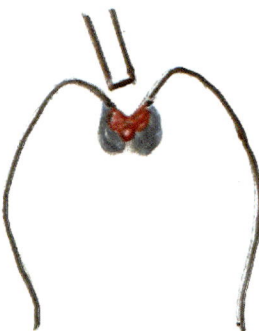

Fig. 6: The tip is angled and aimed at the open tubules beneath the margin at the opposite side to ablate.

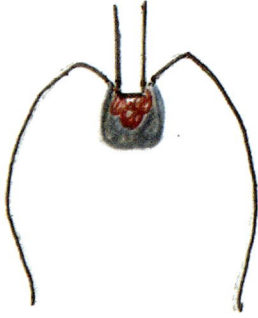

Fig. 7: The tip is perpendicular and
aimed at the pulp floor to ablate.

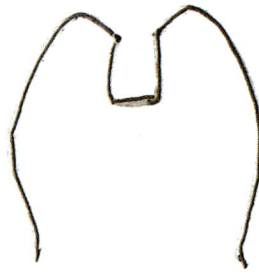

Fig. 8: The finished preparation.

Class I Cavity Prep – Modified Turtle Technique

To start the Modified Turtle Technique, a similar protocol as the Turtle Technique is used.

Laser Parameters, Set 1: Pre-Conditioning

Waterlase MD laser system settings: MG-6 tip, 2.00W, 60% Water, 80% Air, 30 Hz
Other Er,Cr:YSGG laser system settings: G-6 tip, 1.25W, 15% Water, 15% Air

> Keeping the fiber tip in focused mode at all times (1.5-2mm), direct the fiber tip perpendicular towards the fissure, down the long axis of the tooth. When ablating, the motion used is semi-circular and back-and-forth, but primarily aiming at the area where the lesion is located. Move slowly along the length of the lesion. Fire the laser at starting settings for 30 seconds.

Laser Parameters, Set 2: Continue Pre-Conditioning

Waterlase MD laser system settings: 3.00W, 60% Water, 80% Air, 30 Hz
Other Er,Cr:YSGG laser system settings: 2.00W, 30% Water, 30% Air

> Continue to direct the fiber tip in focused mode towards the fissure and down the long axis of the tooth for a further 30 seconds. At this stage, not much ablation will be noticed.

Laser Parameters, Set 3: Enamel Ablation

Waterlase MD laser system settings: 4.50W, 60% Water, 80% Air, 30 Hz
Other Er,Cr:YSGG laser system settings: 4.00W, 60% Water, 65% Air

> Continue to direct the fiber tip in focused mode towards the fissure and down the long axis of the tooth for a further 30 seconds. After 30 seconds, the patient should be sufficiently prepared for the high-speed handpiece with a new ¼, ½ or #1 carbine round bur, which is then used to remove enamel in a light shaving motion, in order to remove a rough outline of enamel in the fissure area.

> For large lesions, a slow-speed round bur may then be used to remove decay and soft dentin, and perform a caries check.

Laser Parameters, Set 4: Complete Preparation

Waterlase MD laser system settings: 2.00W, 30% Water, 35% Air, 30 Hz
Other Er,Cr:YSGG laser system settings: 2.00W, 30% Water, 30% Air

> To finish the cavity preparation, resume using the laser. Move the tip over the cavity surface in focused mode to remove any smear layer or debris. Dry the surface with an air syringe to visualize the completeness of the preparation and

etching, and to check if there is any sclerotic dentin left. Any remaining sclerotic dentin should be removed using the above settings.

Case 1: Class I, Turtle Technique

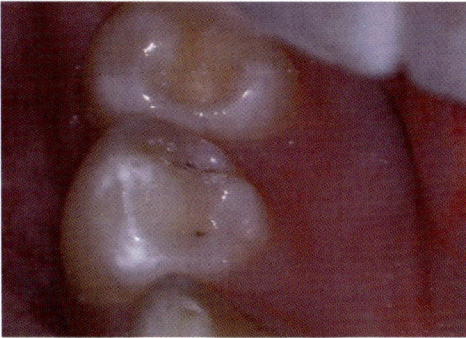

Fig. 1: Pre-op. Distal pit of #28 has an occlusal caries.

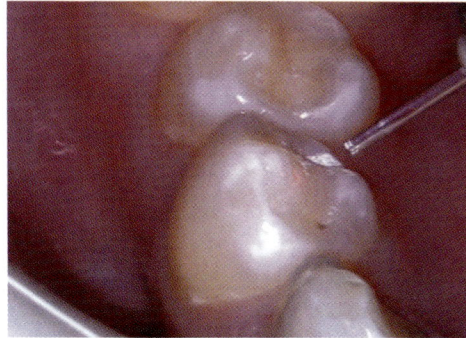

Fig. 2: The tip is focused at caries to precondition the pulp. The setting is 2.00W, 60% Water, 80% Air, 30 Hz.

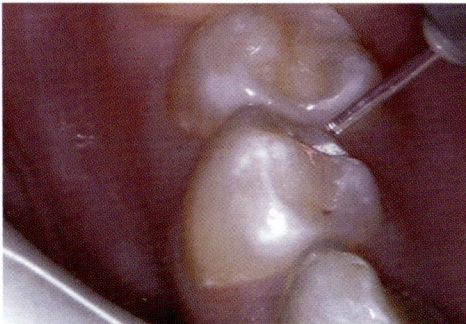

Fig. 3: The tip is focused and angled aiming at the buccal border of caries. The setting is 3.50W 60% Water, 80% Air, 15 Hz.

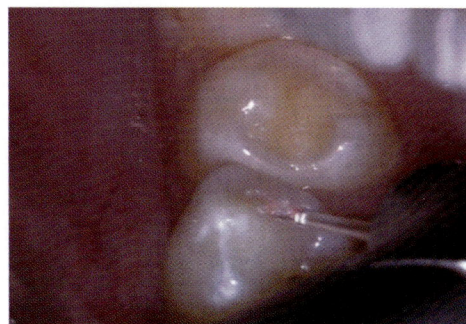

Fig. 4: The tip is focused and angled aiming at another border of caries.

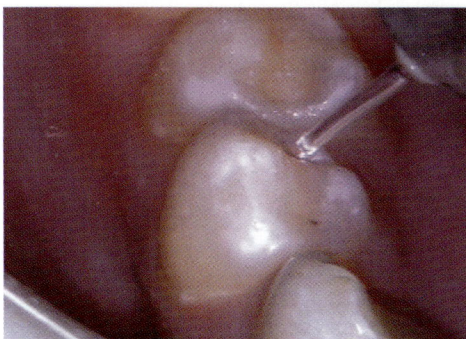

Fig. 5: The tip focused and aimed at the pulp floor to deepen the pulpal floor.

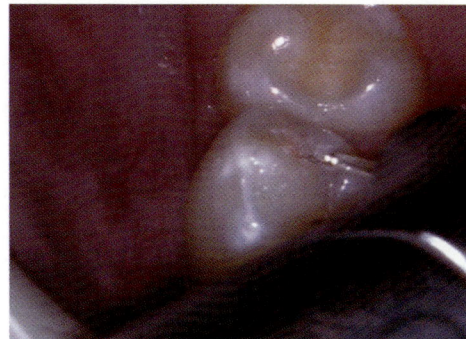

Fig. 6: The tip is focused and angled aiming at sides of tubules underneath the border of caries.

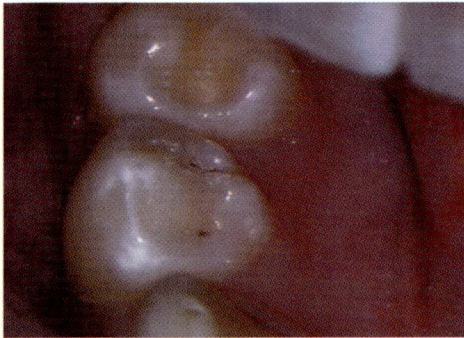
Fig. 7: Post-op. Completion of occlusal prep.

Case 2: Class I, Turtle Technique

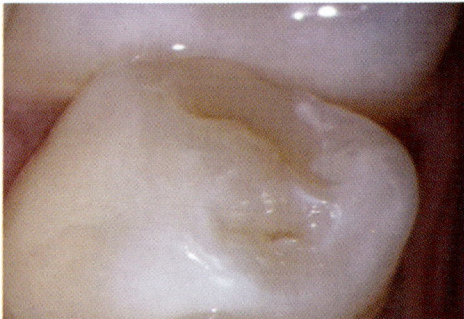
Fig. 1: Pre-op, an occlusal caries is present at the mesial fossa of #28.

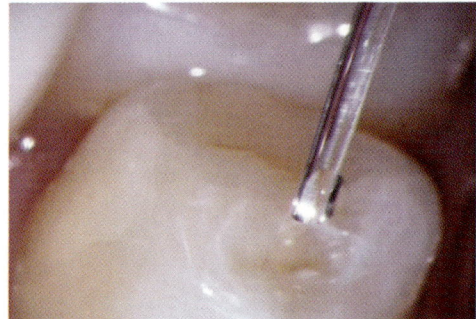
Fig. 2: A MG- 6 tip is focused at 1-2mm from the lesion. The initial setting is 2.00W, 60% Water, 80% Air, 30 Hz to pre-condition the pulp.

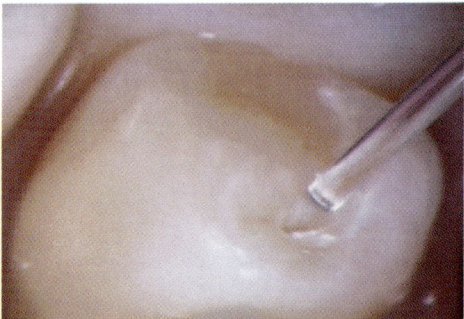
Fig. 3: The tip is focused and angled to aim to extend the border of the caries. The setting is 4.50W, 60% Water, 80% Air, 30 Hz.

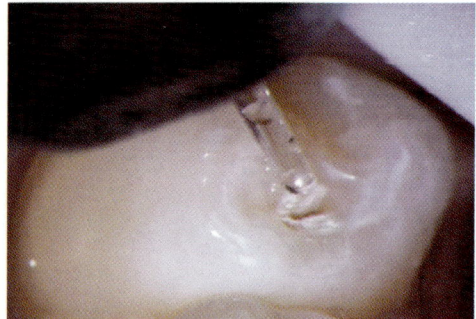
Fig. 4: The tip is focused and angled to aim to extend the other border of caries. Similar setting as in Fig. 3 is used.

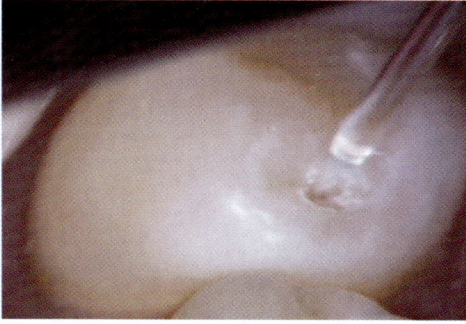

Fig. 5: The tip is placed perpendicular to the pulpal floor to deepen the cavity prep.

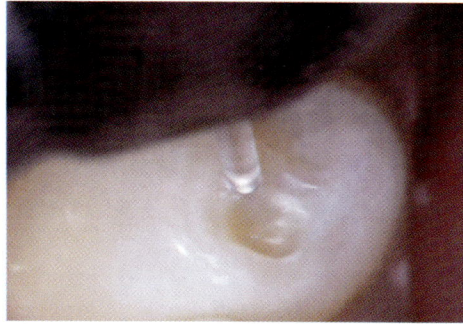

Fig. 6: Caries removal is done by laser energy. The setting is 3.00W, 60% Water, 80% Air, 30 Hz.

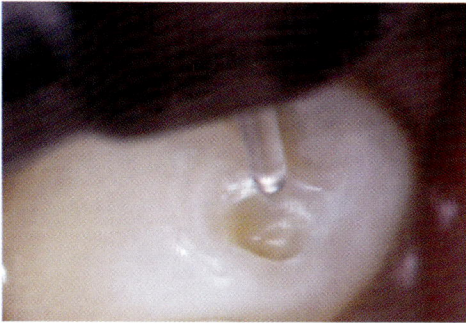

Fig. 7: The cavity is finished with 2.00W, 60% Water, 80% Air, 30 Hz.

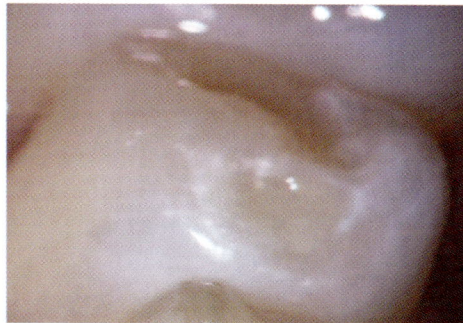

Fig. 8: Post-op, composite restoration is placed.

Class II Preparation – Modified Turtle Technique – Slot Design – Small to Moderate Caries

Laser Parameters, Set 1: Pre-Conditioning

Waterlase MD laser system settings: MG-6 tip, 2.00W, 60% Water, 80% Air, 30Hz
Other Er,Cr:YSGG laser system settings: G-6 tip, 1.25W, 15% Water, 15% Air

When starting this preparation, keep the fiber tip perpendicular to the ridge and down the long axis of the tooth, ensuring that the tip is also parallel to the proximal surface of the adjacent tooth.

Laser Parameters, Set 2: Continue Pre-Conditioning

Waterlase MD laser system settings: 3.00W, 60% Water, 80% Air, 30Hz
Other Er,Cr:YSGG laser system settings: 2.00W, 30% Water, 30% Air

After directing the laser over the treatment site for 30 seconds, change the settings. Aim the laser beam outside the peripheral rim of enamel, directing the energy into where the proximal box will form, for a further 30 seconds.

Laser Parameters, Set 3: Pre-Conditioning and Enamel Ablation

Waterlase MD laser system settings: 4.50W, 60% Water, 80% Air, 30Hz
Other Er,Cr:YSGG laser system settings: 4.00W, 60% Water, 65% Air

Change settings for ablation of the enamel on the marginal ridge. You should see ablation of enamel at this point. Be careful not to ablate the adjacent tooth.

After approximately 30 seconds, switch to a high-speed ¼ to ½ round bur to break the enamel. The high-speed drill is then also used to reach the dentin, until an outline of the proximal slot is established.

Laser Parameters, Set 4: Dentin Ablation

Waterlase MD laser system settings: 2.00W, 60% Water, 80% Air, 30Hz
Other Er,Cr:YSGG laser system settings: 2.00W, 15% Water, 15% Air

Switch back to the laser using the above setting to continue the cavity preparation in the dentin. A slow buccal-lingual (back and forth) sweeping motion is used to continue preparation of a proximal box. Use a slow-speed round bur to remove any remaining caries and perform a caries check. This is followed by one final laser treatment using the current settings to remove any smear layer on the enamel and etch the cavity. Dry the surface with an air syringe to visualize the completeness of the preparation and etching, and to check if there is any sclerotic dentin left. Any remaining sclerotic dentin should be removed using the above settings.

Class II Preparation – Rabbit Technique – Slot Design

Laser Parameters, Set 1: Pre-Conditioning

Waterlase MD laser system settings: MG-6 tip, 3.00-4.50W, 60% Water, 80% Air, 10-15 Hz
Other Er,Cr:YSGG laser system settings: G-6 tip, 5.50-6.00W, 75% Water, 90% Air

Defocus the fiber tip to 6-10mm from the tooth surface, aiming laser energy towards the marginal ridge. Spend 90 seconds going back and forth over the marginal ridge, keeping the defocused distance as constant as possible.

Laser Parameters, Set 2: Ablation

After 90 seconds, focus the fiber tip by bringing it in to within 2-3mm from the peripheral rim of enamel to ablate enamel at the marginal ridge. Aim the laser beam outside the peripheral rim of enamel, directing the energy into where the proximal box will form, for a further 30 seconds.

Use a slow buccal-lingual (back and forth) sweeping motion of the fiber tip to lower the proximal box. Advance the tip downwards, following the preparation into the box.

Once the marginal ridge is removed down to the level of the pulpal occlusal floor, prepare the walls of the box by aiming into the sides. A slow-speed round bur may be used to complete removal of any remaining caries and for caries check. To finish the preparation, defocus the fiber tip to approximately 5mm and etch the cavity surface.

Dry the surface with an air syringe to visualize the completeness of the preparation and etching, and to check if there is any sclerotic dentin left. Any remaining sclerotic dentin should be removed using the above settings.

Class II Slot Preparation (Supplementary Drawings)

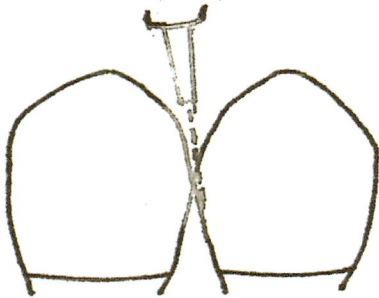

Fig. 1: The tip is placed to aim at the proximal area where the Class II decay is located (buccal view).

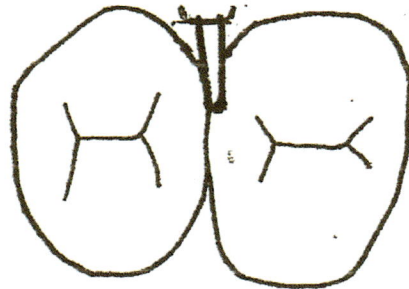

Fig. 2: The tip is placed to aim at the proximal area where the Class II decay is located (occlusal view).

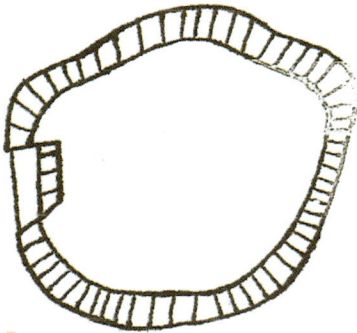

Fig. 3: The slot preparation is complete (occlusal view).

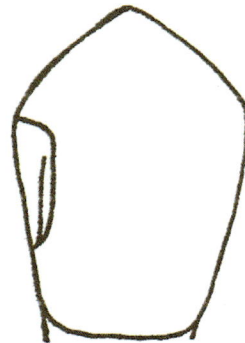

Fig. 4: The slot preparation is complete (buccal view).

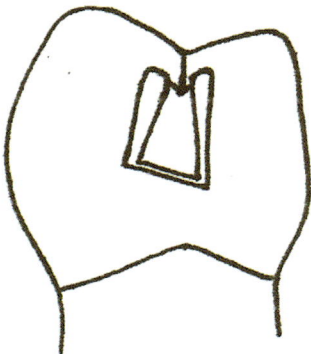

Fig. 5: The slot preparation is complete (proximal view).

Case 1: Class II, Modified Turtle, Slot Design

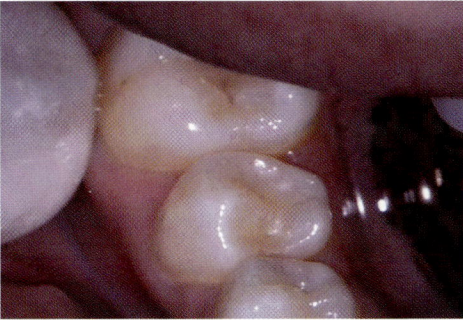

Fig. 1: Pre-op. Distal proximal surface has a Class II caries.

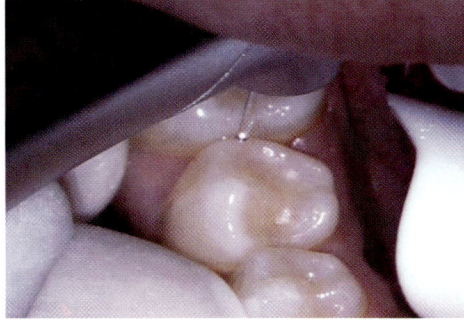

Fig. 2: The tip is focused and aimed at the ridge where the proximal caries are located. To pre-condition the tooth, the setting is 2.00W, 60% Water, 80% Air, 30 Hz.

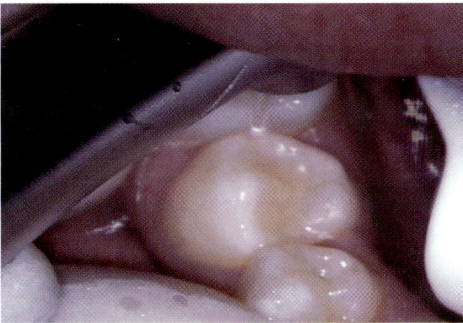

Fig. 3: Ablation of the enamel of the distal ridge. The setting is 3.50W, 60% Water, 80% Air, 15 Hz.

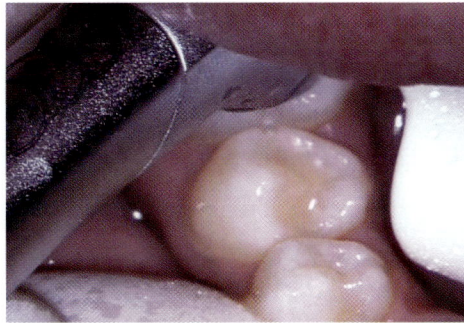

Fig. 4: The tip is angled to extend the cavity prep.

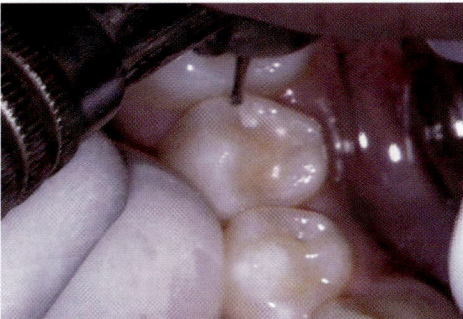

Fig. 5: A ¼ high speed is used to quickly outline the slot prep.

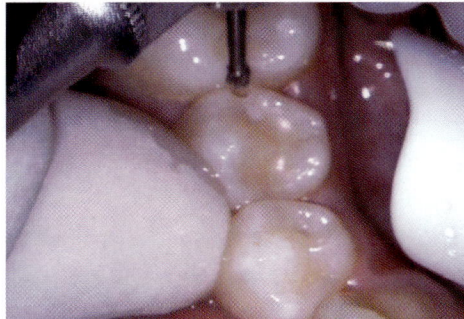

Fig. 6: Slow speed round bur is used to make sure all decay is removed.

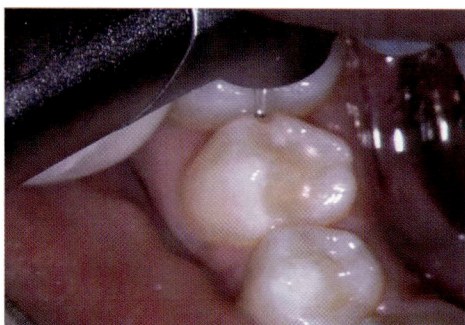

Fig 7: The tip is focused to remove smear, debris, and complete preparation. The setting is 2.00W, 60% Water, 80% Air, 30 Hz.

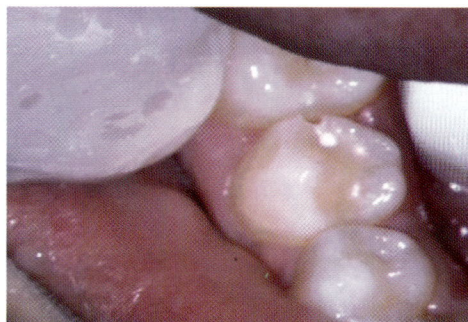

Fig 8: Post-op. The Class II slot prep is complete.

Case 2: Class II, Modified Turtle, Slot Design, Gold Handpiece

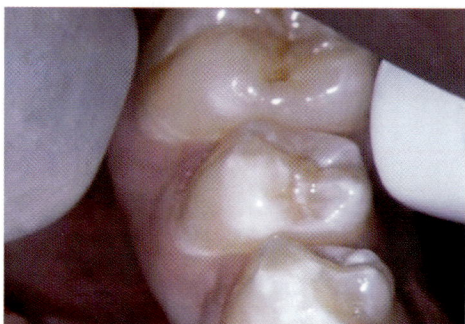

Fig. 1: Pre-op. A small DO lesion is present in #29.

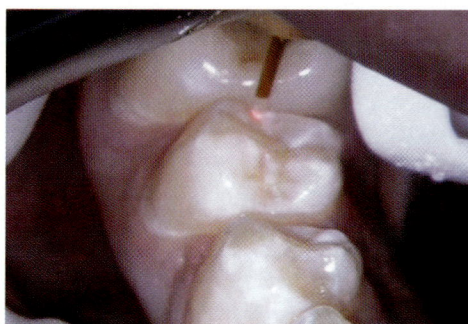

Fig. 2: A MZ-5 tip in a MD Gold handpiece is used to pre-condition #29. The tip is focused at 1.5mm from the distal ridge. The setting is 2.00W 60% Water, 80% Air, 30 Hz.

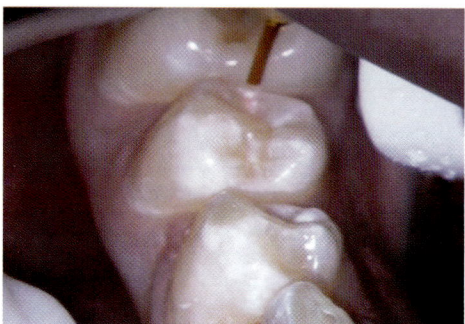

Fig. 3: Pre-conditioning continues with 3.00W and 4.50W, 60% Water, 80% Air, 30 Hz. Ablation of enamel into about ½ the depth of the slot box by laser.

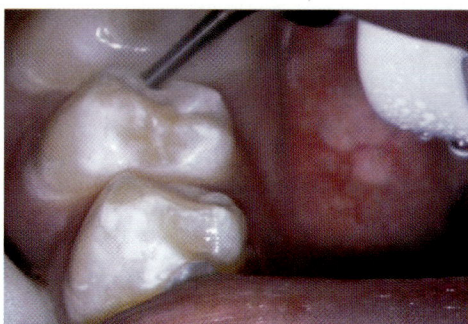

Fig. 4: A high-speed ¼ round bur is used with plenty of water to outline the slot.

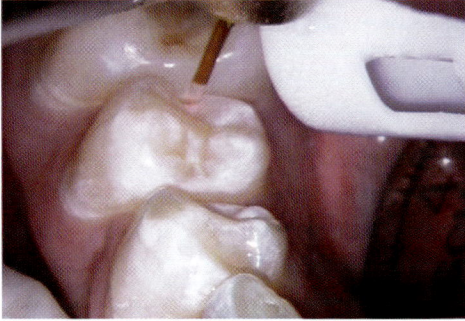

Fig. 5: Laser energy is used to continue ablation and cleaning of the slot.

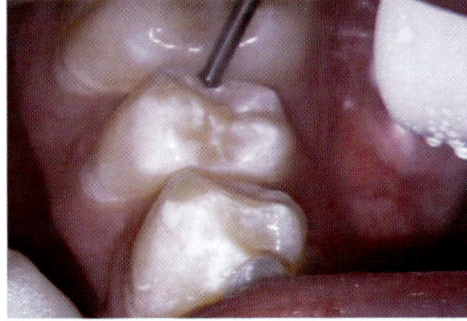

Fig. 6: A slow-speed round bur is used to remove and check caries.

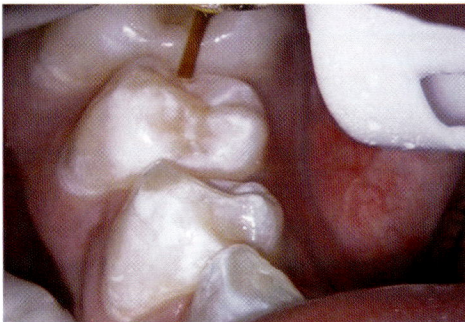

Fig. 7: The cavity preparation is finished with laser energy. The setting is 2.00W, 60% Water, 80% Air, 30 Hz.

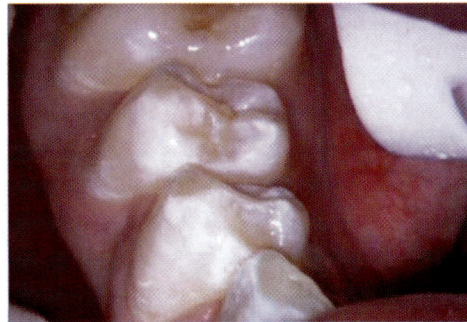

Fig. 8: Post-op. A DO slot prep is complete.

Case 3: Class II, Modified Turtle, Slot Design, Gold Handpiece

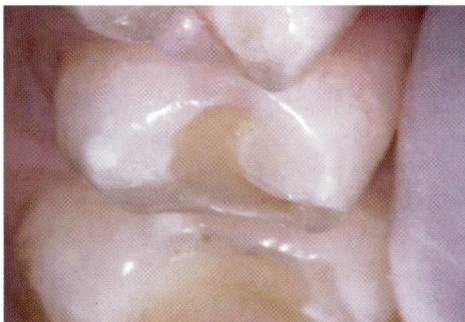

Fig. 1: Pre-op. MO lesion is present in #3.

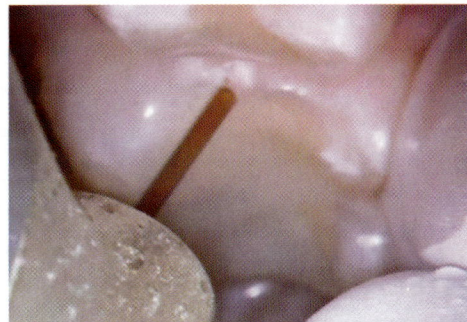

Fig. 2: A MZ-5 tip in a MD gold handpiece is used. It is focused at 1mm aiming at the mesial ridge. The setting is 2.00W, 60% Water, 80% Air, 30 Hz.

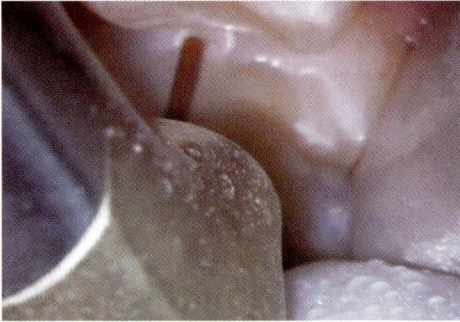

Fig. 3: Pre-conditioning continues with 3.00W and 4.50W, 60% Water, 80% Air, 30 Hz.

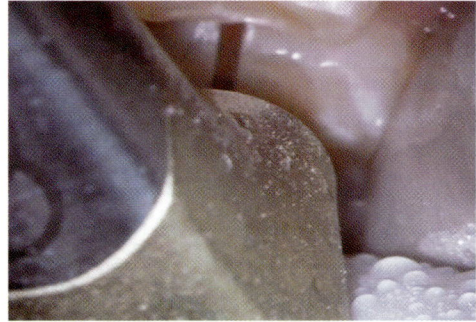

Fig. 4: A slot prep is started by laser energy into the dentin.

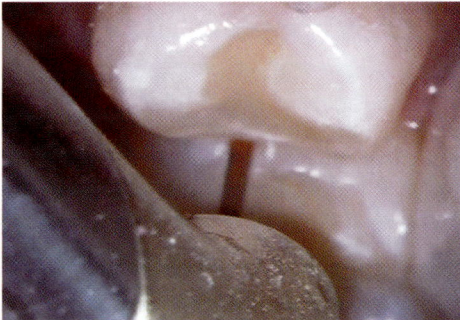

Fig. 5: More efficient ablation is done at 3.50W 60% Water, 80% Air, 15 Hz. Caries removal and slot preparation is being completed.

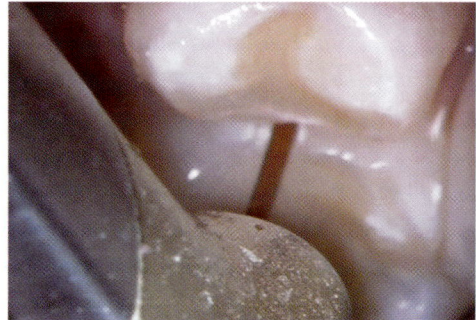

Fig. 6: 2.00W, 60% Water, 80% Air, 30 Hz is used to finish the preparation.

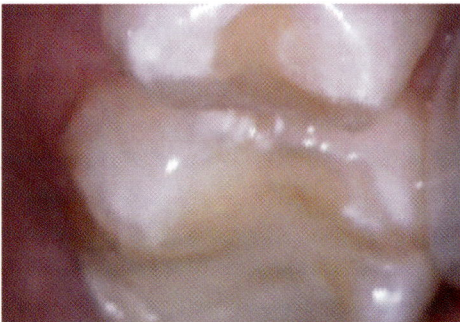

Fig. 7: The MO slot prep is complete.

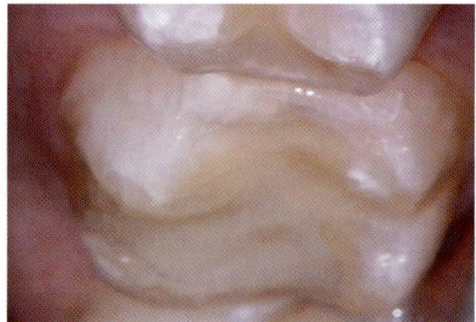

Fig. 8: Immediate post-op after composite restoration.

Case 4: Class II, Modified Turtle, Slot Design

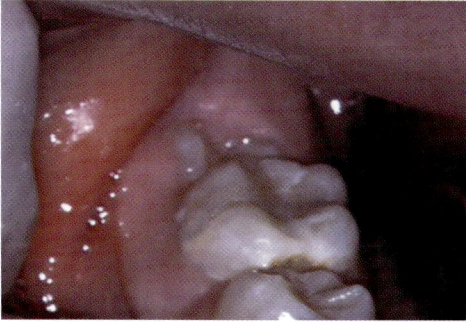

Fig. 1: Pre-op. A moderate size caries is present at the mesial surface of #30.

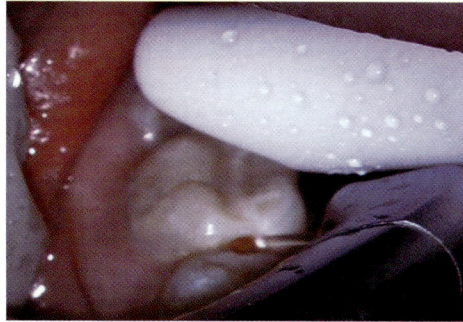

Fig. 2: A MG-6 in a MD standard handpiece is used. Pre-conditioning of the tooth is done at 2.00W, 60% Water, 80% Air, 30 Hz.

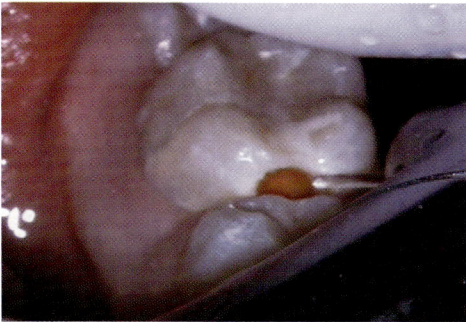

Fig. 3: More pre-conditioning and some caries removal is done at 3.00W and 4.50W, 60% Water, 80% Air, 30 Hz.

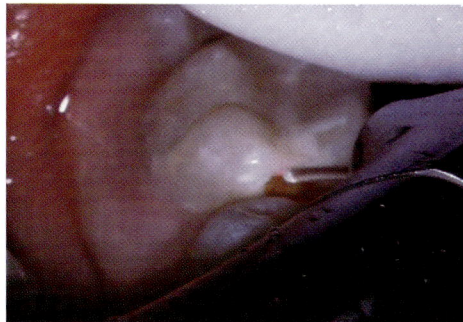

Fig. 4: The preparation continues with 3.50W 60% Water, 80% Air, 15 Hz.

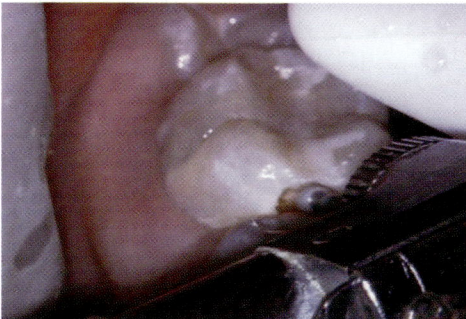

Fig. 5: Caries removal and check is done by a slow-speed round bur.

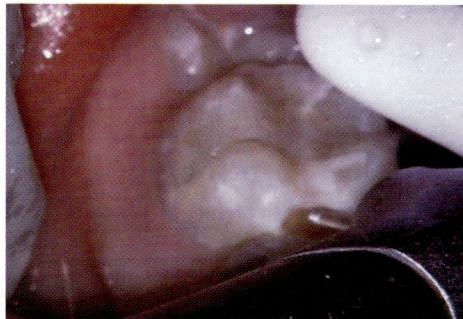

Fig. 6: The preparation is finished with laser energy. The setting is 2.00W, 60% Water, 80% Air, 30 Hz.

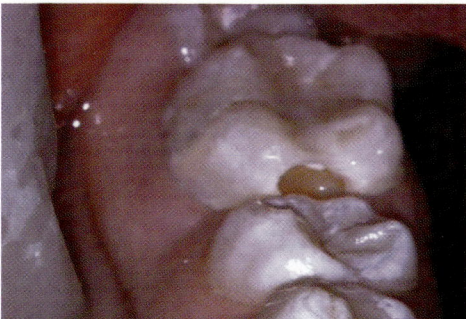

Fig. 7: The MO slot preparation is complete.

Class II Cavity Preparation – Modified Turtle Technique – Tunnel Design

To start the Modified Turtle Technique, a similar protocol as the Turtle Technique is used. Keep the fiber tip in focused mode at all times (1.5-2mm).

Laser Parameters, Set 1: Pre-Conditioning

Waterlase MD laser system settings: MG-6 tip, 2.00W, 60% Water, 80% Air, 30Hz
Other Er,Cr:YSGG laser system settings: G-6 tip, 1.25W, 15% Water, 15% Air

Direct the fiber tip perpendicular towards the fissure, down the long axis of the tooth. When ablating, the motion used is semi-circular, and back-and-forth, but primarily aiming at the area where the lesion is located. Move slowly along the length of the lesion. Fire the laser at starting settings for 30 seconds.

Laser Parameters, Set 2: Continue Pre-Conditioning

Waterlase MD laser system settings: 3.00W, 60% Water, 80% Air, 30Hz
Other Er,Cr:YSGG laser system settings: 2.00W, 30% Water, 30% Air

After directing the laser over the treatment site for 30 seconds, change the settings. Aim the laser beam outside the peripheral rim of enamel for a further 30 seconds.

Laser Parameters, Set 3: Enamel Ablation

Waterlase MD laser system settings: 4.50W, 60% Water, 80% Air, 30Hz
Other Er,Cr:YSGG laser system settings: 4.00W, 60% Water, 65% Air

Change settings to 4.50W, 60% Water, 80% Air, 30 Hz for ablation of the enamel on the marginal ridge. You should see ablation of enamel at this point.

After approximately 30 seconds, switch to a high-speed ¼ to ½ round bur to shave its way into a rough tunnel without breaking the proximal enamel. Switch back to the laser at current settings, and clean the rough tunnel cavity. This is followed by using a slow-speed round bur to break the proximal enamel and remove caries. Laser energy is used to clean the cavity, removing the smear layer and etching the surface.

Note: At least 2mm of tooth structure should be preserved above a tunnel preparation. Even though it is a more conservative preparation than a slot preparation or conventional Class II design, the tunnel preparation may still take more time to complete.

Laser Parameters, Set 4: Complete Preparation

Waterlase MD laser system settings: 2.00W, 60% Water, 80% Air, 30 Hz
Other Er,Cr:YSGG laser system settings: 2.00W, 30% Water, 30% Air

Energy is used to remove smear, debris and etch the cavity before restoration.

Class II Preparation – Rabbit Technique – Tunnel Design

Laser Parameters, Set 1: Pre-Conditioning

Waterlase MD laser system settings: MG-6 tip, 3.00-4.50W, 60% Water, 80% Air, 10-15Hz
Other Er,Cr:YSGG laser system settings: G-6 tip, 5.50–6.00W, 75% Water, 90% Air

> The fiber tip is placed perpendicular towards the fossa and along the long axis of the tooth. Defocus the tip 6-10mm from the tooth surface and spend 90 seconds going back and forth over the fossa, keeping the defocused distance as constant as possible.

Laser Parameters, Set 2: Enamel/Dentin Ablation

> After approximately 90 seconds, the tip is focused to 1-2mm to ablate enamel. Retain the same settings as above. Establish a Class I prep at the fossa before starting a tunnel towards the caries in the proximal surface.
>
> A tunnel outline is established to just shy of breaking the enamel at the proximal area. Use a slow-speed round bur to break the proximal enamel and remove caries. After that, laser energy in a defocused mode is used to clean the cavity, removing smear and etching the surface. Note that about 2mm of the marginal ridge needs to be preserved.

Class II Preparation – Tunnel Design Supplementary Drawings

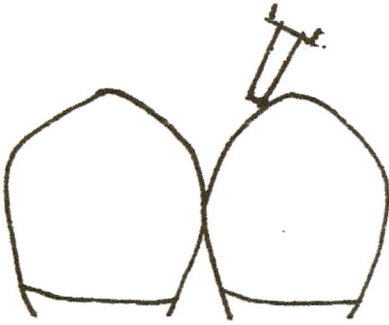

Fig. 1: The tip is placed to aim at the fossa next to the decay (buccal view).

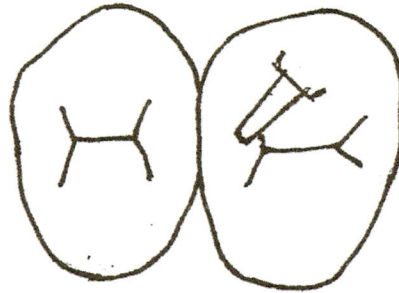

Fig. 2: The tip is placed to aim at the fossa next to the decay (occlusal view).

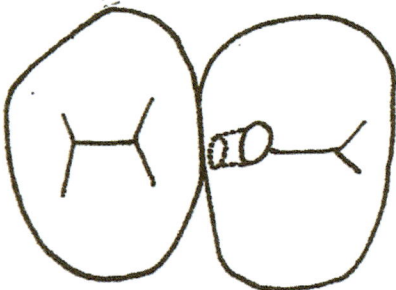

Fig. 3: The tunnel is being prepared (occlusal view).

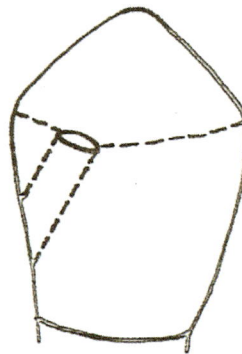

Fig. 4: The tunnel preparation is complete (buccal view).

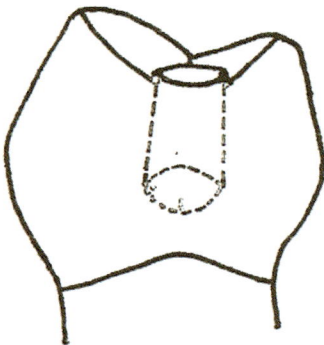

Fig. 5: The tunnel preparation is complete (proximal view).

Case 1: Class II, Modified Turtle, Tunnel Design

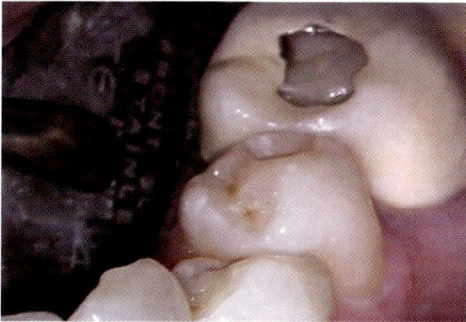

Fig. 1: Pre-op. Caries is present at distal surface and the central and mesial fossa of # 20.

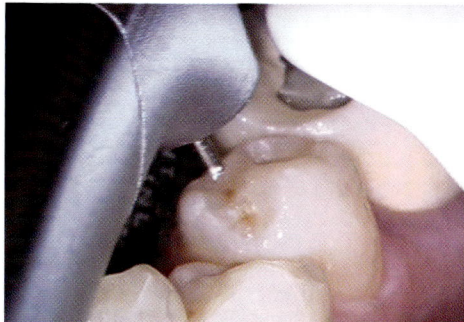

Fig. 2: The tip is focused and aimed at the central fossa to precondition the pulp. The setting is 2.00W, 60% Water, 80% Air, 30 Hz.

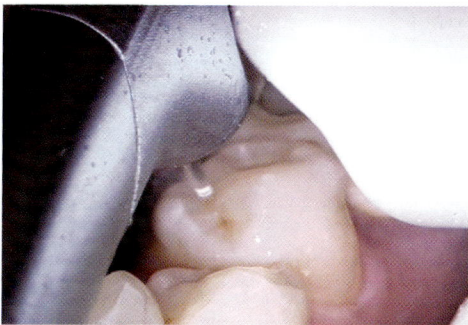

Fig. 3: Class I "dot design" of the central fossa is prepared with the laser. The setting is 3.50W, 60% Water, 80% Air, 15 Hz.

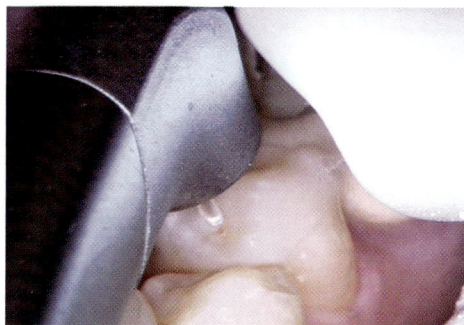

Fig. 4: Class I "dot design" of the mesial fossa is prepared with the laser.

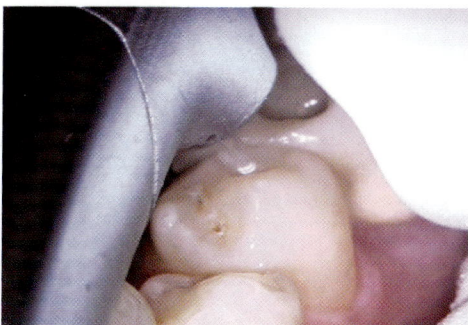

Fig. 5: The tip is focused and aimed at the distal fossa.

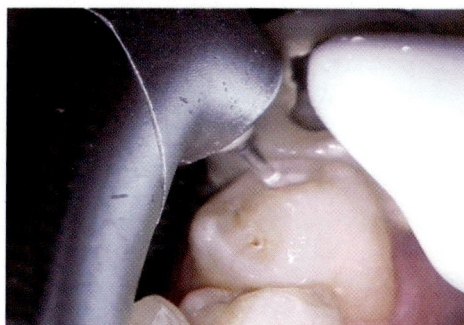

Fig. 6: A conservative occlusal prep is established with the laser.

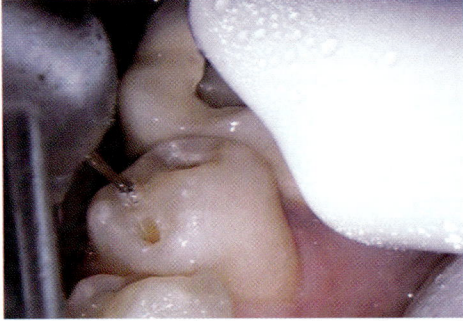

Fig. 7: A ¼ round high-speed is used to outline a tunnel to the distal surface. This is done short of breaking through the enamel at the distal surface.

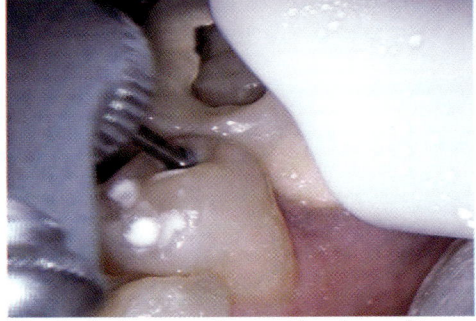

Fig. 8: A slow-speed round bur is used to remove enamel at the distal surface where the caries is. It is also used to complete caries removal.

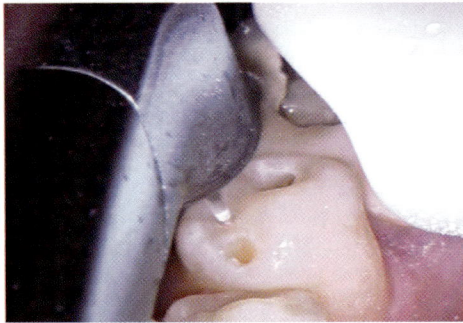

Fig. 9: The "tunnel prep" is completed with laser energy removing smear, debris and etching the cavity. The setting is 2.00W, 60% Water, 80% Air, 30 Hz.

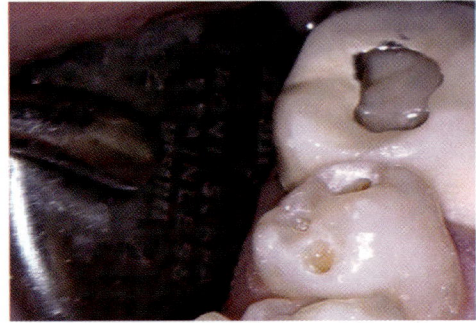

Fig. 10: Post-op. Completion of Class II "tunnel prep" at the distal surface of #20 and Class I "dot prep" at the central and mesial fossa.

Case 2: Class II, Modified Turtle, Tunnel Design

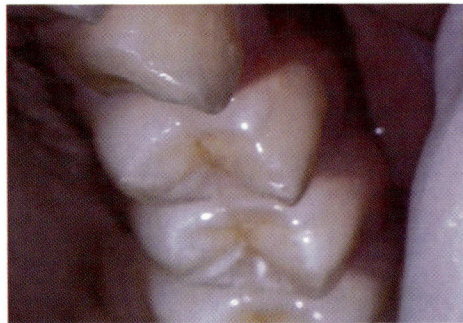

Fig. 1: Pre-op. An occlusal lesion at the mesial fossa and a small DO lesion is present just under the contact in #5.

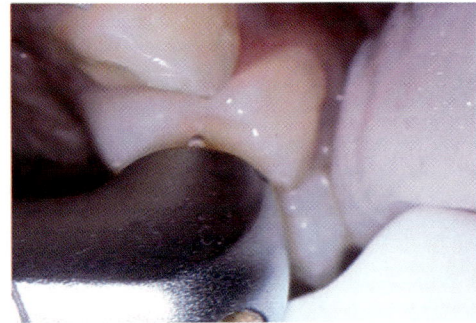

Fig. 2: A MG-6 tip is used to prepare a "dot" prep in the mesial fossa.

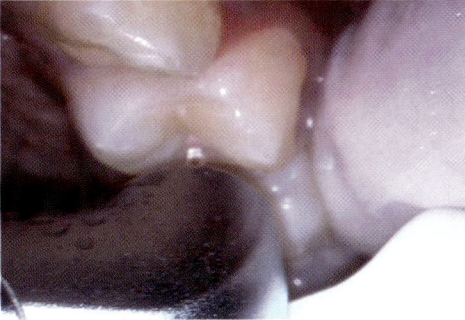

Fig. 3: Another occlusal prep is done by laser at the distal fossa. The setting is 4.50W, 60% Water, 80% Air, 30 Hz.

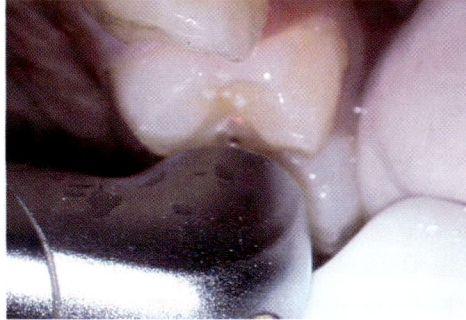

Fig. 4: The tip is angled to start a tunnel prep at the distal.

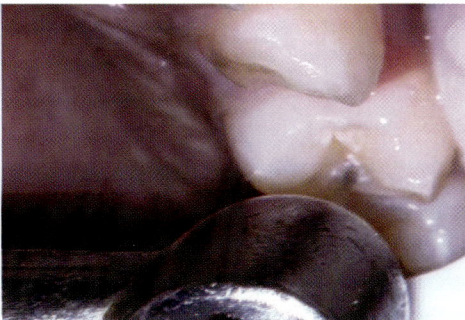

Fig. 5: After laser pre-conditioning of the tooth, a high-speed ½ round bur is used to outline the tunnel to the proximal caries. This is short of breaking the contact.

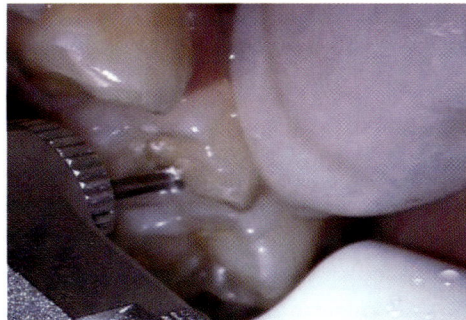

Fig. 6: A slow-speed round bur is used to break the distal contact. It is also used to remove and check caries.

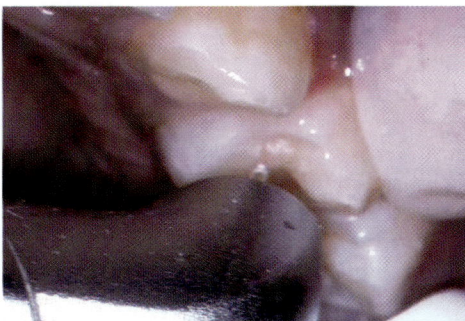

Fig. 7: Laser is used to finish preparation. The setting is 2.00W, 60% Water, 80% Air, 30 Hz.

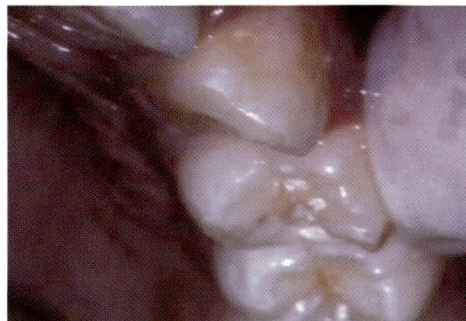

Fig. 8: Post-op. The DO tunnel prep is complete.

Class III – Turtle Technique

Laser Parameters, Set 1: Pre-Conditioning

Waterlase MD laser system settings: MG-6 tip, 2.00W, 60% Water, 80% Air, 30 Hz
Other Er,Cr:YSGG laser system settings: G-6 tip, 2.00W, 15% Water, 15% Air.

Focus the fiber tip towards the lesion on the lingual surface. The tip should be pointed perpendicular to the surface.

Either use a slow circular motion, or an up-and-down motion, concentrating on one particular spot, and advance slowly into the carious lesion for 30 seconds.

Laser Parameters, Set 2: Continue Pre-Conditioning

Waterlase MD laser system settings: 2.50W, 60% Water, 80% Air, 30Hz
Other Er,Cr:YSGG laser system settings: 2.50W, 15% Water, 15% Air

Increase the power by 0.50W and continue ablation for 30 seconds. Laser enamel ablation and separation along the marginal ridges occurs anteriorly until the contact between the adjacent teeth is broken.

This incremental (+0.50W) increase in power continues every 30 seconds until satisfactory enamel ablation speed occurs, without hurting the patient. The power should increase only until speed of ablation is satisfactory or the patient feels discomfort. Normally the highest power needed for the ablation of anterior teeth enamel is between 2.50-3.50W for the Waterlase MD or 2.25-3.00W for other Er,Cr:YSGG laser systems.

Laser Parameters, Set 3: Dentin Ablation

Waterlase MD laser system settings: 2.00-2.5W, 60% Water, 80% Air, 30 Hz
Other Er,Cr:YSGG laser system settings: 2.00-2.5W, 30% Water, 30% Air

Once the preparation reaches the dentin, the power setting is lowered; any ablation in dentin using the laser should take place in a defocused mode, about 2.5-4.0mm away from the target. This is sufficient to remove decay. For large lesions, and/or to ensure all soft caries are removed, use a slow-speed round bur (#2 or #4) to check and/or remove gross soft caries. The cavity should have a sound dentin floor and walls that do not have caries.

Laser Parameters, Set 4: Final Preparation

Waterlase MD Laser system settings: 2.00W, 60% Water, 80% Air, 30 Hz
Other Er,Cr:YSGG laser system settings: 2.00W, 30% Water, 30% Air

To finish the cavity preparation, use the laser at the same settings and in focused mode to remove any smear layer or debris, and prepare the surface for stronger bonding with composite. Dry the surface with an air syringe to visualize the completeness of the preparation and etching, and to check if there is any sclerotic dentin left. Any remaining sclerotic dentin should be removed using the above settings.

Class III – Rabbit Technique

Laser Parameters, Set 1: Pre-Conditioning

Waterlase MD laser system settings: MG-6 tip, 3.00-3.50W, 60% Water, 80% Air, 15Hz
Other Er,Cr:YSGG laser system settings: G-6 tip, 4.00W, 60% Water, 65% Air

> Note: Due to thinner enamel in anterior teeth, the initial high power setting used in this technique is lower than would be used for enamel in other locations.

> Defocus the fiber tip to 6-10mm from the tooth surface, aiming laser energy towards the fissure. Spend 90 seconds going back and forth over the fissure, keeping the defocused distance as constant as possible.

Laser Parameters, Set 2: Enamel Ablation

> After 90 seconds, focus the tip towards the lesion to start ablation of enamel. As the tip gets close to the caries and ablation is noticed, keep the tip at the same defocused distance, advancing slowly into the caries.

> A slow circular or back-and-forth motion is used over the surface. Extend the preparation anteriorly along the marginal ridge area until the contact is broken.

> Care needs to be taken to make sure the tip is defocused to avoid using too much power that may cause discomfort. A slow-speed round bur may be used to complete caries removal and for caries check.

> Finally, use the laser in defocused mode at about 5mm from the tooth surface to etch of the cavity preparation.

Case 1: Class III, Turtle Technique

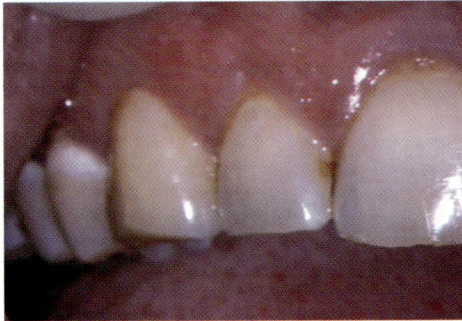

Fig. 1: Pre-op showing a Class III lesion at the mesial surface of #7.

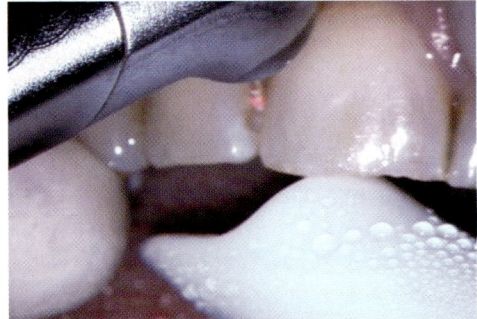

Fig. 2: A MG-6 (or MZ-6) is used, defocused and aimed at the mesial lesion of #7. The setting is 2.00W, 60% Water, 80% Air, 30 Hz.

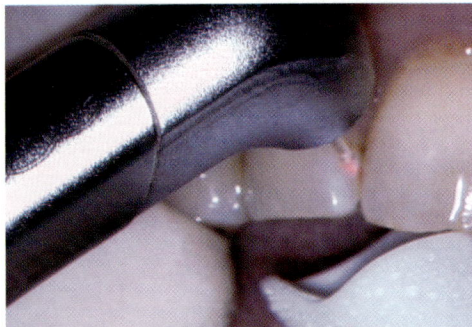

Fig. 3: The power setting is raised 0.25W at a time until enamel ablation is efficient. The setting should be 2.50-3.50W, 60% Water, 80% Air, 30 Hz.

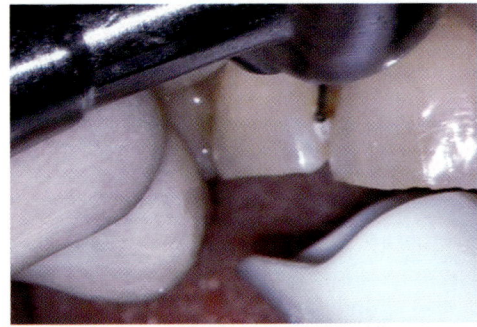

Fig. 4: A slow-speed round bur is used for caries check.

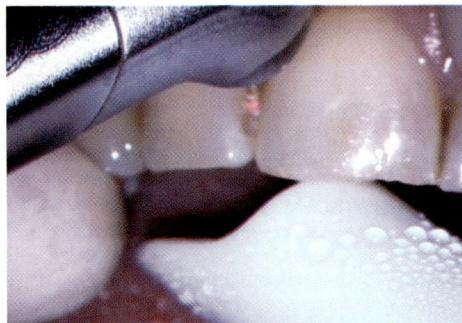

Fig. 5: The Class III preparation is finished with laser debridement and cleaning at 2.00W, 60% Water, 80% Air, 30 Hz.

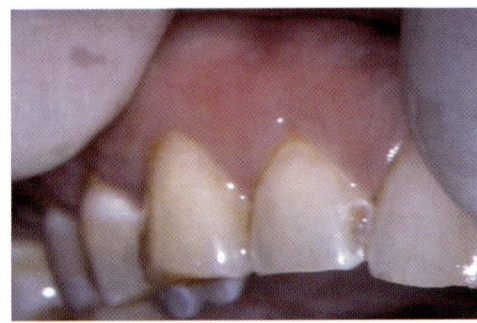

Fig. 6: Immediate post-op of Class III preparation.

Class III Cavity Preparation – Modified Turtle Technique

Laser Parameters, Set 1: Pre-Conditioning

Waterlase MD laser system settings: MG-6 tip, 2.00W, 60% Water, 80% Air, 30Hz
Other Er,Cr:YSGG laser system settings: G-6 tip, 2.00W, 30% Water, 30% Air

Focus the fiber tip towards the lesion on the lingual surface. The tip should be pointed perpendicular to the surface.

Either use a slow circular motion, or an up-and-down motion, concentrating on one particular area, and advance slowly into the carious lesion.

Laser Parameters, Set 2: Continue Pre-Conditioning

Waterlase MD laser system settings: 2.50W, 60% Water, 80% Air, 30Hz
Other Er,Cr:YSGG laser system settings: 2.50W, 30% Water, 30% Air

The power setting is increased by 0.25W every 30 seconds. This incremental increase in power continues every 30 seconds until satisfactory enamel ablation speed occurs, without hurting the patient. The power should increase only until speed of ablation is satisfactory or the patient feels discomfort. The highest power setting for this procedure can range from 1.50-3.50W for the Waterlase MD or 1.25-3.00W for other Er,Cr:YSGG laser systems.

Laser Parameters, Set 3: Complete Preparation

Waterlase MD laser system settings: 2.00W, 60% Water, 80% Air, 30 Hz
Other Er,Cr:YSGG laser system settings: 2.00W, 30% Water, 30% Air

To finish the cavity preparation, use the laser at the same settings and in focused mode to remove any smear layer or debris, and prepare the surface for stronger bonding with composite. Dry the surface with an air syringe to visualize the completeness of the preparation and etching, and to check if there is any sclerotic dentin left. Any remaining sclerotic dentin should be removed using the above settings.

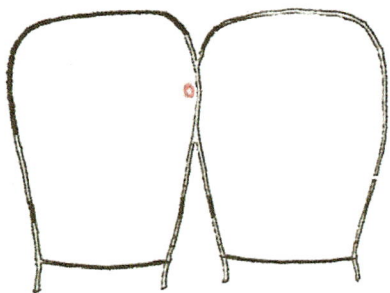

Fig. 1: Pre-operative caries is present in the proximal surface of the anterior tooth and extends to the lingual surface (lingual view).

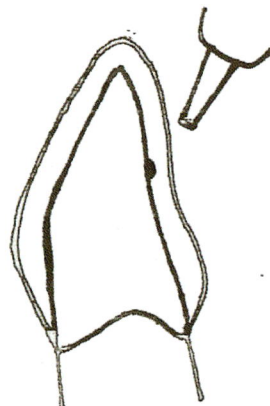

Fig. 2: The tip is focused and aimed at the caries for ablation (proximal view).

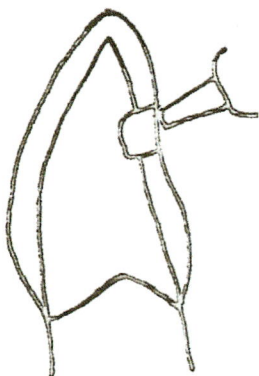

Fig. 3: About ½ of the Class III preparation is done by laser (proximal view).

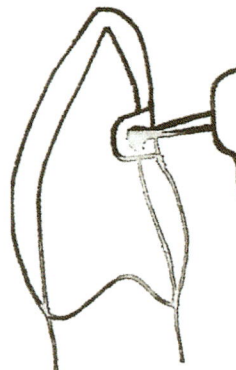

Fig. 4: A ½ round high-speed round bur is used to roughly prepare the Class III preparation (proximal view).

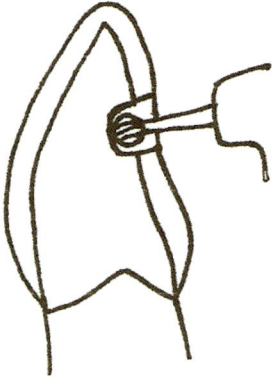

Fig. 5: Slow-speed round bur is used to remove and check caries (proximal view).

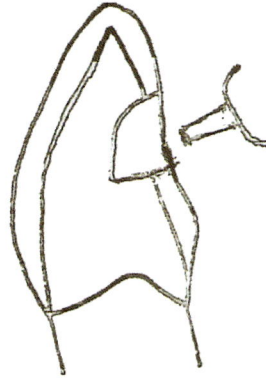

Fig. 6: Laser is used to finish the Class III preparation (proximal view).

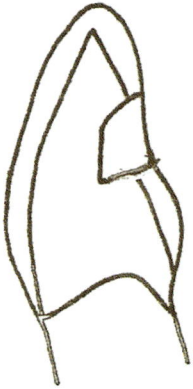

Fig. 7: Class III preparation is complete (proximal view).

Class IV – The Turtle Technique

Laser Parameters, Set 1: Pre-Conditioning

Waterlase MD laser system settings: MG-6 tip, 1.50W, 60% Water, 80% Air, 30Hz
Other Er,Cr:YSGG laser system settings: G-6 tip, 1.25W, 15% Water, 15% Air

The settings used in Class IV preparation are similar to the settings used in Class V. In focused mode, the laser is aimed at the lesion on the lingual surface.

Use a slow circular of back-and-forth motion over the surface and advance slowly into the carious lesion.

Laser Parameters, Set 2: Continue Pre-Conditioning and Enamel Ablation

Waterlase MD laser system settings: 1.75W, 60% Water, 80% Air, 30Hz
Other Er,Cr:YSGG laser system settings: 1.50W, 15% Water, 15% Air

The power setting is increased by 0.25W every 30 seconds. This incremental increase in power continues every 30 seconds until satisfactory enamel ablation speed occurs, without hurting the patient – the power should increase only until speed of ablation is satisfactory, or the patient feels discomfort. The preparation is continued along the marginal ridge continuing anteriorly until the contact is broken. The tip is then placed vertically to remove incisal or cuspal edge enamel and the preparation is extended into the previously prepared proximal region.

The maximum power setting is between 1.50-3.50W for the Waterlase MD and between 1.25-3.25W with other Er,Cr:YSGG laser systems.

Laser Parameters, Set 3: Remove Caries and Complete Preparation

Waterlase MD laser system settings: 1.50-2.00W, 60% Water, 80% Air, 30Hz
Other Er,Cr:YSGG laser system settings: 1.25-1.75W, 15% Water, 15% Air

Reduce the power setting to remove caries and clean and etch the surface of the tooth. Use a slow-speed round bur to complete the removal of caries and for caries check.

Because the tooth is made weaker by the removal of an angle of the tooth, retention is made by beveling the enamel on the facial and lingual surfaces to have a wider area for bonding.

Class IV – Rabbit Technique

Laser Parameters, Set 1: Pre-Conditioning

Waterlase MD laser system settings: MG-6 tip, 4.50W, 60% Water, 80% Air, 30Hz
Other Er,Cr:YSGG laser system settings: G-6 tip, 4.00W, 60% Water, 65% Air

Due to thinner enamel in anterior teeth, the highest power setting needed to ablate tooth tissue is only about 4.00-4.50W. Higher power levels should not be needed.

Aim the tip in a defocused mode 6-10mm at enamel from the lingual surface. After allowing 90 seconds for laser anesthesia, focus the tip towards the lesion to ablate enamel.

As the tip gets close to the caries, it is defocused to reduce power, advancing slowly into caries.

Laser Parameters, Set 2: Ablation

A slow circular or back-and-forth motion is used over the surface. The preparation extends anteriorly along the marginal ridge until the contact is broken. Then the tip is placed vertically to remove incisal or cuspal edge enamel, and the preparation is extended with the previously prepared proximal region.

Care needs to be taken to make sure the tip is defocused to avoid using too much power that may cause discomfort. A slow-speed round bur is used to complete the removal of caries and for caries check. To finish the preparation, laser energy is used to clean and etch the surface.

Case 1: Class IV, Turtle Technique

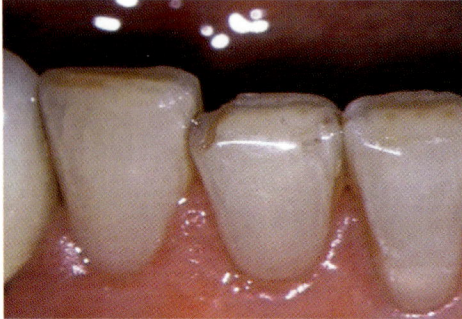

Fig. 1: Pre-op. #25 has caries and fracture at both the mesial and distal incisal angles.

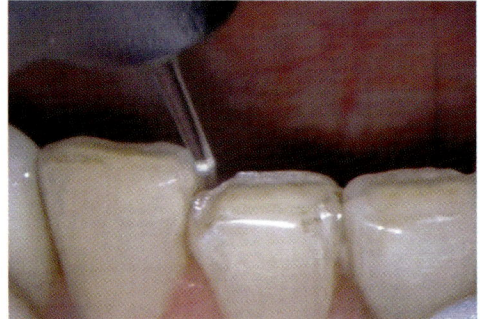

Fig. 2: The tip is focused and aimed at the distal incisal angle lesion. With lower power settings the tooth is treated with laser pre-conditioning. The setting is 1.50W, 60% Water, 80% Air, 30 Hz.

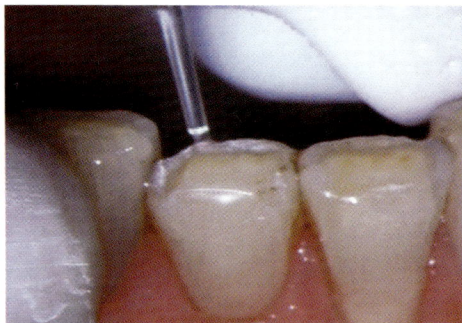

Fig. 3: The tip is focused and the Class IV cavity prep is extended into the incisal area. The setting is 2.00W, 60% Water, 80% Air, 30 Hz.

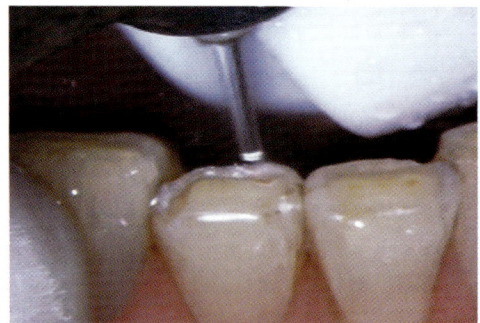

Fig. 4: The tip is focused and the preparation is extended further on the incisal area.

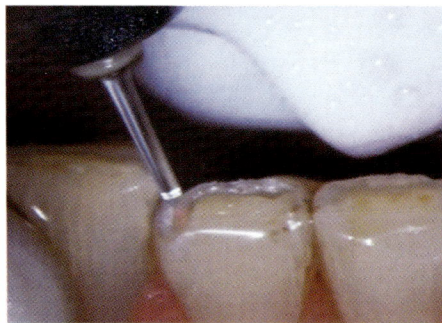

Fig.5: The tip is focused and aimed at the distal lesion to remove caries.

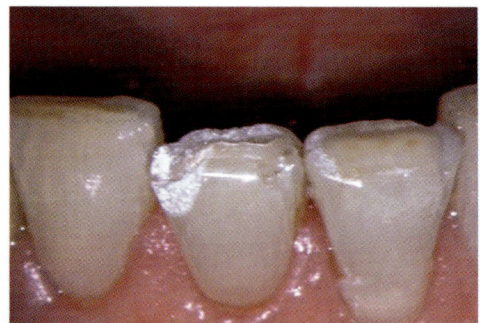

Fig. 6: After initial preparation of the distal lesion is completed, the air-dried surface reveals a chalky white appearance.

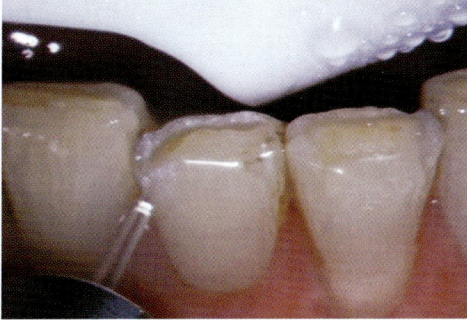

Fig. 7: Change of laser setting to a 40 Hz frequency to smooth away the chalky white rough surface.

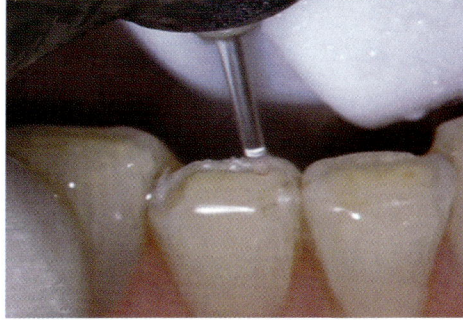

Fig. 8: The tip is focused and aimed at the mesial lesion for preparation.

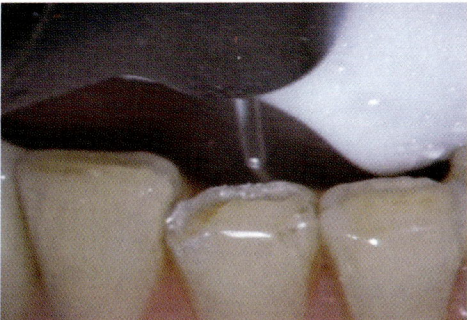

Fig. 9: The preparation of the mesial lesion is completed with 40 Hz frequency to smooth the mesial prep.

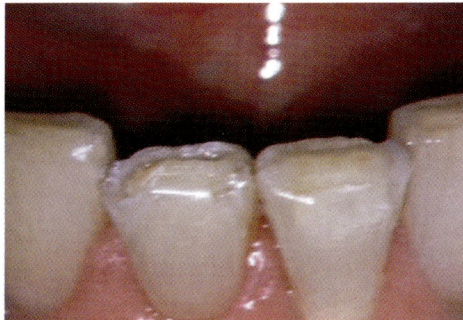

Fig. 10: Post-op Class IV preparation is complete.

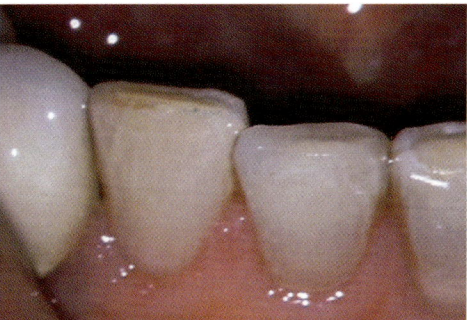

Fig. 11: #25 is restored.

Modified Turtle Technique: Class IV Laser Preparation

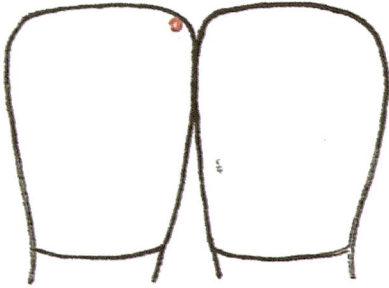

Fig. 1: Pre-operative caries is present in the angle of the incisor at the lingual surface (lingual view).

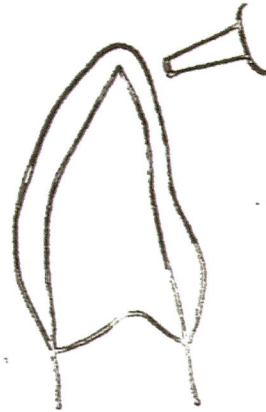

Fig. 2: The tip is aimed at where the caries are located (proximal view).

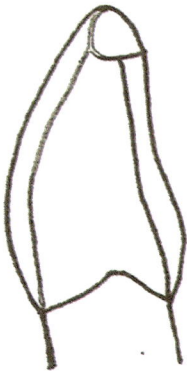

Fig. 3: The preparation after initial laser ablation is complete (proximal view).

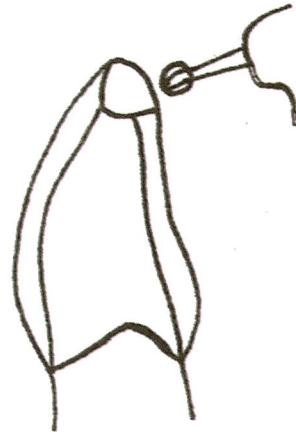

Fig. 4: A slow-speed round bur is used to remove and check caries (proximal view).

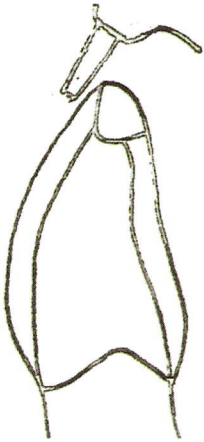

Fig. 5: The tip is aimed to prepare a bevel (proximal view).

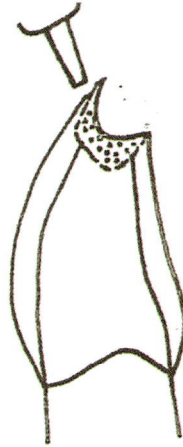

Fig. 6: The tip is aimed to finish the preparation (proximal view).

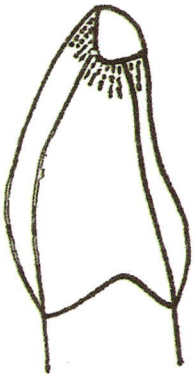

Fig. 7: The Class IV preparation is complete (proximal view).

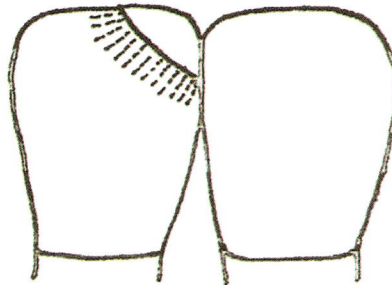

Fig. 8: The Class IV preparation is complete (lingual view).

Class V (Sensitive Lesions) – Turtle Technique

Laser Parameters, Set 1: Pre-Conditioning
(Optional first step should be considered particularly for patients with sensitive lesions –
otherwise, you may start with Laser Parameters, Set 2)

Waterlase MD laser system settings: MG-6 tip, 0.25W, 1% Water, 1% Air, 50 Hz
Other Er,Cr:YSGG laser system settings: G-6 tip, 0.25W, 15% Water, 15% Air

>If the cervical lesion (of erosion or abrasion nature) is sensitive, a procedure using a low-power laser to desensitize the lesion is done first. If the patient is extremely sensitive, increase the Hz setting to about 50, and then come back down to 20Hz with the final treatment settings.

>The tip is focused at 1-2mm from the lesion. The total treatment time for this setting is about 40 seconds.

>The patient should be informed that there are a few seconds of discomfort because water is used. A little time is needed to allow laser analgesia to be effective. This is expected to occur in under 30 seconds.

>In the majority of cases, the patient does not have any complaints about sensitivity during the therapy with the second setting, but if there is, repeat the above procedure for another 40 seconds.

Laser Parameters, Set 2: Pre-Conditioning

Waterlase MD laser system settings: MG-6 tip, 0.25W, 0% Water, 0% Air, 20 Hz
Other Er,Cr:YSGG laser system settings: G-6 tip, 0.25W, 7% Water, 7% Air

>Use a slow circular back-and-forth motion over the surface for 30 seconds and advance slowly into the carious lesion.

Laser Parameters, Set 3: Caries Removal and Cavity Preparation

Waterlase MD laser system settings: 1.25W, 60% Water, 80% Air, 30 Hz
Other Er,Cr:YSGG laser system settings: 1.25W, 15% Water, 15% Air

>Start ablation with the tip defocused at 5mm. After 30 seconds, bring the tip into focus, about 3mm from the lesion. Some patients may have discomfort with this setting. Go back to the second setting and repeat the second protocol for another 30 seconds before using the third setting again. The total treatment time for the third setting is about 30 seconds. (Note: There are patients who still experience some discomfort with 0.25W, 0% Water, 0% Air. Because the lesion is going to be restored and covered, the sensitivity will be gone.) The power setting is increased by 0.25W every 30 seconds until satisfactory enamel ablation occurs, without hurting the patient. Reduce the power setting to remove caries and etch the surface of the cavity.

Dry the surface with an air syringe to visualize the completeness of the preparation and etching, and to check if there is any sclerotic dentin left. Any remaining sclerotic dentin should be removed using the above settings.

Case 1: Class V, Turtle Technique

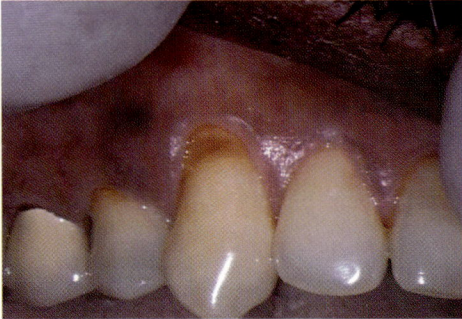

Fig. 1: Pre-op. Class V lesion at the facial surface of #6.

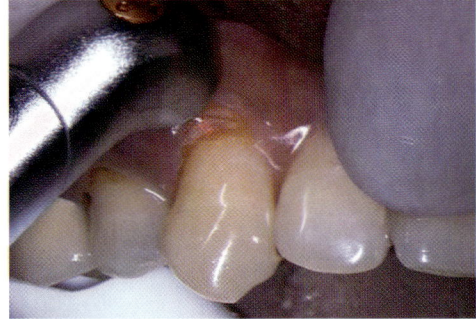

Fig. 2: The tip is focused and aimed at caries to precondition and clean the cavity. The setting is 1.50W, 60% Water, 80% Air, 30 Hz.

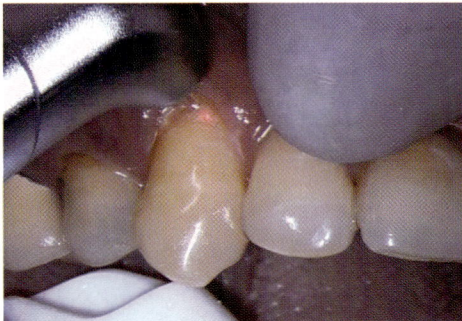

Fig. 3: The tip is focused and the power has been increased to remove enamel caries and dentin. The setting is 1.75W, 60% Water, 80% Air, 30 Hz.

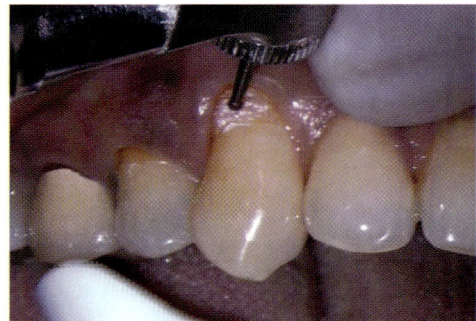

Fig. 4: A slow-speed round bur is used to check caries.

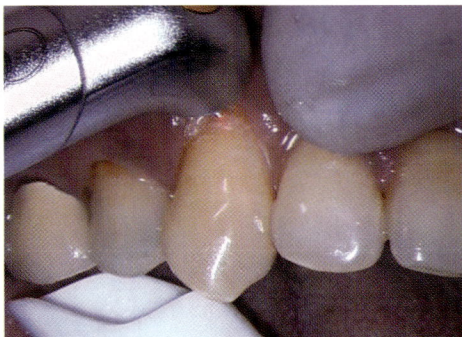

Fig. 5: The tip is focused and laser energy is used to remove smear, debris and complete the preparation.

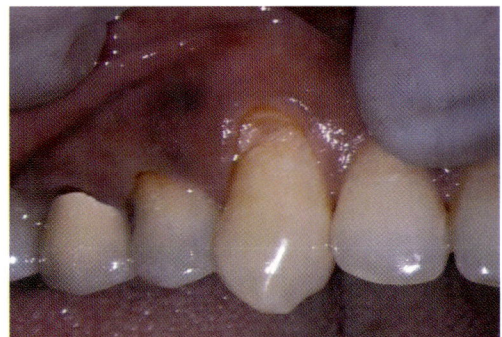

Fig. 6: Post-op. Class V cavity prep is completed.

Class V – Rabbit Technique

Laser Parameters, Set 1: Pre-Conditioning

Waterlase MD laser system settings: MG-6 tip, 2.00W, 60% Water, 80% Air, 15Hz
Other Er,Cr:YSGG laser system settings: G-6 tip, 2.00W, 30% Water, 30% Air

> The tip is defocused at 6-10mm from the lesion, 90 seconds is spent at preconditioning the tooth. The tip is moved slowly from one border of the lesion to the other, and this is done in a back-and-forth fashion.

Laser Parameters, Set 2: Enamel Ablation

Waterlase MD laser system settings: MG-6 tip, 2.00W, 60% Water, 80% Air, 15 Hz
Other Er,Cr:YSGG laser system settings: G-6 tip, 2.00W, 30% Water, 30% Air

> The tip is focused at 1-2mm from the lesion. This is aimed at removing enamel. The tip can be at a slight angle aiming at the lesion for faster ablation. Again, a slow back-and-forth motion over the surface is used.

Laser Parameters, Set 3: Dentin and Caries Removal

Waterlase MD laser system settings: MG-6 tip, 2.00W, 60% Water, 80% Air, 15 Hz
Other Er,Cr:YSGG laser system settings: G-6 tip, 2.00W, 30% Water, 30% Air

> The tip is defocused at 3-5mm from the pulpal floor. Dentin and caries removal is performed. A slow-speed round bur is used to check caries and to complete removal of caries. A light shaving motion is used with the slow-speed rotary instrument. The tip is defocused at 3-5mm from the pulp floor to finish preparation by removing smear, debris, and etching surface.

Case 2: Class V, Rabbit Technique

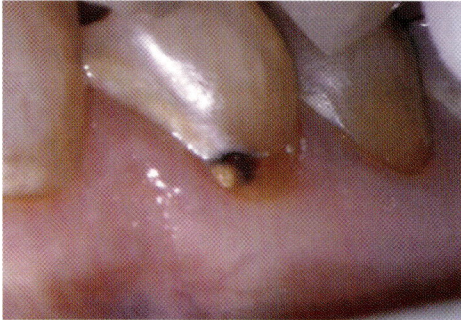

Fig. 1: Pre-op. A Class V caries with the gingival margin in the subgingival area.

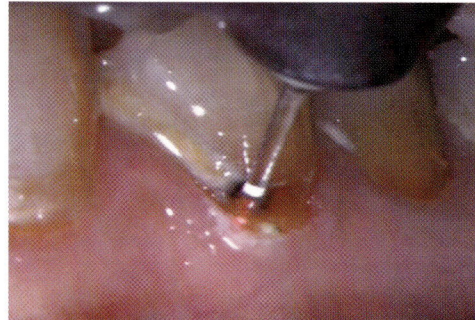

Fig. 2: Gingivectomy is performed to reveal the subgingival caries. The tip used is MG-6. The setting is 1.25W, 11% Water, 11% Air, 30 Hz.

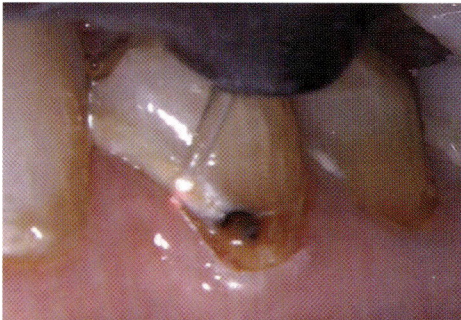

Fig. 3: Gingivectomy continues until the subgingival caries is revealed.

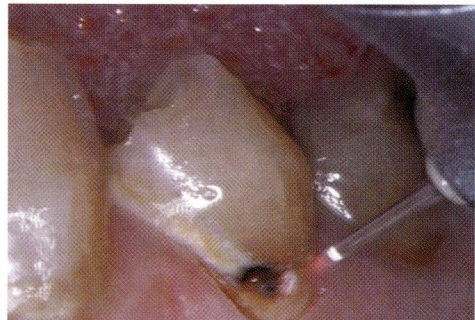

Fig. 4: A hard tissue setting is used to remove caries and prepare the Class V cavity prep. The setting is 2.00W, 60% Water, 80% Air, 15 Hz.

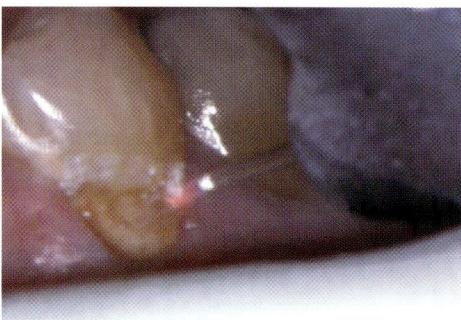

Fig. 5: To finish the prep, smear and debris are removed. Same settings used as in Fig. 4, in a defocused mode.

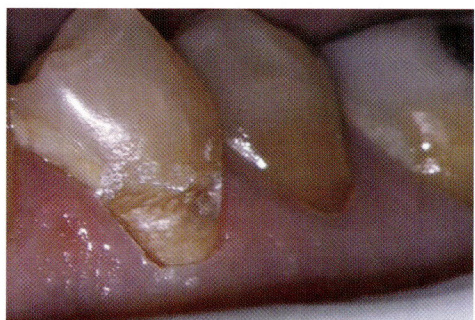

Fig. 6: Immediate post-op.

Pediatric Dentistry

Introduction

Dentistry has not traditionally been popular with patients because many patients find the experience traumatic. Fear of the needle keeps some patients from seeking preventive care, as many wait for a toothache to develop before visiting the dentist. These patients do not like the experience of having a needle injected into the oral cavity. They do not enjoy the numb feeling that dental anesthesia leaves them, even after they have left the dental chair. They associate the high-speed drill with vibrations, smell and the "fire engine" sound. They also fear the post-operative bleeding, swelling, and pain from oral surgery.

With the advancement of laser dentistry, patients' experience during and after dental treatment is very different than in conventional dentistry. Procedures such as cavity preparation, frenectomy, pulpotomy, operculectomy, and even extractions can be done without the use of needle injection, without the post-operative dysfunction of numbness and complications. The "never-before-traumatized" pediatric patients have a chance to experience dentistry more comfortably. Their impression of laser dental care is typically very different from their impression of traditional dental care, which can be characterized by fear of the dentist and dental treatment. The pediatric patient can now accept a dental visit as a painless, gentle exercise. Without years of fear and dislike of dentistry, these new, young patients will have a chance to enjoy their routine visits to a dental office. The high percentage of success in performing "no shot", "no pain" dentistry makes a great case that laser dentistry is revolutionary.

The Importance of Educating Patients on How the Er,Cr:YSGG Laser System Works

It is important to illustrate the gentleness of the Er,Cr:YSGG laser system to pediatric patients by showing them the sound of the laser and by demonstrating how the water sprayer works on one's hand. We also explain how the laser system works to pediatric patients by using phrases such as, "The Er,Cr:YSGG laser system uses water to wash away the cavity bugs" and "The laser popping sounds are like Woody Woodpecker (for slightly older patients) or popcorn popping." The show-and-tell education session is essential to gain the confidence and trust from the young patient. Providing entertainment during dental treatment is a good way to distract the pediatric patient. For example, we sometimes use headphones and I-Glass (virtual-reality glasses in which a patient can enjoy audio-visual display of a movie or program). These modalities provide a good distraction to the patients while dentistry is being performed. Some young patients even look forward to dental visits as opportunities catch up on entertainment. The distraction modality also works well on adult patients, of course.

Pediatric Class I – Cavity Preparation

Laser Parameters, Set 1: Pre-Conditioning

Waterlase MD laser system settings: MG-6 tip, 2.00W, 60% Water, 80% Air, 30 Hz
Other Er,Cr:YSGG laser system settings: G-6 tip, 1.25W, 15% Water, 15% Air

> Keep tip 1-2mm from the tissue surface throughout the procedure. Use a slow circular back-and-forth motion over the surface and advance slowly into the carious lesion.

Laser Parameters, Set 2: Continue Pre-Conditioning and Enamel Ablation

Waterlase MD laser system settings: 3.00W, 60% Water, 80% Air, 30 Hz
Other Er,Cr:YSGG laser system settings: 2.00W, 30% Water, 30% Air

> After directing laser energy towards the treatment site for about 30 seconds, change the laser settings. The tip remains focused at 1-2mm from the fossa or groove. More pre-conditioning with the laser and the enamel will continue to be softened by laser energy.

Laser Parameters, Set 3: Enamel Ablation

Waterlase MD laser system settings: 4.50W, 60% Water, 80% Air, 30 Hz
Other Er,Cr:YSGG laser system settings: 4.00W, 60% Water, 65% Air

> At this setting, enamel ablation may take place. The tip is focused at 1-2mm and is at an angle aiming at the edge of the fossa. This will extend one side of the lesion. The tip is then aimed at the other side of the lesion at an angle. This will extend the other side of the lesion. This is followed by the tip placed perpendicular to the pulpal floor to deepen the cavity prep. Now tubules of the tooth are better exposed in the cavity for more efficient ablation of the caries and dentin. The maximum power setting for the Waterlase MD should be around 4.00-4.50W, and approximately 4.50W for other Er,Cr:YSGG laser systems.

Laser Parameters, Set 4: Caries and Dentin Ablation

Waterlase MD laser system settings: 3.00W, 60% Water, 80% Air, 30 Hz
Other Er,Cr:YSGG laser system settings: 2.50W, 30% Water, 30% Air

> After 30 seconds, use the Modified Turtle Technique to remove enamel and outline the cavity preparation into the dentin. After 30 seconds at 4.5W, the patient should be sufficiently prepared for the high-speed handpiece, which is then used to remove enamel in a light shaving motion, in order to remove a rough outline of enamel in the fissure area. A slow-speed round bur is used to check caries and to complete caries removal.

Laser Parameters, Set 5: Complete Preparation

Waterlase MD laser system settings: 2.00W, 60% Water, 80% Air, 30 Hz
Other Er,Cr:YSGG laser system settings: 2.00W, 30% Water, 30% Air

To finish the cavity preparation, use the laser at the same settings to remove the smear layer and debris and to etch the cavity. Dry the surface with an air syringe to visualize the completeness of the preparation and etching, and to check if there is any sclerotic dentin left. Any remaining sclerotic dentin should be removed using the above settings or using ¼ round high-speed in shaving motion. Whenever rotary instrumentation is applied, laser energy will be used to clean and complete preparation.

Case 1: Deciduous 1st Molar, Class I, "Modified Turtle Technique"

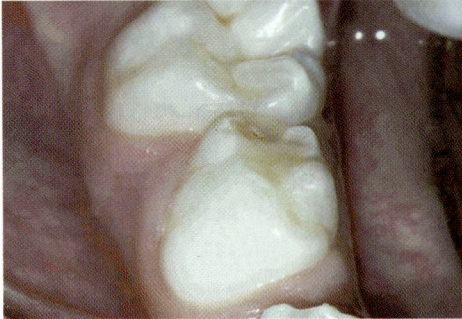

Fig. 1: Pre-op. An occlusal Class I caries is found in #S distal fossa.

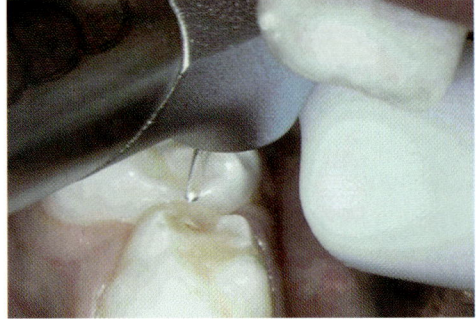

Fig. 2: A MG-6 (or MZ-6) tip is used. The initial setting is 2.00W, 60% Water, 80% Air, 30 Hz.

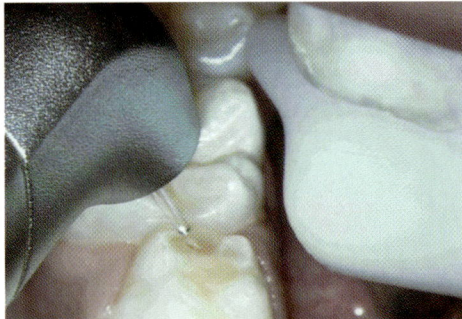

Fig. 3: The tip is angled to extend the border of the carries lingually. The setting is the same as in Fig. 2.

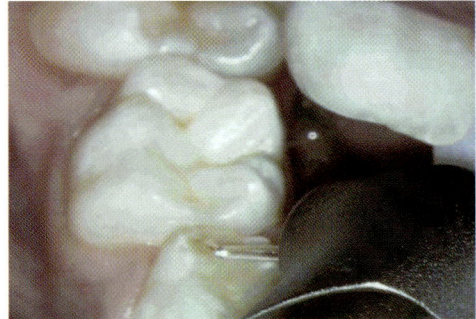

Fig. 4: The tip is angled and aimed at the buccal margin to extend the preparation buccally.

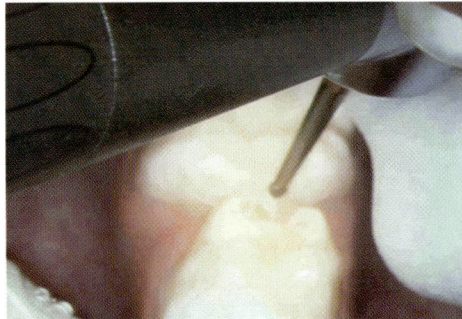

Fig. 5: A slow-speed round bur is used to remove and check caries.

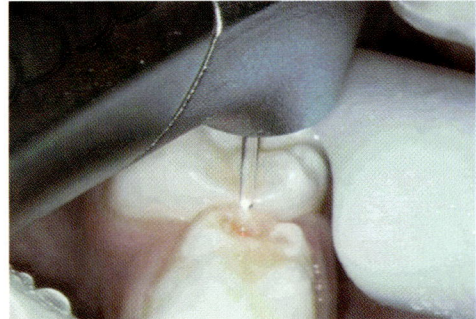

Fig. 6: Laser is used to remove smear, debris and finish the preparation. The setting is 2.00W 60% Water, 80% Air, 30 Hz.

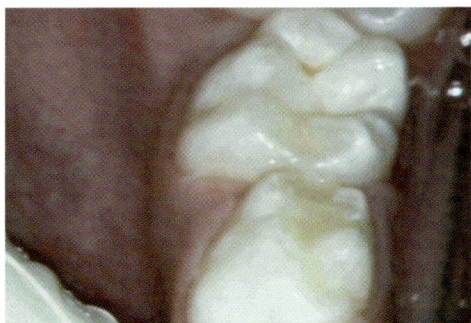

Fig. 7: Immediate post-op.

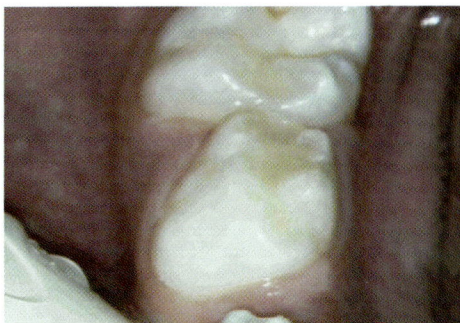

Fig. 8: Post-op with composite restoration placed.

Pediatric Class II – Slot Design

Slot Design: The fiber tip is focused at all times. Direct the energy perpendicular to the ridge and parallel to the proximal surface of the adjacent tooth.

Laser Parameters, Set 1: Pre-Conditioning

Waterlase MD laser system settings: MG-6 tip, 2.00W, 60% Water, 80% Air, 30Hz
Other Er,Cr:YSGG laser system settings: G-6 tip, 1.25W, 15% Water, 15% Air

Aim the laser beam outside the peripheral rim of enamel ridge and direct laser energy towards the rim for about 30 seconds.

Laser Parameters, Set 2: Continue Pre-Conditioning

Waterlase MD laser system settings: 3.00W, 60% Water, 80% Air, 30 Hz
Other Er,Cr:YSGG laser system settings: 2.00W, 30% Water, 30% Air

Change the laser settings and continue to direct laser energy towards the rim for about 30 seconds. Continue to pre-condition the tooth. In some cases enamel ablation is noted.

Laser Parameters, Set 3: Enamel Ablation

Waterlase MD laser system settings: 4.50W, 60% Water, 80% Air, 30 Hz
Other Er,Cr:YSGG laser system settings: 4.00W, 60% Water, 65% Air

Use a high-speed ¼ to ½ round bur to break the enamel and quickly outline the proximal box in the dentin. Switch back to the laser to continue the cavity preparation. A slow buccal-lingual (back-and-forth) sweeping motion is used. The tip is placed at an angle on one side of the cavity fossa. Ablation of enamel will take place after a few seconds. Next, use a slow-speed round bur to complete caries removal and for caries check.

Laser Parameters, Set 4: Complete Preparation

Waterlase MD laser settings: 2.00W, 60% Water, 80% Air, 30 Hz
Other Er,Cr:YSGG laser system settings: 2.00W, 30% Water, 30% Air

To finish the cavity preparation, use the laser at 2.00W to remove the smear layer and debris and to etch the cavity. Dry the surface with an air syringe to visualize the completeness of the preparation and etching, and to check if there is any sclerotic dentin left. Any remaining sclerotic dentin should be removed using the above settings.

Case 1: Deciduous 1st Molar, Class II, Slot Prep, "Modified Turtle Technique"

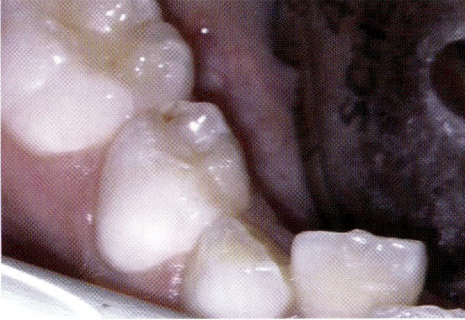

Fig. 1: Pre-op. A DO caries is noted in #S.

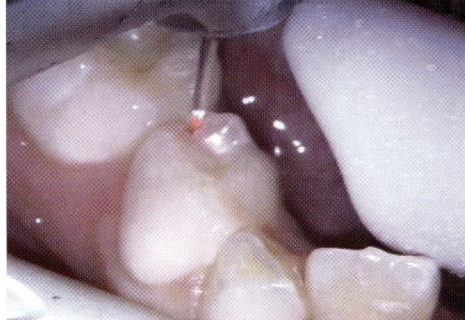

Fig. 2: Pre-conditioning and initial preparation of the tooth is done by laser fiber tip aiming at the ridge where the slot prep is to be prepared. The tip is MG-6 (or MZ-6). The setting is 2.00W, 60% Water, 80% Air, 30 Hz.

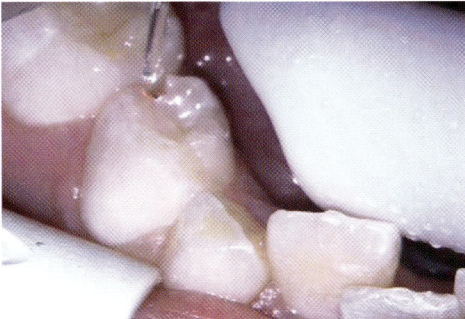

Fig. 3: The setting is raised from 2.00W to 3.00W, and then to 4.50W. Ablation of the slot prep proceeds into the dentin about ½ distance into the slot prep.

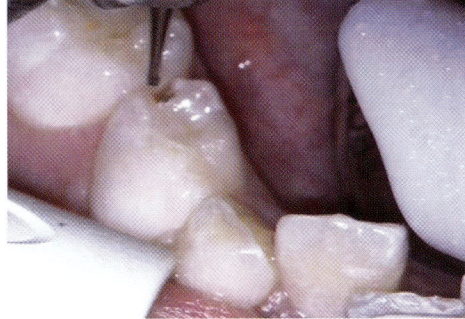

Fig. 4: A ½ round high-speed round bur is used to outline the slot prep. This is done with abundance of water and in light touches of the bur on tooth tissue (in a shaving motion).

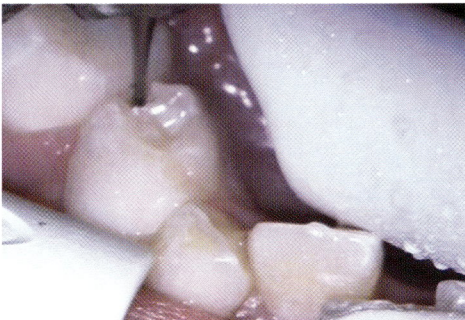

Fig. 5: A slow-speed round bur is used to remove and check caries.

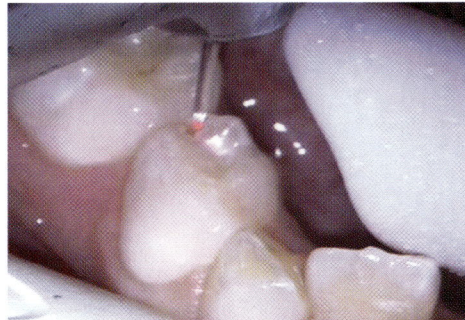

Fig. 6: Laser is used to finish the preparation to remove smear and debris.

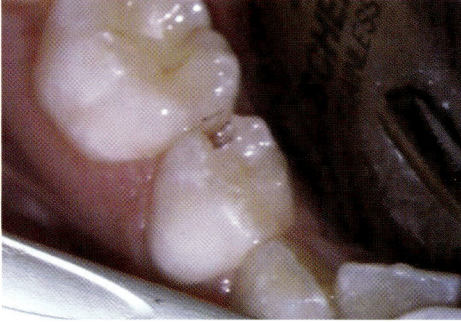

Fig. 7: Post-op. The class II DO slot prep is complete and ready for composite restoration.

Pediatric Class II – Tunnel Design

Laser Parameters, Set 1: Pre-Conditioning

Waterlase MD laser system settings: MG-6 tip, 2.00W, 60% Water, 80% Air, 30 Hz
Other Er,Cr:YSGG laser system settings: G-6 tip, 1.25W, 15% Water, 15% Air

The fiber tip is focused at 1-2mm from the fossa. Sub-ablative power is used to precondition the tooth.

Laser Parameters, Set 2: Continue Pre-Conditioning

Waterlase MD laser system settings: 3.00W, 60% Water, 80% Air, 30 Hz
Other Er,Cr:YSGG laser system settings: 2.00W, 30% Water, 30% Air

Continue in a focused mode aiming at the fossa, further pre-conditioning and softening of the enamel is being performed.

Laser Parameters, Set 3: Enamel Ablation

Waterlase MD laser system settings: 4.50W, 60% Water, 80% Air, 30 Hz
Other Er,Cr:YSGG laser system settings: 4.00W, 60% Water, 65% Air

With this power setting, laser energy is high enough to ablate enamel of most deciduous molars. The tip is angled to aim at extending the fossa on opposing sides of the fossa. This is followed by deepening of the pulpal floor. The tunnel prep to the proximal caries is started by laser energy. Then, a high-speed ¼ round bur is used to quickly outline a tunnel to the proximal lesion without breaking the enamel. The preparation of the tunnel is completed by using a slow-speed round bur to remove the proximal enamel.

Laser Parameters, Set 4: Dentin and Caries Removal

Waterlase MD laser system settings: 2.00W, 60% Water, 80% Air, 30 Hz
Other Er,Cr:YSGG laser system settings: 2.00W, 30% Water, 30% Air

The tunnel prep is cleaned and caries removed by this laser setting. Caries check can be done by gentle slow-speed round bur or caries indicator.

To finish the cavity preparation, use the laser in a focused mode to remove the smear layer and debris and to etch the cavity. Dry the surface with an air syringe to visualize the completeness of the preparation and etching, and to check if there is any sclerotic dentin left. Any remaining sclerotic dentin should be removed using the above settings.

Case 1: Deciduous 2nd Molar, Class II, Tunnel Prep, "Modified Turtle Technique"

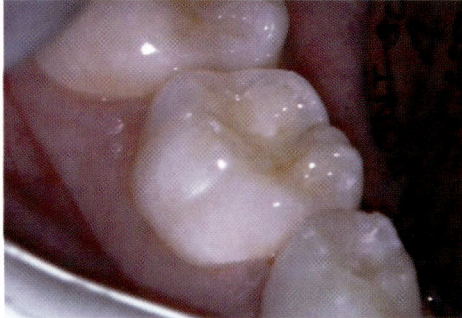

Fig. 1: Pre-op. A Class II MO caries lesion is present in #T.

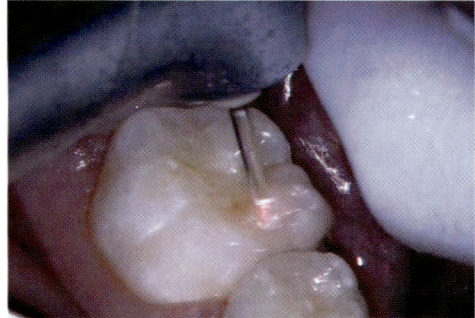

Fig. 2: Pre-conditioning and initial preparation is done by a MG-6 (Or MZ-6) tip. The setting is 2.00W, 60% Water, 80% Air, 30 Hz.

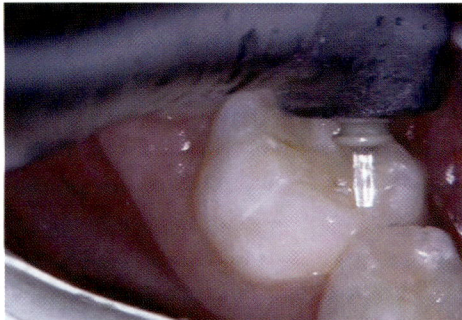

Fig.3: The setting is raised from 2.00W to 3.00W, and then to 4.50W. Half of the tunnel prep is established.

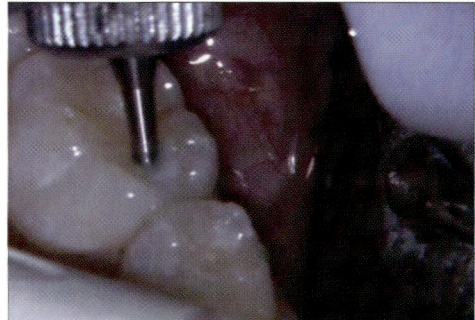

Fig. 4: After using a ½ round high-speed bur to outline the tunnel prep, a low-speed round bur is used to remove and check caries.

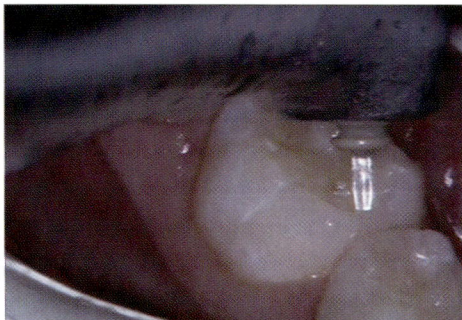

Fig. 5: The MO slot prep is finished with 2.00W, 60% Water, 80% Air, 30 Hz to remove smear and debris.

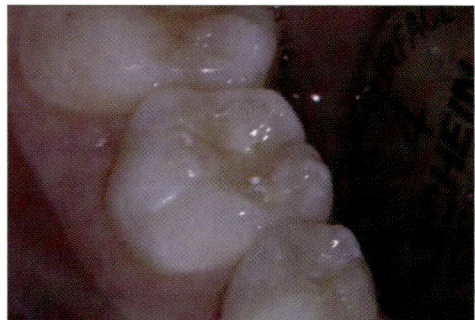

Fig. 6: Post-op. Composite restoration is placed on the MO of #T.

Pediatric Class III – Cavity Preparation

Laser Parameters, Set 1: Pre-Conditioning

Waterlase MD laser system settings: MG-6 tip, 2.00W, 60% Water, 80% Air, 30 Hz
Other Er,Cr:YSGG laser system settings: G-6 tip, 1.25W, 15% Water, 15% Air

> The fiber tip is focused at 1-2mm from the lingual surface. Use a slow circular, back-and-forth motion over the surface. Advance slowly into the carious lesion.

Laser Parameters, Set 2: Continue Pre-Conditioning and Enamel Ablation

Waterlase MD laser system settings: MG-6 tip, 2.50-4.00W, 60% Water, 80% Air, 30 Hz
Other Er,Cr:YSGG laser system settings: G-6 tip, 3.50W, 60% Water, 65% Air

> Increase the power setting is by 0.50W at a time. This incremental (+0.50W) increase in power continues every 30 seconds until satisfactory enamel ablation speed occurs, without hurting the patient. Normally the highest power needed for the ablation of anterior teeth enamel is up to 4.00W for the Waterlase MD, or up to 3.50W for other Er,Cr:YSGG laser systems.

> After initial preparation, a high-speed ¼ or ½ bur is used to outline the Class III preparation; includes breaking the contact. A slow-speed round bur is used to remove caries and for caries check. A gentle shaving motion should be used when using rotary instrument.

Laser Parameters, Set 3: Complete Preparation

Waterlase MD laser system settings: 2.00W, 60% Water, 80% Air, 30 Hz
Other Er,Cr:YSGG laser system settings: 2.00W, 30% Water, 30% Air

> To finish the cavity preparation, use the laser at 1.25W to remove the smear layer and debris and to etch the cavity. Dry the surface with an air syringe to visualize the completeness of the preparation and etching, and to check if there is any sclerotic dentin left. Any remaining sclerotic dentin should be removed using the above settings.

Case 1: Deciduous Cuspid, Class III, MD Gold HP with MZ-5 Tip

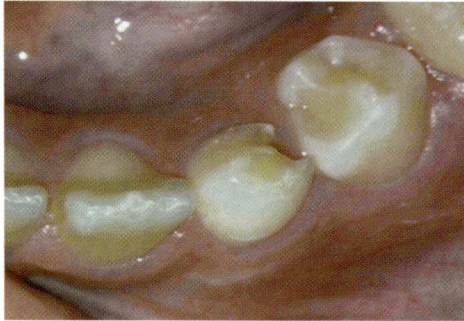

Fig. 1: Pre-op. #M has a distal lesion.

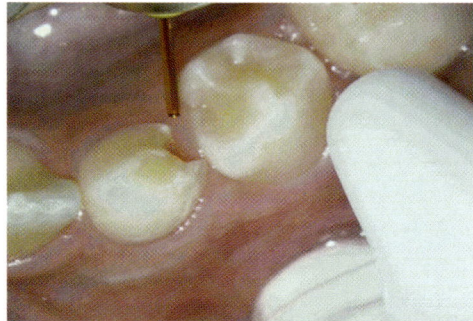

Fig. 2: A MZ-2 tip (or MG-6, or MZ-6) and MD Gold Handpiece is used. The setting is 2.00W, 60% Water, 80% Air, 30 Hz.

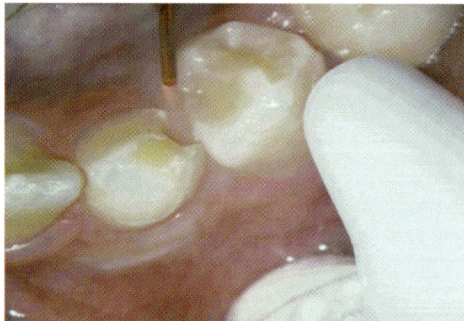

Fig. 3: Cavity preparation is continued with 2.00W, 60% Water, 80% Air, 30 Hz.

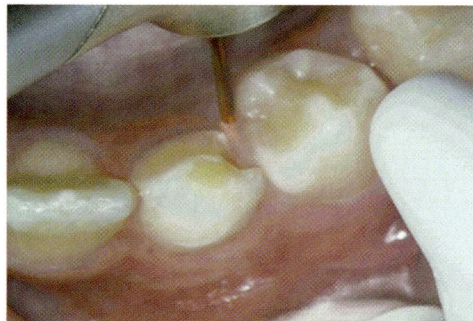

Fig. 4: Caries enamel is done with 2.00W, 30 Hz.

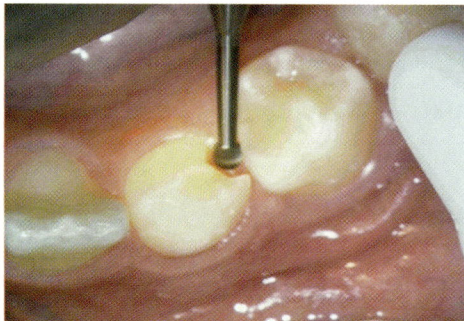

Fig. 5: A slow-speed round bur is used to check and remove caries.

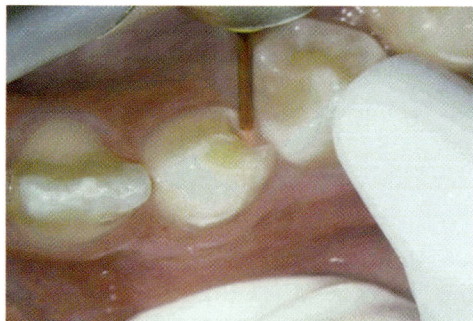

Fig. 6: Laser is used to finish the preparation. The setting remains 2.00W, 60% Water, 80% Air, 30 Hz.

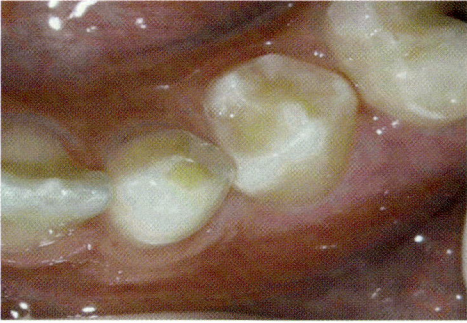

Fig. 7: Immediate post-op. Class III composite restoration is placed.

Pediatric Class IV – Cavity Preparation

Laser Parameters, Set 1: Pre-Conditioning

Waterlase MD laser system settings: MG-6 tip, 2.00W, 60% Water, 80% Air, 30 Hz
Other Er,Cr:YSGG laser system settings: G-6 tip, 1.25W, 15% Water, 15% Air

The fiber tip is focused at 1-2mm from lingual surface. Use a slow circular or back-and-forth motion over the surface and advance slowly into the carious lesion for 30 seconds.

Laser Parameters, Set 2: Continue Pre-Conditioning and Enamel Ablation

Waterlase MD laser system settings: MG-6 tip, 2.25W, 60% Water, 80% Air, 30 Hz
Other Er,Cr:YSGG laser system settings: G-6 tip, 1.50W, 15% Water, 15% Air

Increase the power setting and continue moving over the surface. This incremental increase in power is continued by 0.25W every 30 seconds, until it reaches 2.00W or until enamel ablation is noted.

Laser Parameters, Set 3: Complete Enamel Ablation

Waterlase MD laser system settings: 2.00W, 60% Water, 80% Air, 30 Hz
Other Er,Cr:YSGG laser system settings: 1.75W, 15% Water, 15% Air

Using the laser, remove incisal or cuspal edge enamel. Extend the preparation into the previously prepared proximal region.

Laser Parameters, Set 4: Caries Removal and Dentin Preparation

Waterlase MD laser system settings: 2.00W, 60% Water, 80% Air, 30 Hz
Other Er,Cr:YSGG laser system settings: 1.50W, 15% Water, 15% Air

Reduce the power setting and ablate caries. Use a slow-speed round bur for caries check.

Laser Parameters, Set 5: Complete Preparation

Waterlase MD laser system settings: 2.00W, 60% Water, 80% Air, 30 Hz
Other Er,Cr:YSGG laser system settings: 1.50W, 15% Water, 15% Air

To finish the cavity preparation, use the laser to remove the smear layer and debris and to etch the cavity. Dry the surface with an air syringe to visualize the completeness of the preparation and etching, and to check if there is any sclerotic dentin left. Any remaining sclerotic dentin should be removed using the above settings.

Because the tooth is made weaker by the removal of an angle of the tooth, retention is made by beveling the enamel on the facial and lingual surfaces to create a wider area for bonding.

<u>Case 1</u>: Deciduous Lateral Incisor, Class IV, MD Regular HP with MG-6 Tip

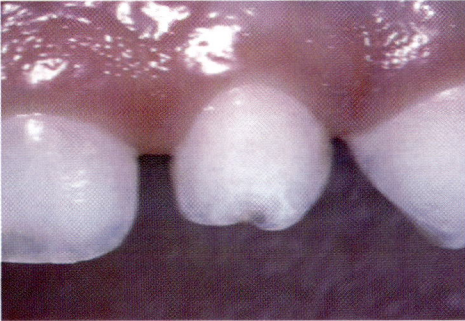

Fig. 1: Pre-op. A Class IV lesion is present in Tooth #G.

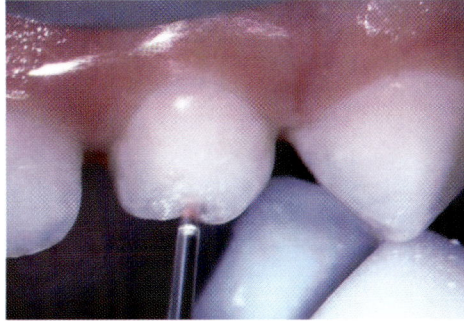

Fig. 2: Pre-conditioning and initial preparation is done by a MG-6 (or MZ-6) tip. The setting is 1.50W, 60% Water, 80% Air, 30 Hz.

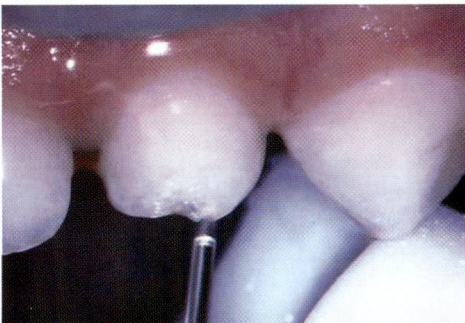

Fig. 3: The Class IV preparation continues with the power raised 0.25W at a time until efficient ablation of enamel is noted.

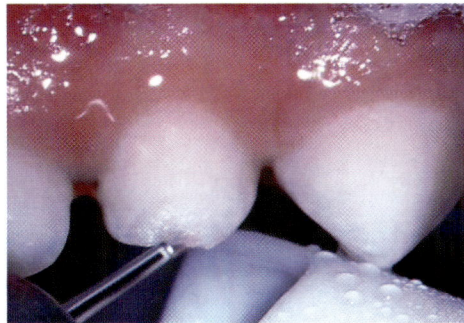

Fig. 4: More efficient ablation is done by angling the tip to go after sides of the tubules. The setting is 1.75W, 60% Water, 80% Air, 30 Hz.

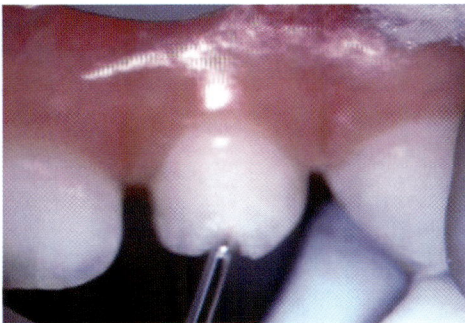

Fig. 5: The preparation is finished with the setting of 1.50W, 60% Water, 80% Air, 30 Hz.

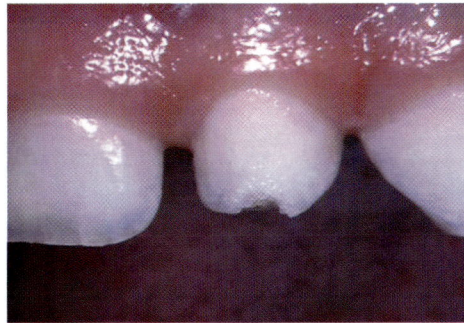

Fig. 6: Immediate post-op before composite restoration is placed.

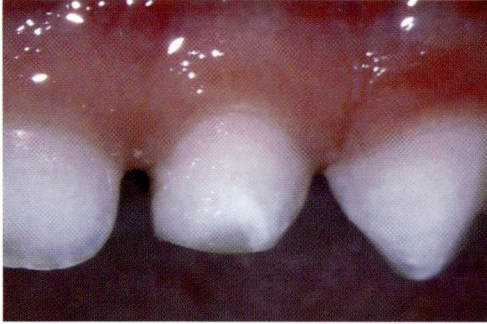

Fig. 7: Post-op. Composite restoration is placed.

Pediatric Class V – Cavity Preparation

Laser Parameters, Set 1: Pre-Conditioning

Waterlase MD laser system settings: MG-6 tip, 1.50W, 60% Water, 80% Air, 30 Hz
Other Er,Cr:YSGG laser system settings: G-6 tip, 1.25W, 15% Water, 15% Air

> The technique involves placing the tip in a position perpendicular to the surface. Use a slow sweeping motion, move the tip back-and-forth or in a circular fashion over the enamel. The tip is moved sideways to cover the entire lesion, including the margins. This setting is aimed at pre-conditioning the pulp.

Laser Parameters, Set 2: Continue Pre-Conditioning

Waterlase MD laser system settings: MG-6 tip, 2.00W, 60% Water, 80% Air, 30 Hz
Other Er,Cr:YSGG laser system settings: G-6 tip, 2.00W, 30% Water, 30% Air

> Increase the power setting 0.25W every 30 seconds. This incremental increase in power continues every 30 seconds until efficient enamel ablation takes place, without hurting the patient. Normally the highest power needed for the ablation of anterior teeth enamel is about 2.00W for the Waterlase MD, or 2.00W for other Er,Cr:YSGG laser systems.

> Use a slow-speed round bur to complete caries removal and for caries check.

Laser Parameters, Set 3: Complete Preparation

Waterlase MD laser system settings: 1.75W, 60% Water, 80% Air, 30 Hz
Other Er,Cr:YSGG laser system settings: 1.75W, 15% Water, 15% Air

> To finish, use the laser to clean smear and debris and to etch the cavity. Dry the surface with an air syringe to visualize the completeness of the preparation and etching, and to check if there is any sclerotic dentin left. Any remaining sclerotic dentin should be removed using the above settings.

Case 1: Deciduous Cuspid, Class V MD Regular HP with MG-6 Tip

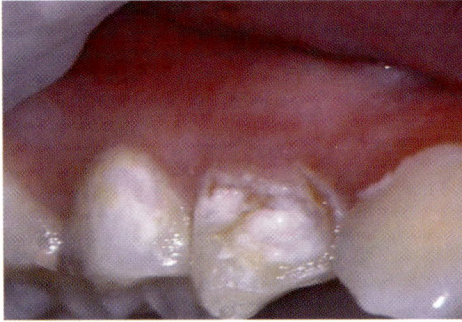

Fig. 1: Pre-op. A large Class V lesion is present in #C.

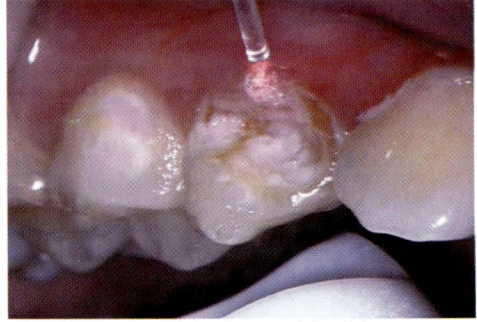

Fig. 2: Pre-conditioning and initial preparation is done by a MG-6 (or MZ-6) tip. The setting is 1.50W, 60% Water, 80% Air, 30 Hz.

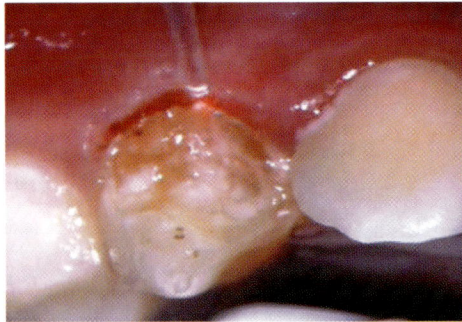

Fig. 3: Gingival recontouring to reveal subgingival caries is done with a setting of 1.25W, 7% Water, 11% Air, 30 Hz.

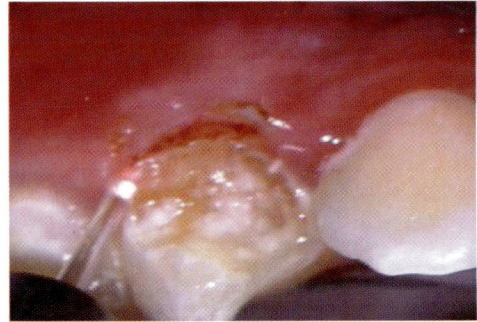

Fig. 4: Hemostasis is done by a setting of 2.25W, 1% Water, 11% Air, 50 Hz, S mode.

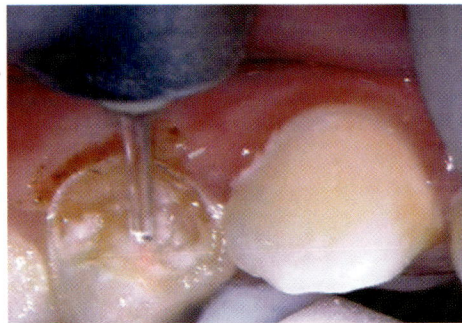

Fig. 5: The Class V preparation is continued by raising the power 0.25W, at a time until efficient ablation of the caries is observed. The setting used here is 2.00W, 60% Water, 80% Air, 30 Hz.

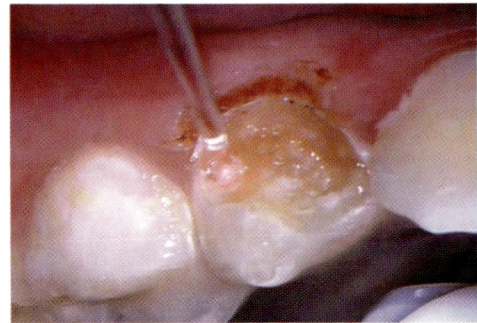

Fig. 6: After caries removal and cheek is done by a slow-speed round bur. Laser is used to finish the Class V prep. The setting is 1.75W, 60% Water, 80% Air, 30 Hz.

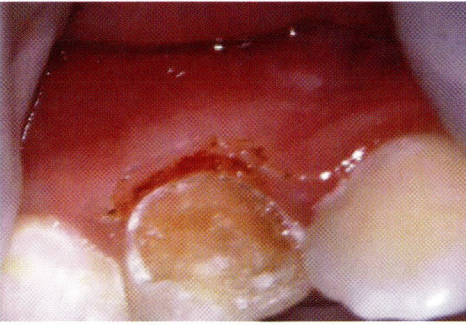

Fig. 7: Immediate post-op before composite restoration is placed.

Pulpotomy

Laser Parameters, Set 1: Pre-Conditioning

Waterlase MD laser system settings: MG-6 tip, 0.25W, 0% Water, 0% Air, 50 Hz
Other Er,Cr:YSGG laser system settings: G-6 tip, 0.25W, 15% Water, 15% Air

> Aim the fiber tip at the cervical-sulcus area, at either the buccal or the lingual. With a sweeping back-and-forth motion, low level laser energy is aimed towards the pulp chamber for 120 seconds. When using a Millennium 2 system, spend at least 30 seconds per site (an average size molar has four sites, mesio-buccal, mesio-lingual, disto-buccal, and disto-lingual).

> Note: There are two sites in anterior and bi-cuspids, the facial and lingual sites. In an average molar, there are four sites. Two sites are on the buccal surface and the other two sites on the lingual surface. In a large molar, there are six sites for laser anesthesia.

> After pre-conditioning the tooth, buccal and lingual gingival sulcus are pre-conditioned with the same setting. This is followed by placing rubber dam clamp and rubber dam. Make sure the patient is comfortable before proceeding to the next step.

Laser Parameters, Set 2: Enamel Ablation

Waterlase MD laser system settings: 4.50W, 60% Water, 80% Air, 15 Hz
Other Er,Cr:YSGG laser system settings: 4.50W, 60% Water, 65% Air

> Aim the tip at an angle to the border of the cavity (in focused mode). This will break down the enamel quickly and establish an outline of the cavity.

Laser Parameters, Set 3: Caries Removal and Dentin Preparation

Waterlase MD laser system settings: 3.00W, 60% Water, 80% Air, 15 Hz
Other Er,Cr:YSGG laser system settings: 3.00W, 60% Water, 65% Air

> Continue treatment to remove caries and dentin. The cavity preparation is extended to include the area next to the pulp chamber.

Laser Parameters, Set 4: Exposure of the Pulp

Waterlase MD laser system settings: 3.00W, 60% Water, 80% Air, 30 Hz
Other Er,Cr:YSGG laser system settings: 2.50W, 30% Water, 30% Air

> When the pulp is close to being exposed, lower the power further to about 3.00W, 30 Hz. With this laser setting, when exposing the pulp, the patient most likely will not feel pain. Continue to extend the exposure of the pulp chamber.

Laser Parameters, Set 5: Pulpotomy

Waterlase MD laser system settings: 1.75-2.50W, 7% Water, 11% Air, 30 Hz
Other Er,Cr:YSGG laser system settings: 1.25W, 7% Water, 11% Air

> Once the pulp is exposed, change the settings to perform the pulpotomy. A high-speed #2 round bur is used to make sure all pulp horns are exposed. This is followed by using laser to complete pulpotomy.

Laser Parameters, Set 6: Hemostasis

Waterlase MD laser system settings: 1.25W, 0% Water, 11% Air, 30 Hz
Other Er,Cr:YSGG laser system settings: 1.00W, 0% Water, 11% Air

> Change the laser setting to perform hemostasis. All bleeding must stop before completion of pulpotomy. IRM is placed as a temporary, or other restorative material is used to complete the procedure. Rubber dam and clamp are removed.

Case 1: Deciduous 1st Molar, Pulpotomy, No Injection Anesthesia, MD Regular HP with MG-6 Tip

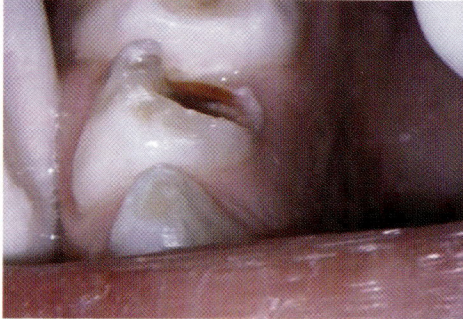

Fig. 1: Pre-op. A very large lesion is present in #S. Pulpotomy is indicated.

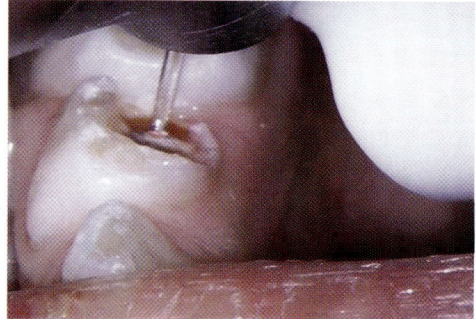

Fig. 2: Pre-conditioning of the tooth is done by a MG-6 (MZ-6) tip at a low level laser dosage of 0.25W, 0% Water, 0% Air, 50 Hz. The tip is aiming at the large cavity directly.

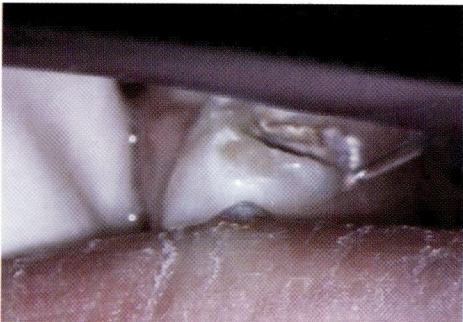

Fig. 3: Pre-conditioning of the lingual sulcus. Same setting as used in Fig. 2.

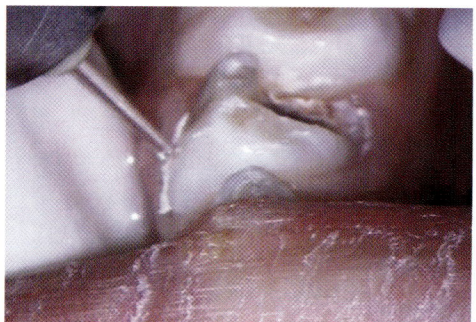

Fig. 4: Pre-conditioning of the buccal sulcus.

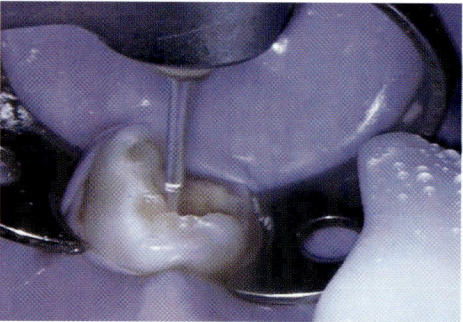

Fig. 5: Ablation of enamel is done with a setting of 4.50W, 60% Water, 80% Air, 15 Hz.

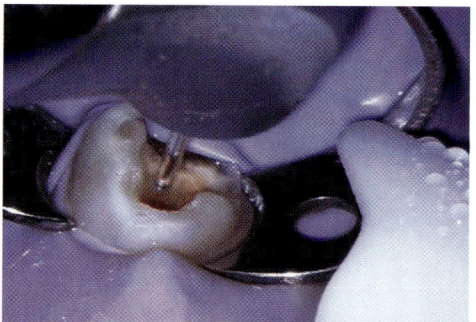

Fig. 6: Ablation of dentin and caries is done with a lower power setting of 3.00W, 60% Water, 80% Air, 30 Hz. The pulp is exposed with this setting.

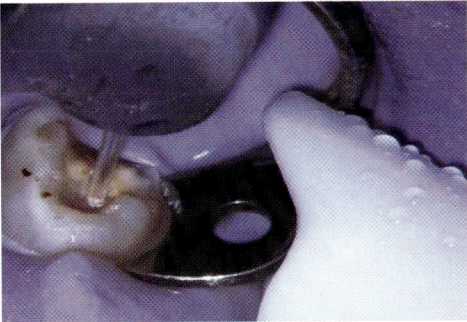

Fig. 7: Pulpotomy is done with a surgical setting of 2.00W, 7% Water, 11% Air, 30 Hz.

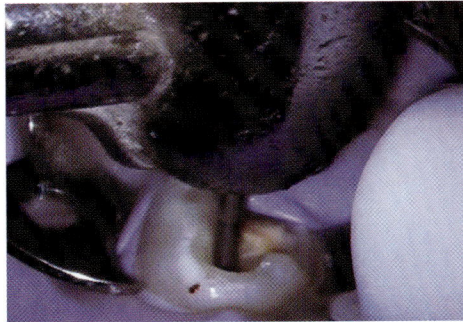

Fig. 8: The exposure of the chamber is complete by using a #2 high-speed round bur.

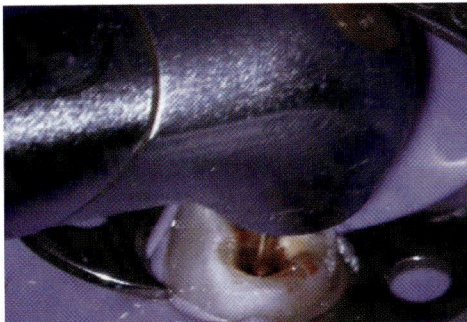

Fig. 9: Pulpotomy is continued with a surgical setting of 2.00W, 7% Water, 11% Air. Hemostasis and bactericidal treatment is performed with a setting of 1.25W, 0% Water, 11% Air, 30 Hz, followed by a setting of 1.25W, 0% Water, 11% Air, 30 Hz, S mode to finish.

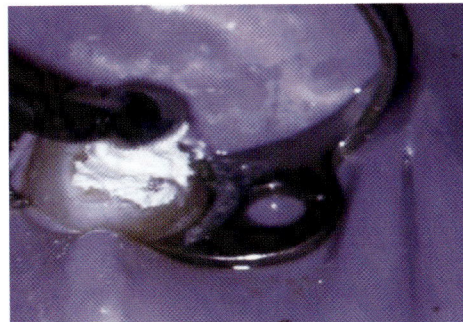

Fig. 10: IRM temporary is placed.

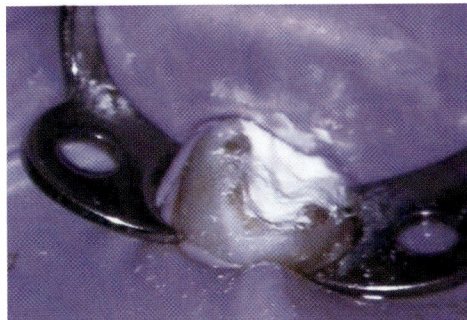

Fig. 11: Immediate post-op.

Case 2: Deciduous 1ˢᵗ Molar, Pulpotomy, No Injection Anesthesia, M2 with G-6 Tip

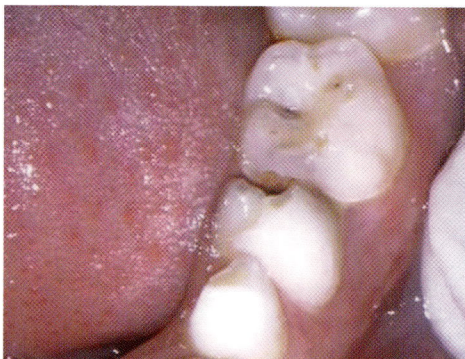

Fig. 1: Pre-op. A deep caries is present in #L with indication for pulpotomy.

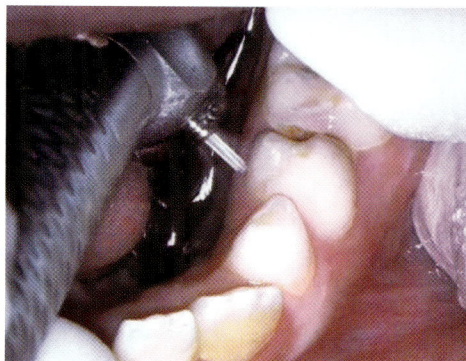

Fig. 2: Pre-conditioning of the sulcus in the lingual is done by laser. The tip used is G-6 (or Z-6). The setting is 0.25W, 15% Water, 15% Air, for 30 seconds.

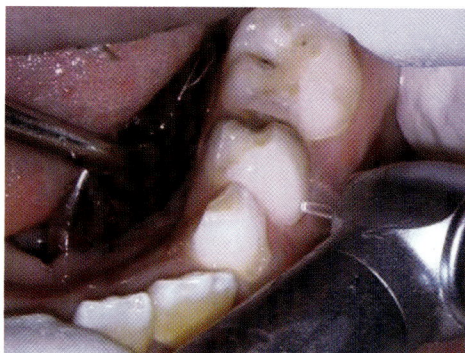

Fig. 3: Pre-conditioning of the sulcus in the buccal is done by the same setting in Fig. 2.

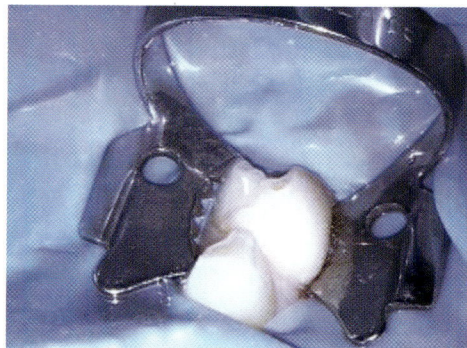

Fig. 4: Rubber dam clamp and rubber dam is in place at #L.

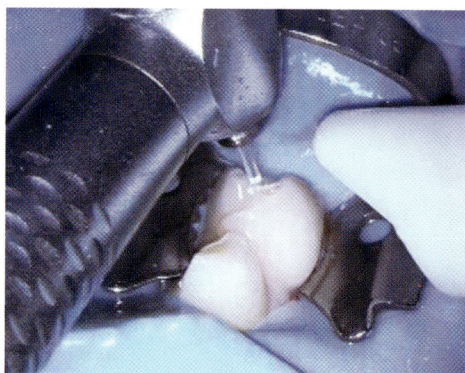

Fig. 5: Pre-conditioning and initial preparation is at 1.25W, 15% Water, 15% Air.

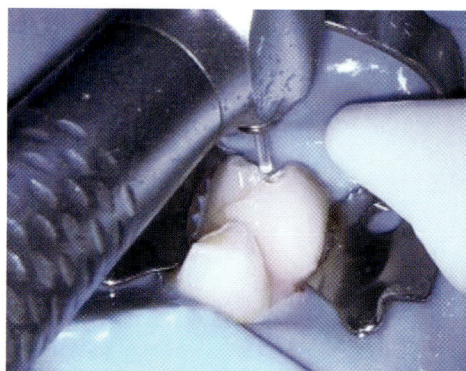

Fig. 6: The power is raised from 1.25W to 2.00W, 30% Water, 30% Air, and then to 4.00W 60% water, 65% air. Efficient enamel ablation should take place at 4.00W.

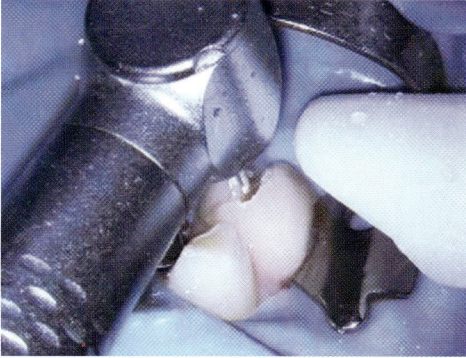

Fig. 7: The power is lowered in ablation of caries and dentin to 2.50W, 30% Water, 30% Air.

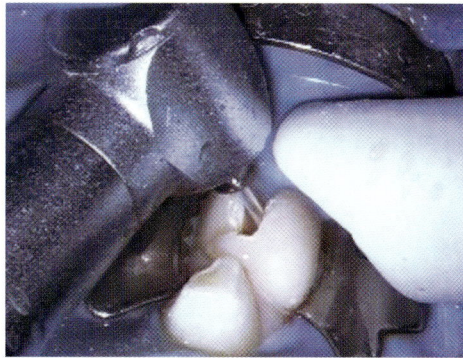

Fig. 8: The pulp is exposed with a setting of 2.00W, 30% Water, 30% Air.

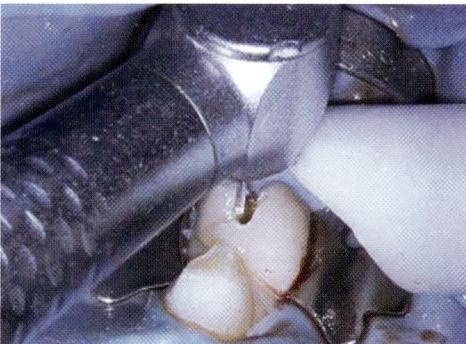

Fig. 9: Pulpotomy is done with a setting of 1.25W, 7% Water, 11% Air. Hemostasis and bactericidal treatment is done with a setting of 0.75W, 0% Water, 11% Air.

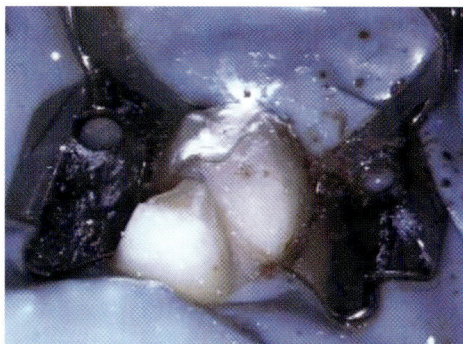

Fig. 10: IRM temporary restoration is placed.

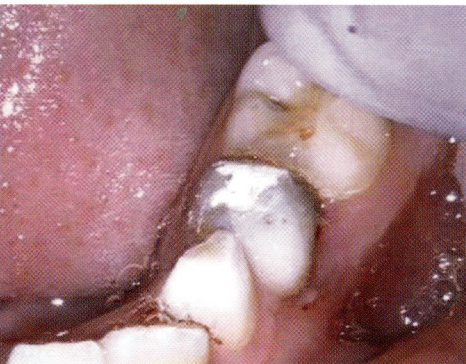

Fig. 11: Immediate post-op.

Extraction of Loose Deciduous Teeth

In a loose deciduous tooth, there are only some ligaments holding the tooth. By using the soft tissue setting, the ligaments can be cut to exfoliate the tooth. Concentrated topical is applied to gingiva in both the facial and lingual areas for 3 minutes before the laser procedure.

Laser Parameters, Set 1: Gingival Ablation

Waterlase MD laser system settings: MG-6 tip, 1.50-2.50W, 7-11% Water, 11% Air, 30Hz

Other Er,Cr:YSGG laser system settings: G-6 tip, 0.50W, 7% Water, 11% Air

Ablate the gingiva around the tooth. Increase the power by 0.25 Watt increments every 30 seconds until the gingiva is being efficiently ablated.

The tip is then placed on the buccal site aiming at the ligaments at 70-80° to the long axis of the tooth.

The gingivectomy of the buccal ligaments is complete. Move the tip to cut the ligaments at the lingual area. Then perform a gingivectomy at the mesial and distal areas. The tip is then placed under the molar from the buccal to cut the ligament under the tooth. The procedure is repeated from the lingual. By now the tooth is very loose. Repeat the procedure underneath the tooth from mesial to distal, back-and-forth several times.

Normally the tooth can be lifted easily on the buccal face. Place the index finger on the occlusal surface; lift the tooth out of the socket by placing an elevator underneath the tooth from the buccal. The tooth should comes out of the socket in an arc-like direction, not a straight line. If done properly, this is a painless procedure.

Laser Parameter Set 2. Biologic Band-Aid

Waterlase MD laser system settings: MG-6 tip, 1.25W, 0% Water, 11% Air, 30 Hz
Other Er,Cr:YSGG laser system settings: G-6 tip, 1.00W, 0% Water, 11% Air

Defocus the tip 3-5mm aiming at the surgical site. Apply laser energy at 1.25W, 0% Water, 11% Air, 30 Hz to coagulate, disinfect and biostimulate the surgical site. This serves as a biologic band-aid to finish the surgery.

Case 1: Laser-assisted Extraction of Deciduous 1st Molar, No Injection Anesthesia, MD Regular HP with MG-6 Tip

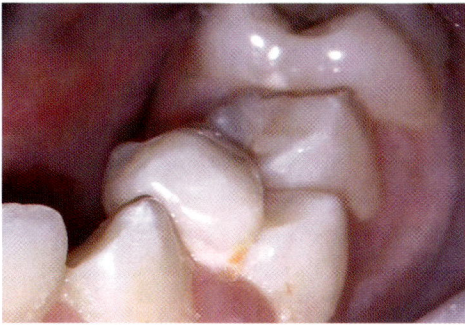

Fig. 1: Pre-op. #L is loose with the erupting #21 present.

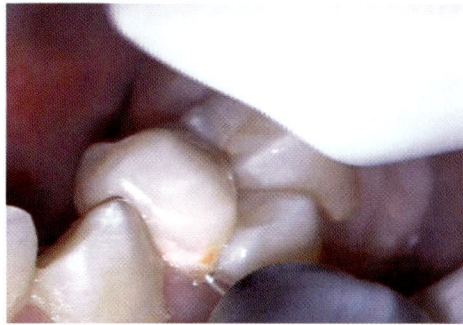

Fig. 2: After tac-gel is applied to both buccal and lingual gingiva for 3 minutes. Laser gingivectomy is performed to cut the ligaments from the buccal aspect holding #L. A MG-6 (or MZ-6) tip is used. The setting is 2.00W, 7% Water, 11% Air, 30 Hz.

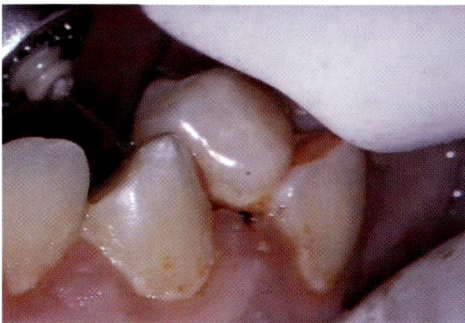

Fig. 3: Laser gingivectomy continues in the lingual until all ligaments to #L is severed.

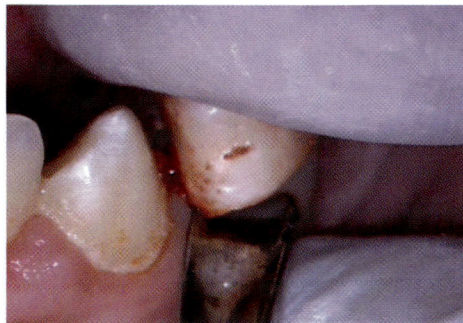

Fig. 4: With the index finger stabilizing #L, an extraction elevator is placed under #L. The loose tooth is removed in an arch-like direction.

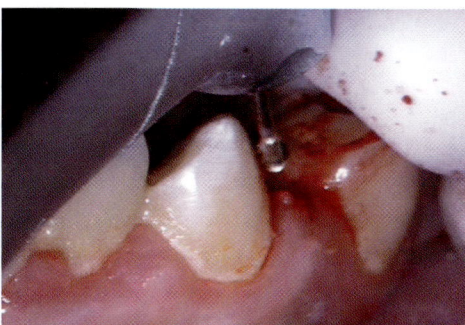

Fig. 5: Laser biologic band-aid is applied to the surgical site. Avoid erupting #21. The setting is 1.25W, 0% Water, 11% Air, 30 Hz, defocused to 3mm.

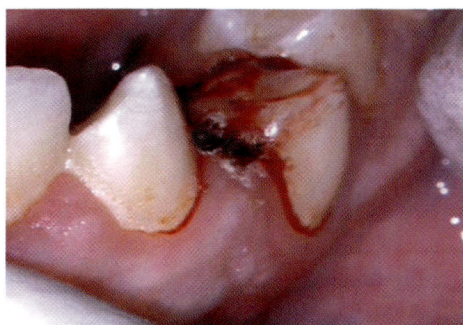

Fig. 6: Immediate post-op.

Soft Tissue Procedures

Introduction

Several advantages of using lasers in dentistry and medicine are best demonstrated in soft tissue applications. These advantages include good hemostasis, an on-site bactericidal effect, decreased post-operative swelling, scaring and damage to soft tissue, a reduction in mechanical trauma, bacteria and post-operative pain, and a more precise and accurate surgery.

There are many reasons to use the Er,Cr:YSGG laser in soft tissue surgery whenever possible. In conventional oral surgeries, cutting soft tissue with a scalpel causes histamine release and results in bleeding, swelling and pain. Sutures are almost always required. On the other hand, when laser surgery is properly performed, the resulting intraoral wounds heal more successfully and often do not require sutures. In addition, use of the laser reduces the histamine release response, which results in increased patient post-operative comfort. Finally, many patients respond well to laser treatment and do not require topical anesthetics during surgery.

The only tradeoff to the advantages of using a laser is operative speed, as the scalpel is naturally faster than the laser. However, the difference in speed is only a matter of seconds of treatment time.

The glossary set forth in the Introduction to this book describes the two pulse widths that the Waterlase MD offers for soft tissue applications: a short pulse setting ("H mode") of 140 microseconds and a long pulse setting ("S mode") of 750 microseconds. For any given power level, a longer pulse width allows the same amount of energy to be deposited over a relatively longer period of time; the result is increased heat deposition that provides the Waterlase MD better capabilities in hemostasis and more precision in soft tissue cutting. Properly handled, there still should be minimal carbonization of target tissues.

Biopsy

This procedure can be performed with or without local anesthesia. Higher power settings should be used when local anesthesia is administered.

Laser Parameters, Set 1: Outline Lesion

Waterlase MD laser system settings: MG-6 tip, 0.50W, 0% Water, 11% Air, 30 Hz
Other Er,Cr:YSGG laser system settings: G-6 tip, 0.50W, 0% Water, 11% Air

To start the procedure, place concentrated topical on the border of the lesion for three to five minutes. This is followed by outlining the lesion by means of a low-power dry cut in a non-contact mode. Make a superficial mark on the surface of the target without deep penetration.

Laser Parameters, Set 2: Incision in Lesion

Waterlase MD laser system settings: 2.25-3.00 W, 7% Water, 11% Air, 30 Hz
or 2.75-3.50 W, 7% Water, 11% Air, 30 Hz, S mode
Other Er,Cr:YSGG laser system settings: 1.25-2.00 W, 7% Water, 11% Air

Change the laser setting and make an incisional cut in the lesion following the outline. The lesion is then grasped by a tissue forceps and is lifted up from the bone. Make an excisional cut into the lesion following the outline. An excisional cut is made to remove the fibroma. Most of the biopsy does not require placement of suture because bleeding and scarring usually are minimized.

Laser Parameters, Set 3: Hemostasis

Waterlase MD laser system settings: 1.25W, 0% Water, 11% Air, 30 Hz
Other Er,Cr:YSGG laser system settings: 1.00-1.25W, 0% Water, 11% Air

To finish, a low-power laser setting is used to coagulate and apply low-level laser therapy on the wound, allowing hemostasis and promoting a faster recovery.

Laser Parameters, Alternative Settings: Location Anesthetic + Soft Tissue Ablation

Waterlase MD laser system settings: MG-6 tip, 2.75-3.50W, 7% Water, 11% Air, 30 Hz
or 3.25-4.00 W, 7% Water, 11% Air, 30 Hz, S mode
Other Er,Cr:YSGG laser system settings: G-6 tip, 1.75-2.50W, 7% Water, 11% Air

If the biopsy is to be performed with local anesthesia, a higher power setting can be used for speedier procedures. The power setting is 2.00-2.50W, 7% Water, 11% Air. In all other respects, the procedure is identical to that described above.

The same technique may be used to remove the following lesions:
1. Papilloma
2. Epulis fissurata
3. Hyperplastic tissue excision

Because a laser is being used to excise the portion, it should be noted for the pathologist prescription that the specimen was prepared by an incision-excisional biopsy and that the preparation was performed with a 2.78 micron wavelength laser.

Case 1: Biopsy, Fibroma, MD Regular HP with MG-6 Tip

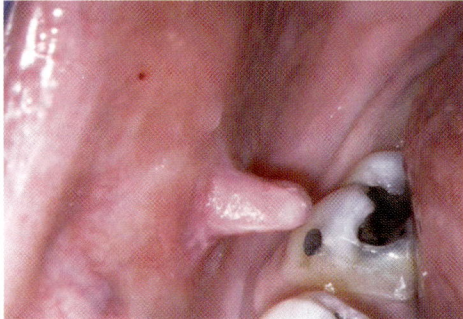

Fig. 1: Pre-op. Fibroma removal is indicated.

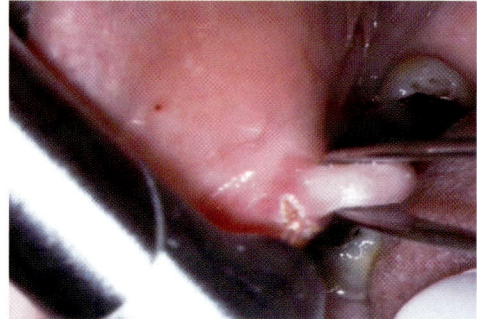

Fig. 2: Grip tissue with forceps; make incision at base using Er,Cr:YSGG.

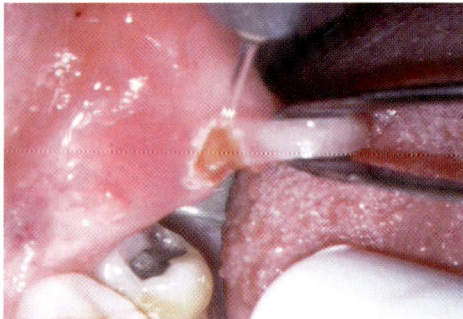

Fig. 3: Continue incision around base, adjusting the position of the laser handpiece as necessary.

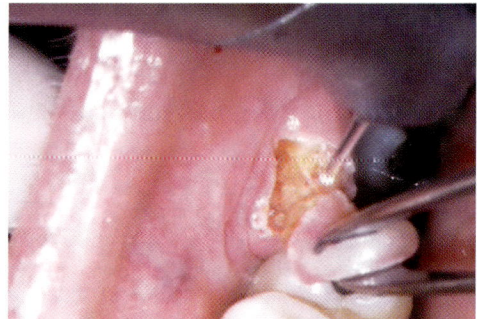

Fig. 4: Maintain pressure on tissue with the forceps, pulling away from tissue as Er,Cr:YSGG ablates the base.

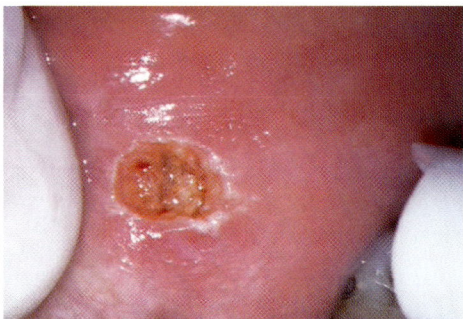

Fig. 5: Immediate post-op treatment site.

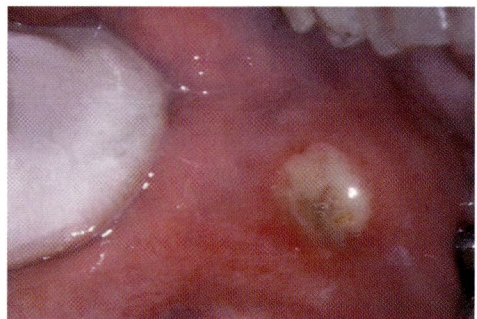

Fig. 6: Post-op, one day later.

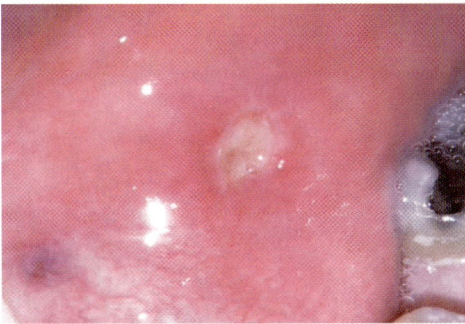

Fig. 7: Post-op. 4 days

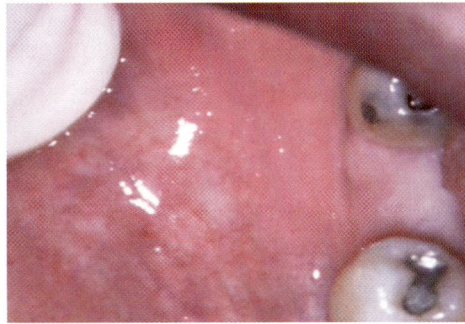

Fig. 8: Post-op. 1 month.

Case 2: Biopsy, Epulis, MD Regular HP with MG-6 Tip

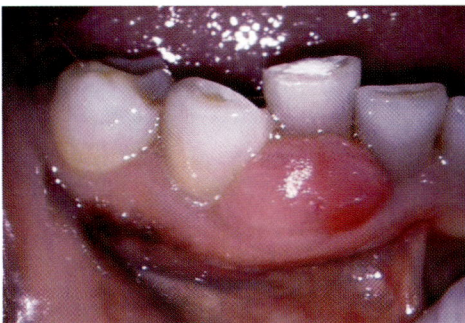

Fig. 1: Pre-op. A large epulis lesion is present at the labial surface from mesial of #27 to distal of #25. Tac-gel is applied to the lesion for approximately 3.5 minutes.

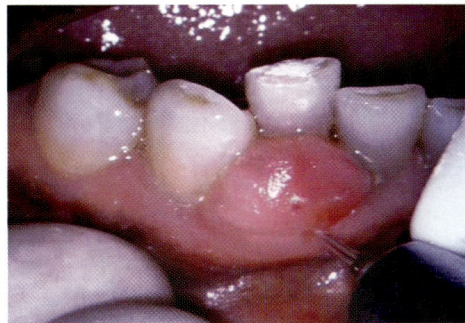

Fig. 2: A MG-6 (or MZ-6) is used to incise at the border of the lesion. The setting is 3.00W 7% Water, 11% Air, 30 Hz.

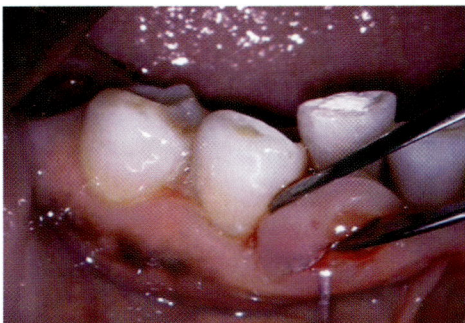

Fig. 3: With a tissue forcep holding the lesion, excision is made at the same setting as in incision. (See Fig. 2)

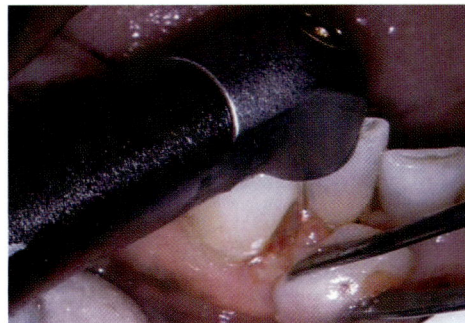

Fig. 4: Completion of the excision of the lesion from the opposite side.

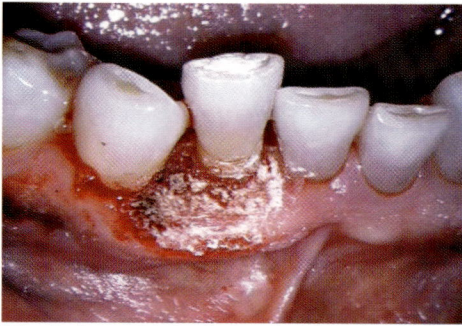

Fig. 5: Laser biologic band-aid is completed using a MC-12 tip at 1.50W, 0% Water, 11% Air, defocused 3-5 mm. No suture is needed due to good hemostasis.

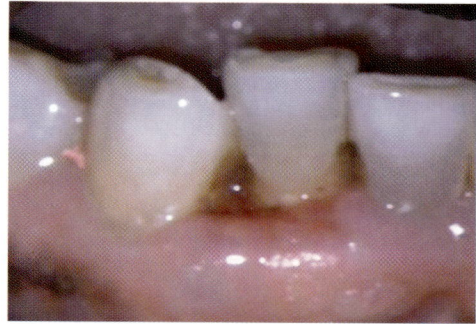

Fig. 6: Post-op. At one week, no complications, remarkable healing.

Case 3: Biopsy, Moderate Size Fibroma on Tongue, MD Regular HP with MG-6 Tip

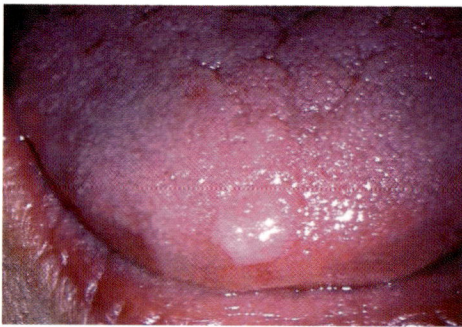

Fig. 1: Pre-op. A moderate size fibroma close to the top of the tongue.

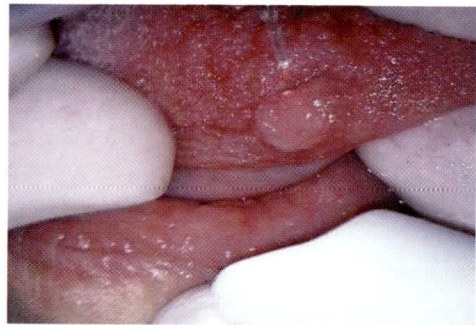

Fig. 2: Tac-gel is applied to lesion for approximately 3.5 minutes.

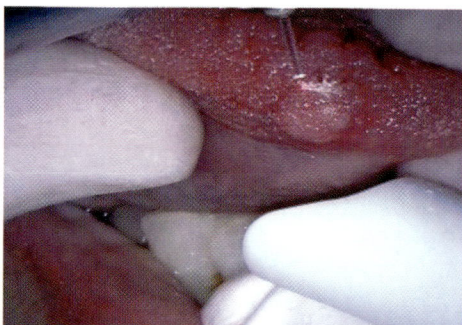

Fig. 3: Laser biopsy starts with an incision using a MG-6 (or MZ-6) tip. The setting is 2.75W, 7% Water, 11% Air, 30 Hz.

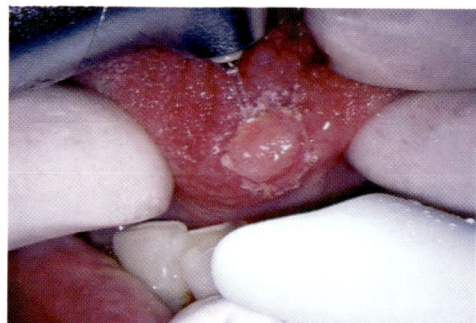

Fig. 4: The incision is made all around the lesion.

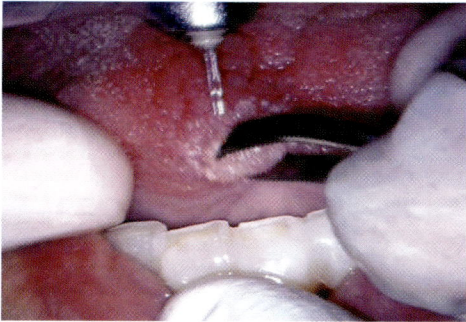

Fig. 5: With tissue forceps holding the lesion excision is made with the laser. Same setting as the incision. (See Fig. 3)

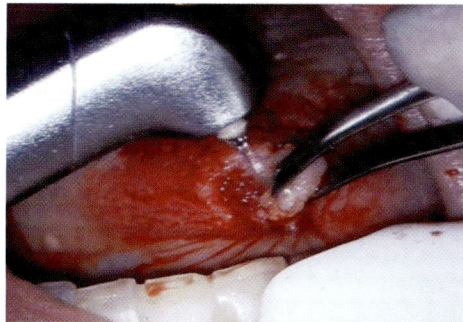

Fig. 6: The excision continues until the lesion is freed from the tongue.

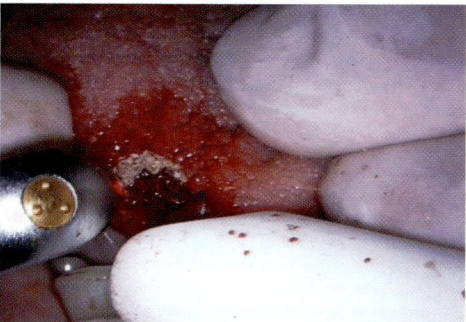

Fig. 7: Laser biologic band aid is performed with the MG-6 (or MZ-6) tip. The setting is 1.25W, 0% Water, 11% Air, 30 Hz, defocused for 3-5 mm.

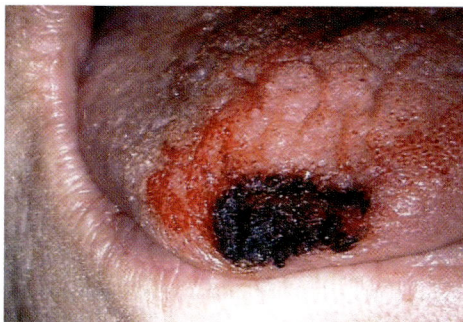

Fig. 8: Post-op complete. Hemostasis is required before dismissing the patient. No suture is needed.

Case 4: Biopsy, Small Fibroma on Tongue, MD Regular HP with MG-6 Tip

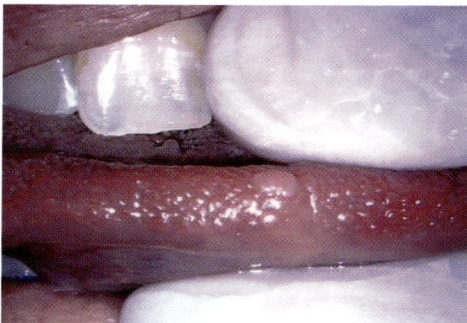

Fig. 1: Pre-op. A small fibroma is present near the tip of the tongue. Tac-gel is applied to the lesion for approximately 3 minutes.

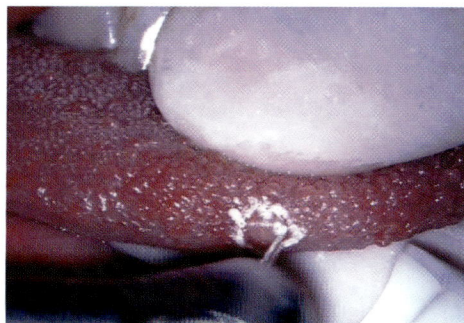

Fig. 2: The tongue is stabilized by firm finger pressure. Marking the lesion is made by laser. A C-6 tip is used. The setting is 0.50W, 0% Water, 11% Air.

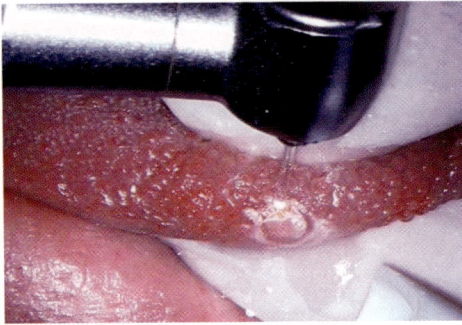

Fig. 3: Laser incision is made with the C-6 tip. The setting is 1.75W, 7% Water, 11% Air.

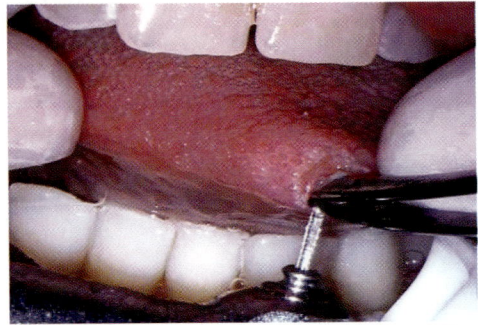

Fig.4: Laser excision is made with tissue forceps holding the lesion. Same setting as the incision is used. (See Fig. 3)

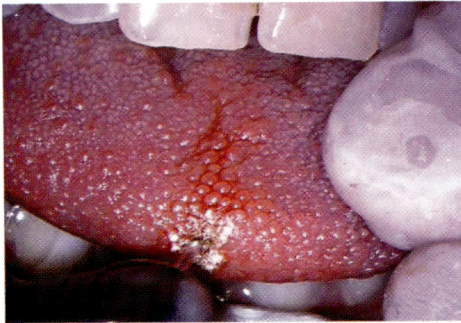

Fig. 5: Laser biologic band aid is applied. The setting is 1.50W, 0% Water, 11% Air, defocused 3 mm.

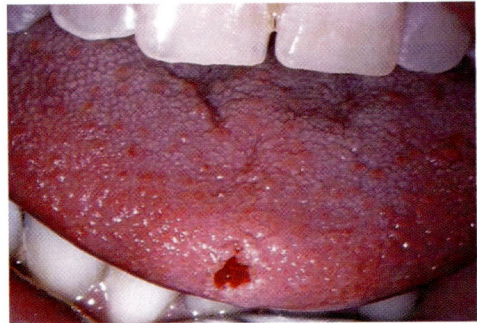

Fig. 6: Immediate post-op.

Labial Frenectomy

When labial frenum impingement causes diastema between the central incisors, rotation of the central incisors, and/or recession of the labial gingival crest that results in tooth elongation and gingival clefting of the crest, a labial frenectomy is indicated.

Before beginning the laser frenectomy procedure, two cotton swabs soaked with concentrated topical anesthetic such as EMLA or Tac-gel are placed at the frenum where the laser cutting will occur. Both sides of the frenum should be treated by the topical anesthetic. During the frenectomy procedure, use one hand to hold the Er,Cr:YSGG laser system handpiece and the other hand to hold the lip. In reflecting the lip, the muscular impingement of the frenum results in blanching of the crestal gingival tissue at the labial area of the centrals. Here a G-6 fiber tip is used.

Laser Parameters, Set 1: Relief of Frenum

Waterlase MD laser system settings: MG-6 tip, 2.25-3.00W, 7% Water, 11% Air, 30 Hz
                    or 2.75-3.50W, 7% Water, 11% Air, 30 Hz, S mode
Other Er,Cr:YSGG laser system settings: 1.25-2.00W, 7% Water, 11% Air

To start the procedure, the tip is placed about parallel with the long axis of the anterior teeth. In a light contact mode with the frenum, laser energy is used to relieve the frenum from the gingival tissue until the relief reaches the mucogingival line.

Laser Parameters, Set 2: Continue Relief of Frenum

Waterlase MD laser system settings: MG-6 tip, 2.25-3.00W, 7% Water, 11% Air, 30 Hz
                    or 2.75-3.50W, 7% Water, 11% Air, 30 Hz, S mode
Other Er,Cr:YSGG laser system settings: 1.25-2.00W, 7% Water, 11% Air

Change the direction of the tip and aim the tip at the frenum perpendicular to the long axis of the anterior teeth. Make a horizontal cut at the mucogingival formation of the frenum. This horizontal cut should extend on each side of the frenum from 1/3 to the total width of the central incisor, until the blanching of the labial crestal gingiva disappears. The depth of the surgical cut should be all the way to the bone. The laser energy cuts deeper into the mucogingival tissue in a deliberate horizontal line, which serves as a scar. This will keep the tissue from reattachment and will avoid muscular impingement.

The starting power should be lower than the suggested power. Raise the power in increments of 0.25W until the surgeon is satisfied with the speed at which the frenum is cut. Keep in mind that several uncontrollable factors determine the maximum speed of the laser. These factors include tissue water concentration, tissue fiber concentration, and the patient's attitude and tolerance of pain. The gradual increase in power will help reach the ideal cutting parameter for each particular patient while building up the patient's tolerance for the Er,Cr:YSGG laser system. Sometimes increasing or decreasing the Water % also helps cater to patients' speed or comfort. The parameters can be customized for each patient intraoperatively to provide the best result. When the soft tissue ablates well and the patient has no discomfort at all, that particular setting should be used to complete the procedure.

The final power setting is normally between 2.00-3.00W. Ensure that you avoid ablating the underlying bone. If you accidentally do so, ensure that there is no charring left on the bone surface by increase the Water % and "washing" the char off. This helps reduce any delays in healing.

Laser Parameters, Set 3: Hemostasis

Waterlase MD laser system settings: 1.25W, 0% Water, 11% Air, 30 Hz
Other Er,Cr:YSGG laser system settings: 1.00W, 0% Water, 11% Air

To complete the procedure, use the laser to coagulate the open wound and to apply low-level laser therapy for the purpose of pain attenuation, anti-inflammatory action and faster wound healing. No suturing is required. Make sure hemostasis has been completed. Again, avoid directing any laser energy at bone.

Post-operative instructions should include the following, if you do not already include these in your recommendations to the patient:

1. Have nothing hot to eat or drink for 24 hours. Food and drink should be at room temperature, at warmest.
2. Do not brush or floss for 24 hours.
3. Do not eat anything spicy or use any sharp instruments in the mouth for 24 hours (i.e., do not eat chips, do not use straws).
4. Do not allow contact with or aggravation of the lips for 24 hours (i.e., no contact sports, strenuous exercise, or kissing).
5. Use over-the-counter pain medication such as Tylenol or ibuprofen, as necessary.
6. If there is bleeding, use gauze and place light pressure on the wound for 15 minutes. If bleeding does not stop, call the doctor.
7. Call the doctor if there is excessive pain, bleeding, and swelling.
8. Make an appointment to be checked by the doctor in 7 days.

Note: In severe cases, especially in the maxilla, frenum attachment may extend between the central incisors into the palate. Large diastema (-3 mm) may be present. The surgical cut should include the vertical component extending all the way into the palate. The fibrous ligaments in the interproximal space should be removed. Care needs to be taken to avoid the nasopalatine foramen.

Case 1: Maxillary Labial Frenectomy, MD Regular HP with MG-6 Tip

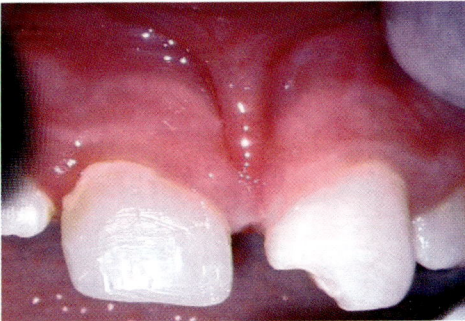

Fig. 1: Maxillary labial frenum causes a large diastema between teeth #8 and #9.

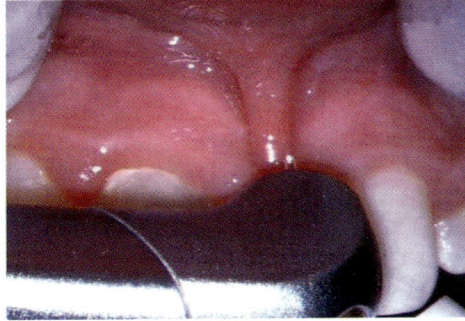

Fig. 2: After concentrated topical has been applied for 3.5 minutes, the tip is placed parallel to the long axis of tooth, and is focused to aim at ablating the border of the impingement at the mesial area.

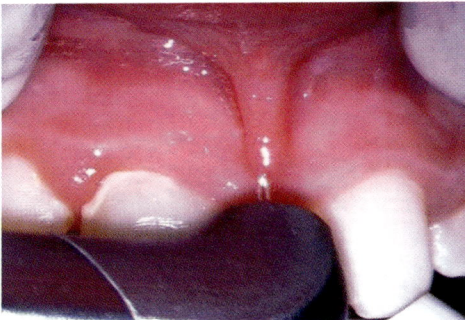

Fig. 3: The relief of the impingement continues by holding the upper lip firmly with the fingers of the left hand and slowly moving the lip up to accelerate the frenectomy by the laser.

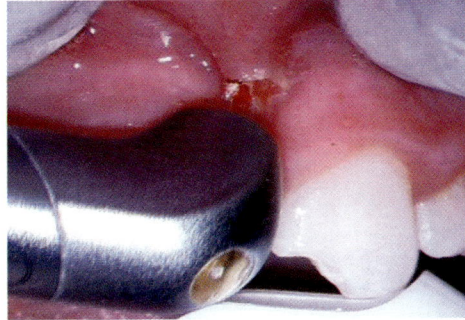

Fig. 4: The frenectomy continues towards the mucogingival line.

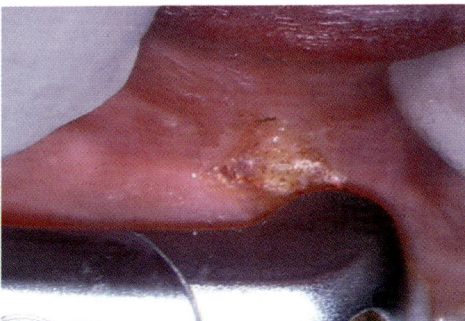

Fig. 5: When the relief of the frenum reaches the mucogingival line, the tip changes direction such that it is perpendicular to the tissue surface. A horizontal cut is made along the mucogingival line towards #8 and #9 on both sides.

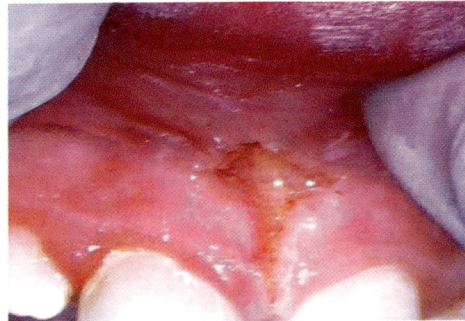

Fig. 6: The extent of the horizontal relief is determined by the changing of color of gingiva of #8 and #9 from bleaching white to normal pinkish white color.

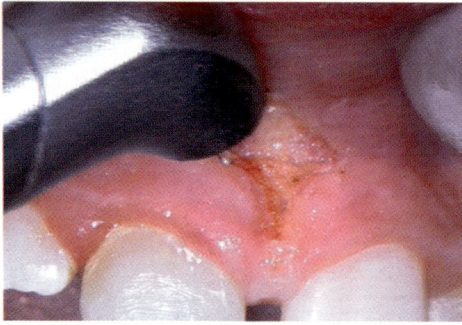

Fig. 7: The horizontal cut is made all the way until it just reaches the bone.

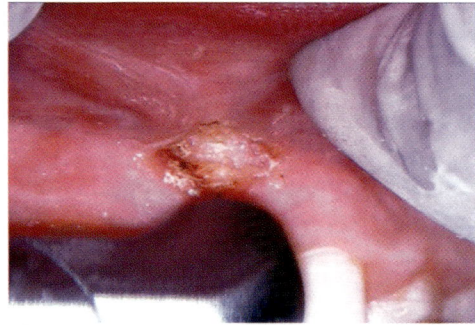

Fig. 8: The tip is defocused and a biologic band-aid setting is used to blanket the surgical site.

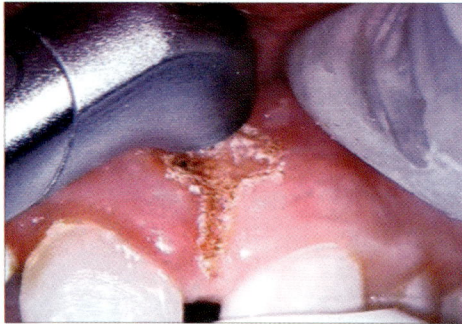

Fig. 9: Hemostasis, bactericidal therapy and low level laser therapy are intended in the biologic band-aid procedure.

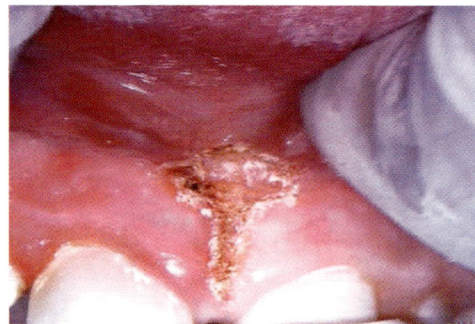

Fig. 10: Post-op. Maxillary labial frenectomy is complete.

Case 2: Mandibulary Labial Frenectomy, MD Gold HP with MZ-5 Tip & S mode

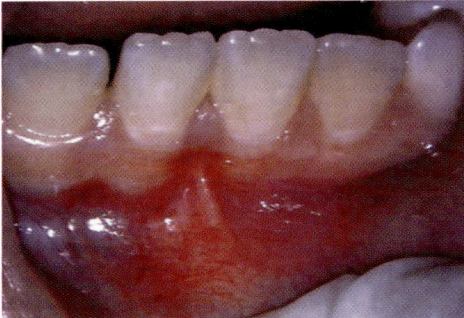

Fig. 1: Pre-op. Mandibular labial muscular impingement causes recession of marginal gingiva of #24 and #25.

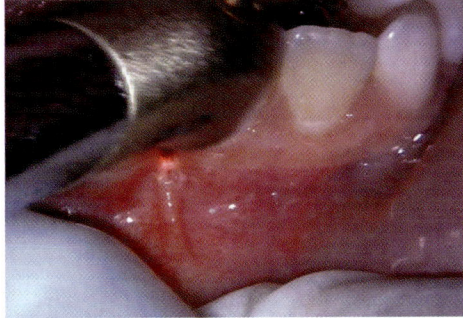

Fig. 2: After 3-minute applications of Tac-gel, a MZ-5 tip in an MD Gold Handpiece is used. The tip is parallel to the long axis of the incisors and the labial frenectomy begins at the base of the frenum attachment. The setting is 2.75W, 7-15% Water, 11% Air, 30 Hz, S mode.

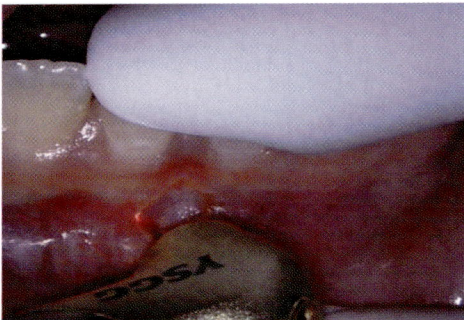

Fig. 3: When the frenectomy reaches the mucogingival line, the tip is placed perpendicular to the long axis of the incisors. A horizontal relief line is established.

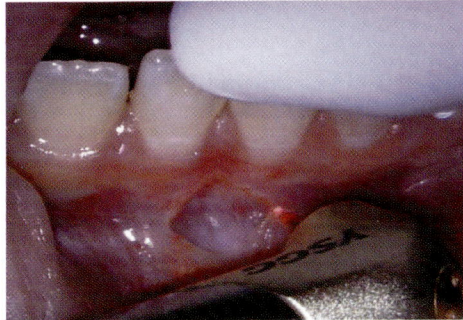

Fig. 4: The horizontal cut continues until it reaches the bone. This scar line serves as a stop for reattachment of the muscle fiber at this position.

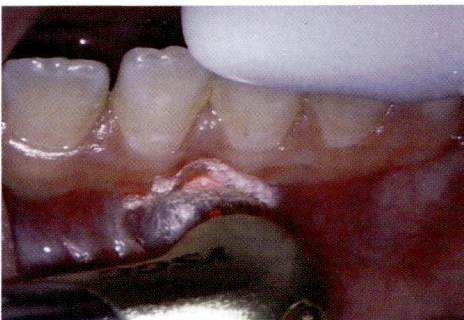

Fig. 5: Biologic band-aid is performed to complete the frenectomy. The setting is 1.25W 0% Water, 11% Air, 30 Hz.

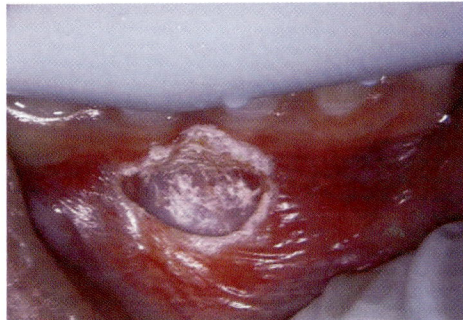

Fig. 6: Immediate post-op.

Case 3: Mandibulary Labial Frenectomy, MD Gold HP with MZ-5 Tip & S mode

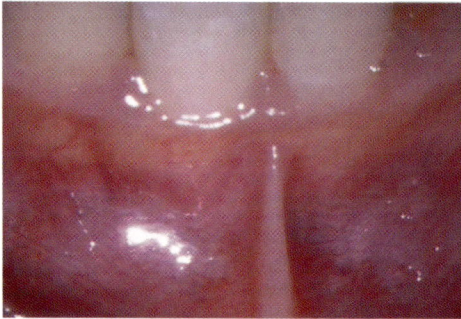

Fig. 1: Recession of marginal gingiva of #24 and #25 is caused by muscular impingement of the labial frenum.

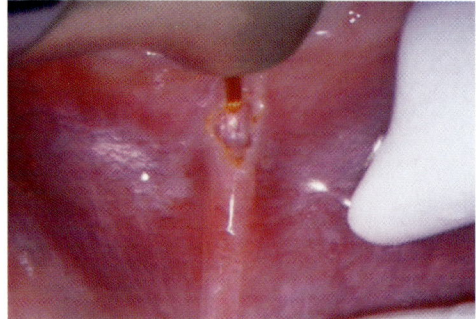

Fig. 2: 3-minute application of Tac-gel. Labial frenectomy begins with the tip placed parallel to the long axis of #24 and 25. A MZ-5 tip in a MD Gold Handpiece is used. The setting is 2.75W 15% Water, 11% Air, 30 Hz, S mode.

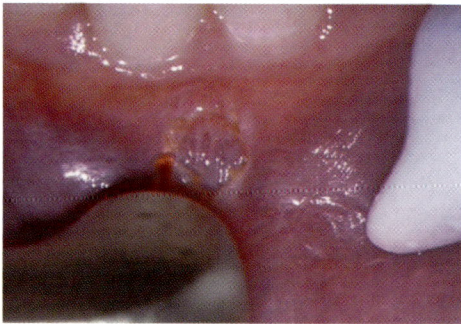

Fig. 3: When the frenectomy reaches the mucogingival line, the tip is placed perpendicular to the #24 and #25 long axis. A horizontal cut is made.

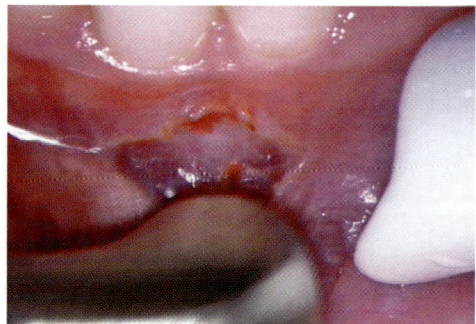

Fig. 4: The horizontal cut continues until it reaches the bone. The relief of the muscular impingement is completed.

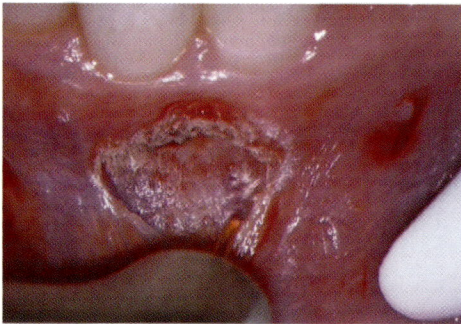

Fig. 5: Biologic band-aid is performed using the MZ-5 tip. The setting is 1.25W, 0% Water, 11% Air, 30 Hz, H mode.

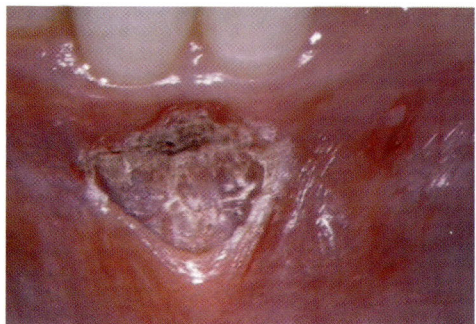

Fig. 6: Immediate post-op.

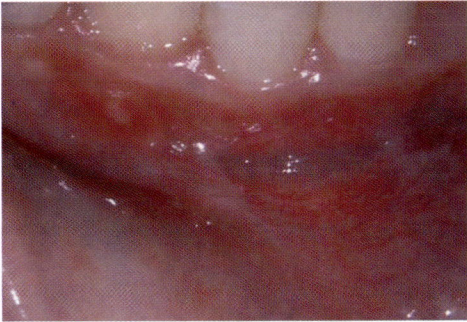

Fig. 7: One week post-op. Significant improvement of the marginal gingiva is noted at #24 and #25.

Case 4: Maxillary Labial Frenectomy, MD Regular HP with MC-3 Tip

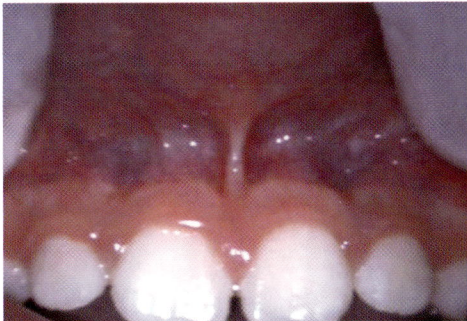

Fig. 1: Pre-op. Diastema between #8 and 9 is caused by the muscular impingement of the labial frenum.

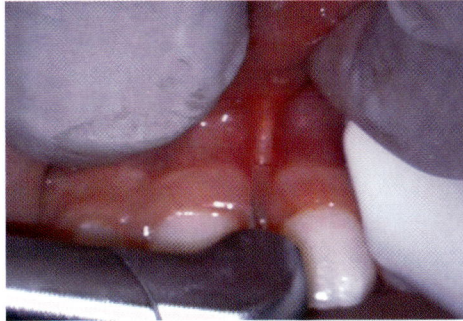

Fig. 2: Labial frenectomy begins with a MC-6 tip. The tip is placed parallel to the long axis of #8 and #9. The setting is 3.25W, 15% Water, 11% Air, 30 Hz, S mode.

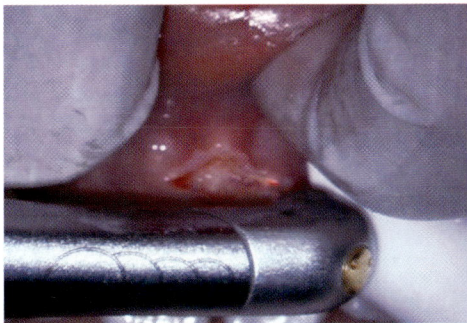

Fig. 3: At the mucogingival line, the tip is now placed perpendicular to the long axis of #8 and #9. A horizontal cut is made along the mucogingival line.

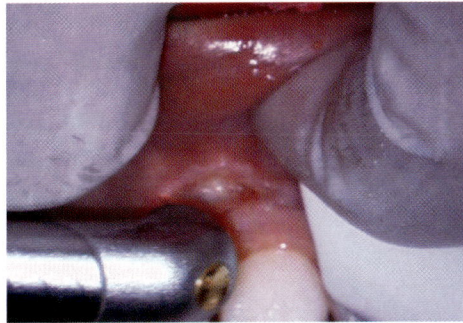

Fig. 4: The horizontal relief continues until it reaches the bone.

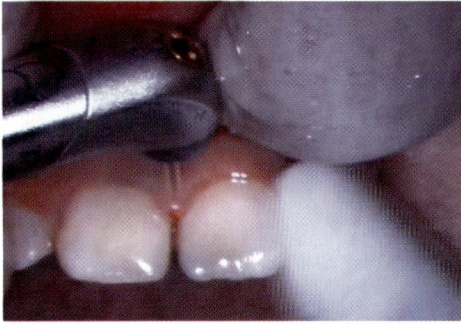

Fig. 5: A MG-6 tip is used to ablate the muscular impingement in the interproximal area of #8 and #9. The setting is 2.75W, 15% Water, 11% Air, 30 Hz, S mode.

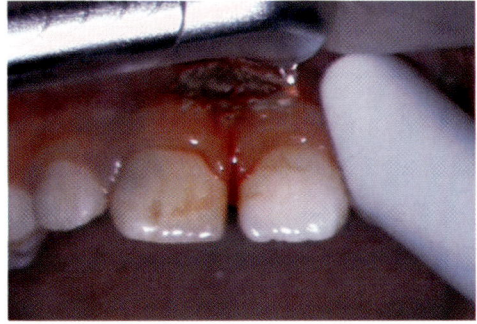

Fig. 6: Biologic band-aid is performed with the MC-3 tip. The setting is 1.50W, 0% Water, 11% Air, 30 Hz.

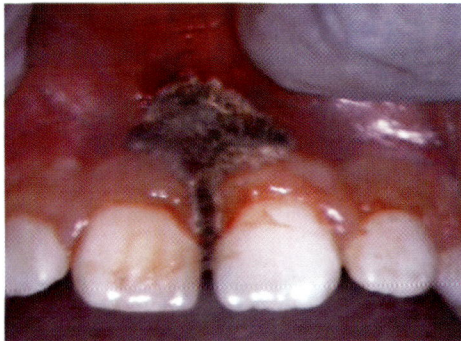

Fig. 7: Immediate post-op.

Lingual Frenectomy

Terminology such as tongue-tied and ankyloglossia are used to describe a condition that restricts the tongue's mobility such that the tongue may not be able to touch the roof of the mouth or lick the lips. This condition may also create a handicap for the patient in speech, swallowing, and eating. A diastema between mandibular anterior teeth may be present.

To begin the procedure, apply concentrated topical such as Emla or Tac-gel. Use two cotton swabs soaked with the concentrated topical gel. Place a cotton swab on each side of the frenum for 3.5 minutes. Please note that the topical should be applied to the surgical sites at different times and at different depths of the surgical site. This will allow the procedure to be performed without discomfort for the patient even at deeper portions of the frenum impingement. A difficult lingual frenectomy may require the use of concentrated topical up to three separate times.

Often there are two components in the lingual frenum. The major restriction in tongue movement stems from the base of the tongue. There is also a fiber that attaches to the lingual gingiva of the anterior area of the mandible.

Laser Parameters, Set 1: Relief of the Lingual Frenum

Waterlase MD laser system settings: MG-6 tip, 2.25-3.00W, 7% Water, 11% Air, 30 Hz
or 2.75-3.50W, 7% Water, 11% Air, 30 Hz, S mode
Other Er,Cr:YSGG laser system settings: G-6 tip, 1.25-2.00W, 7% Water, 11% Air

> Concentrated topical such as Emla or Tac-gel is used by means of two cotton swabs for 3.5 min. This is followed by aiming the tip at the lingual frenum. The laser power is adjusted in increments of 0.25 Watts. Increase the speed of cutting to a speed that the surgeon and the patient are most comfortable with, aiming towards a goal of efficient cutting speed and painless treatment. The final power setting is normally around 2.25-3.00W (H mode) or 2.75-3.50W (S mode).

> It is easier to perform the frenectomy at the lingual surface of the treatment area first. Be aware that there may be several branches of fibers, and all of these branches require relief. The tongue is held and reflected up posteriorly. A horizontal cut is made at the frenum in the base of the tongue. (Note: Avoid the glands in the submandibular area. The cut should be at least 2mm away from the glands.)

Laser Parameters, Set 2: Continue Relief of Lingual Frenum

Waterlase MD laser system settings: MG-6 tip, 2.25-3.00W, 7% Water, 11% Air, 30 Hz
or 2.75-3.50W, 7% Water, 11% Air, 30 Hz, S mode
Other Er,Cr:YSGG laser system settings: G-6 tip, 1.25-2.00W, 7% Water, 11% Air

Apply concentrated topical to the partially relieved lingual frenum for another 3.5 minutes. Again the tongue is held and reflected up posteriorly. The horizontal relief cut is continued deeper in the base of the tongue.

For deeper ablation that is required to relieve a more fibrous lingual frenum, concentrated topical is used a third time before completion of the frenectomy. The tongue reaches the palate at an open position. The surgical wound should appear as a "diamond shape" open wound.

Laser Parameters, Set 3: Hemostasis

Waterlase MD laser system settings: 1.25W, 0% Water, 1% Air, 30 Hz
Other Er,Cr:YSGG laser system settings: 1.00W, 0% Water, 11% Air

To finish the procedure, use the laser to coagulate the open wound and induce hemostasis. No suturing is required. Make sure hemostasis is firmly established before dismissing the patient.

Post-operative instructions should include the following, if you do not already include these in your recommendations to the patient:
1. Have nothing hot to eat and drink for 24 hours. Food and drink should be at room temperature, at warmest.
2. Do not brush or floss for 24 hours.
3. Do not eat anything spicy or use any sharp instruments in the mouth for 24 hours (i.e., do not eat chips, do not use straws).
4. Do not allow contact with or aggravation of the lips for 24 hours (i.e., no contact sports, strenuous exercise or kissing).
5. Use over-the-counter pain medication such as Tylenol or ibuprofen, as necessary.
6. If there is bleeding, use gauze and place light pressure on the wound for 15 minutes. If bleeding does not stop, call the doctor.
7. Call the doctor if there is excessive pain, bleeding, and swelling.
8. Make an appointment to be checked by the doctor in 7 days.
9. After 3 days have passed, practice tongue exercises to ensure proper healing. Place the tongue on the roof of the mouth and extend it to the lips. This exercise should be repeated 20 times a day.

Case 1: Lingual Frenectomy, MD Regular HP with MG-6 Tip

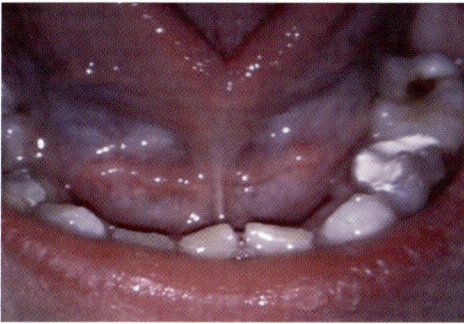

Fig. 1: Pre-op. "Tongue tie" that is indicated for a lingual frenectomy.

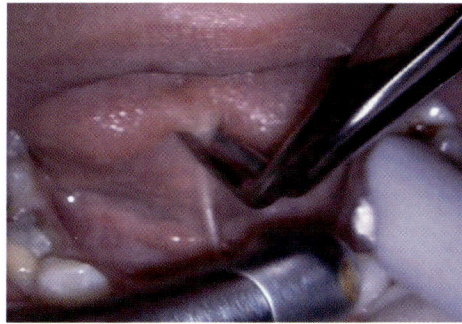

Fig. 2: After Tac-gel is applied to the surgical site for 3.5 minutes, lingual frenectomy starts at the lingual surface of the mandible. A MG-6 (or MZ-6) tip is used. The setting is 2.25W, 7% Water, 11% Air, 30 Hz.

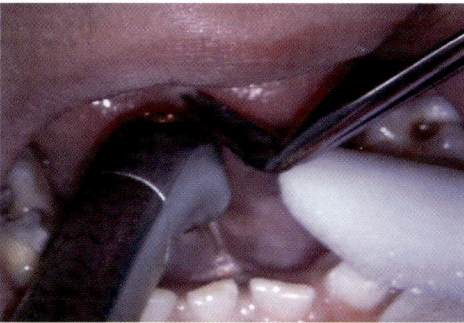

Fig. 3: Lingual frenectomy is performed at the base of the tongue. A horizontal relief is made in the ventral surface of the tongue until a large diamond-shaped opening is made. Same setting is used as in Fig. 2.

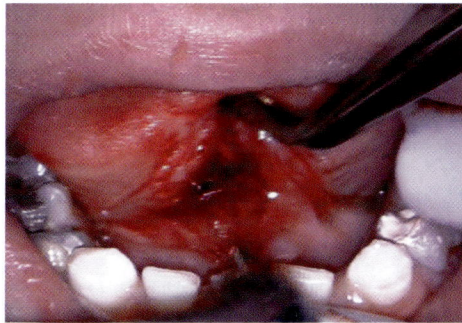

Fig. 4: Laser biologic band aid is made by using a MC-12 tip. The setting is 1.75W, 0% Water, 11% Air, 30 Hz.

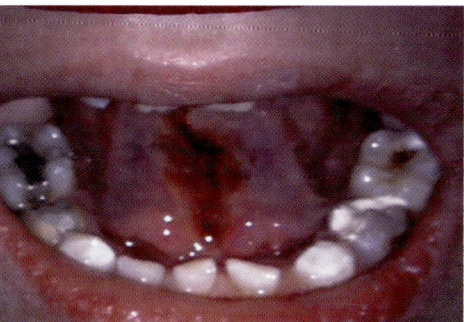

Fig. 5: Immediate post-op.

Case 2: Lingual Frenectomy, MD Regular HP with MG-6 Tip

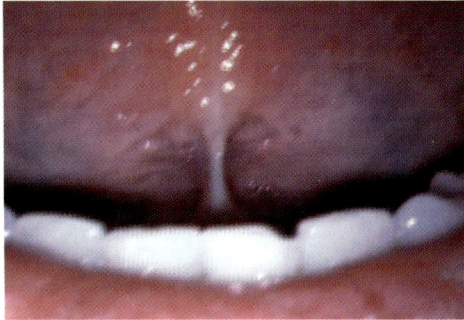

Fig. 1: Pre-op. Lingual frenectomy is indicated due to ankyloglossia.

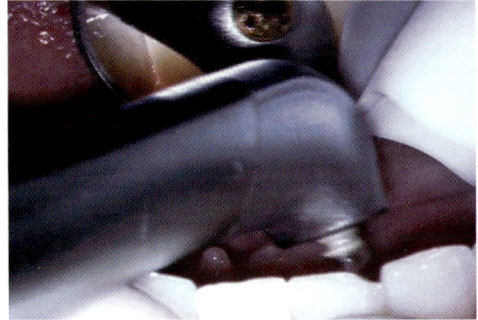

Fig. 2: After 3 minutes of concentrated topical treatment is administered, a MG-6 tip is used with settings of 2.75W, 30 Hz, 15% water, 11 % air, S mode. Laser is used to release the muscle attachments apical to the crowns of the anterior teeth in the lingual surface.

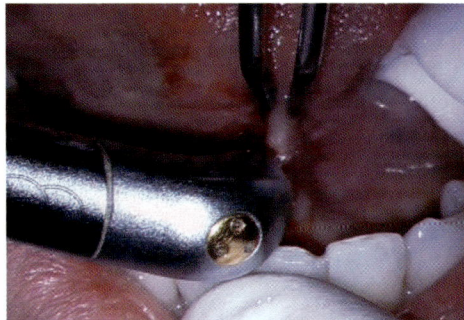

Fig. 3: With the tongue steadied by a forcep, laser is used to start a horizontal release cut of the genioglossus muscles and lingual septum to reduce the muscle impingement that causes the ankyloglossia. Care is to be taken to avoid cutting the submandibular duct, submandibular gland and sublingual gland, sublingual caruncle and lingual artery.

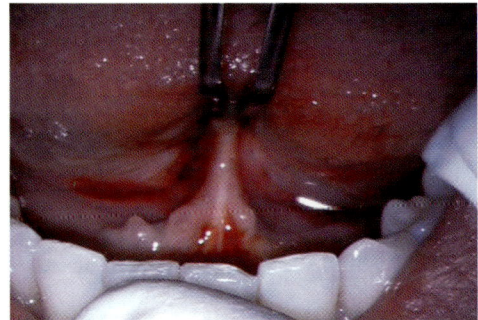

Fig. 4: Concentrated topic is applied the second time after the horizontal release is several mm into the genioglossus muscle.

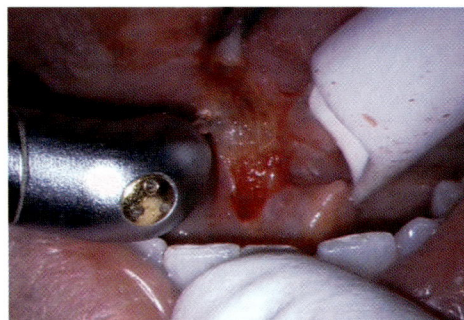

Fig. 5: Lingual frenectomy is continued with the same setting as in Fig. 2.

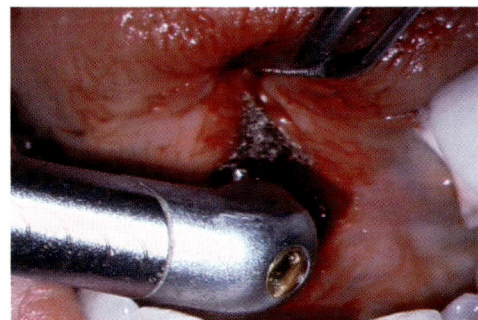

Fig. 6: After a third application of concentrated topical, the lingual frenectomy is performed to finish.

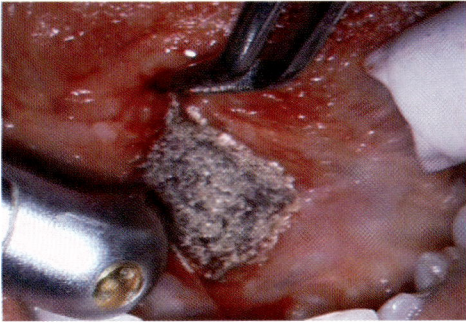

Fig. 7: Biologic band-aid is used to complete the procedure. The setting is 1.25W, 30 Hz, 0% water, 11% air, H mode, defocused 5 mm.

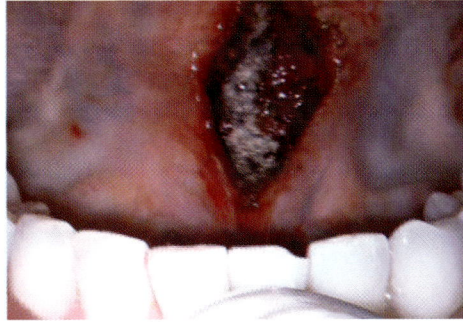

Fig. 8: Immediate post-op.

Aphthous Ulcer Therapy

Laser Parameters, Set 1: Pre-Conditioning

Waterlase MD laser system settings: 0.25W, 1% Water, 11% Air, 50 Hz
Other Er,Cr:YSGG laser system settings: 0.25W, 3-5% Water, 11% Air

Pre-conditioning of the lesion by adding a little water to the laser setting is effective as an alternative to using concentrated topical. It takes approximately 60-120 seconds to pre-condition the lesion.

Laser Parameters, Set 2: Treatment of Aphthous Ulcer

Waterlase MD laser system settings: MG-6 tip, 0.25W, 0% Water, 11% Air, 30 Hz
Other Er,Cr:YSGG laser system settings: G-6 tip, 0.25W, 3-5% Water, 11% Air

Aim the laser at the lesion and defocus the tip to 3-5mm away. Using 5% Water and a slow circular motion, apply laser energy to the lesion. The tissue will gradually turn from pink to white as the laser therapy continues. Lower the Water setting 1% every 15 seconds, until the ulcer is completely white in color. The final Water setting should be 1-2% for the Waterlase MD, and about 3-5% for other Er,Cr:YSGG laser systems.

Laser Parameters, Set 3: Completion of Treatment

Waterlase MD laser system settings: MG-6 tip, 0.25W, 0% Water, 11% Air, 20 Hz
Other Er,Cr:YSGG laser system settings: G-6 tip, 0.25W, 3-5% Water, 11% Air

At a defocused distance of 3-5mm and using a similar slow circular motion, laser energy is used to cover the lesion a second time. This is normally sufficient to remove all sensitivity for nearly all patients. There may be some who have not quite obtained total relief. In that case, the above procedure may be repeated once more. In the last sequence of treatment, laser energy is used to cover 1-2mm of area beyond the border of the lesion.

Case 1: Aphthous Ulcer Therapy on Border of Tongue, MD Regular HP with MG-6 Tip

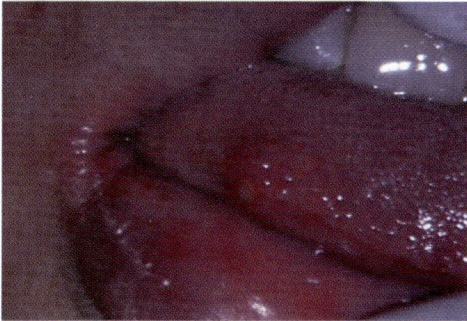

Fig. 1: Pre-op. An aphthous ulcer is present at the right border of the tongue.

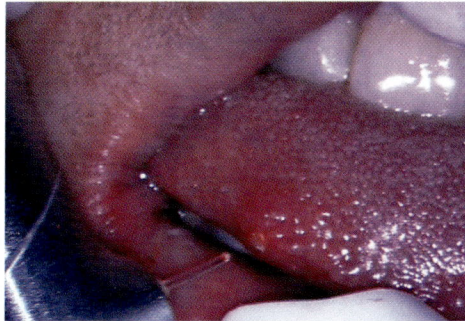

Fig. 2: A MG-6 (or MZ-6) tip is used. The starting setting is 0.25W, 1% Water, 11% Air, 50 Hz.

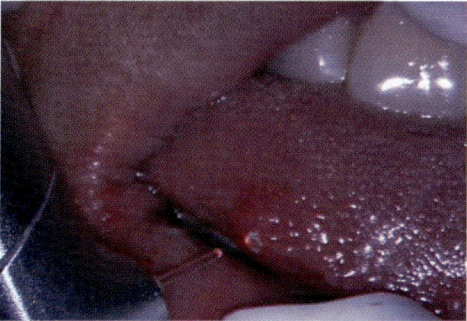

Fig. 3: The second setting is 0.25W, 0% Water, 11% Air, 30 Hz, defocused.

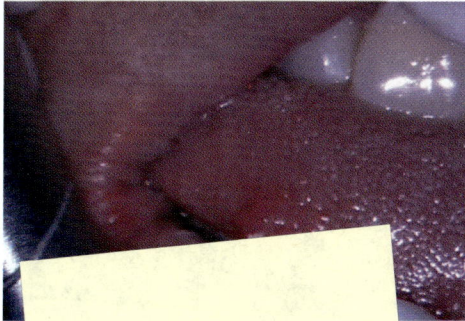

Fi... ...Water, 11...

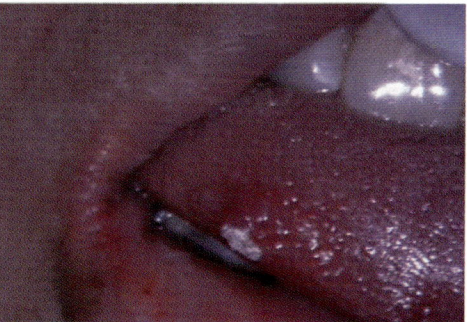

Fig. 5: Immediate post-op.

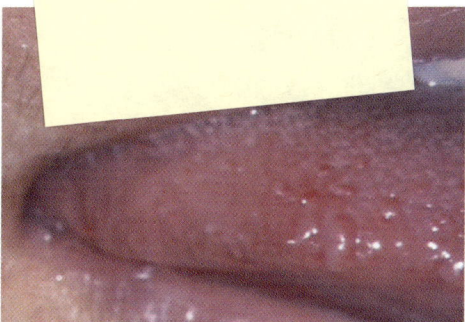

Fig. 6: One week post-op.

Case 2: Aphthous Ulcer Therapy at Mucogingival Tissue, MD Regular HP with MG-6 Tip

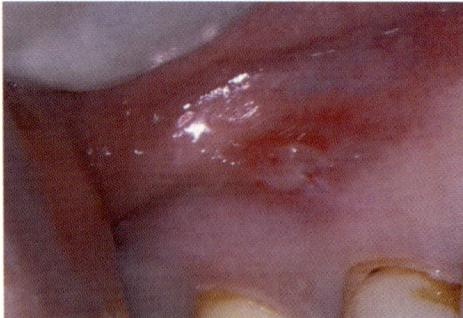

Fig. 1: 6x10 mm aphthous ulcer is present at the buccal mucogingival area of #2 and #3.

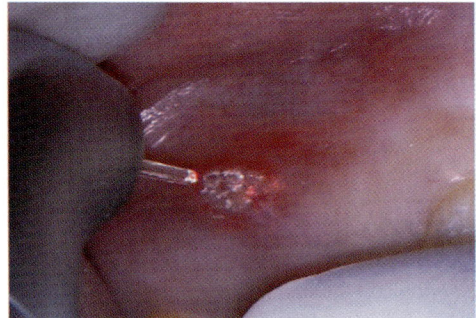

Fig. 2: A MG-6 fiber tip is used at 1mm from the aphthous ulcer. Laser energy is applied for the treatment. The setting is 0.25W, 1% Water, 11% Air, 50 Hz, (for preconditioning).

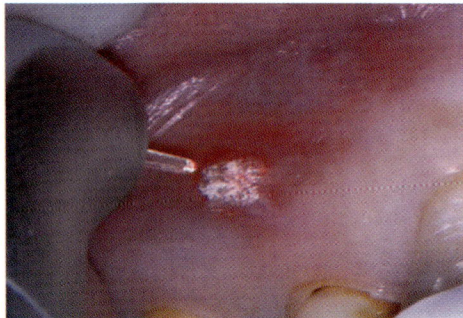

Fig. 3: Aphthous ulcer therapy continues on with 0.25W, 0% Water, 11% Air, 30 Hz, defocused.

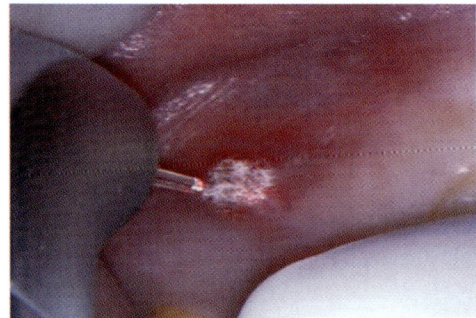

Fig. 4: Final settings are 0.25W, 0% Water, 11% Air, 20 Hz, defocused.

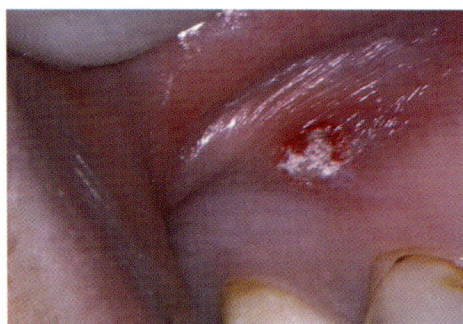

Fig. 5: Immediate post-op.

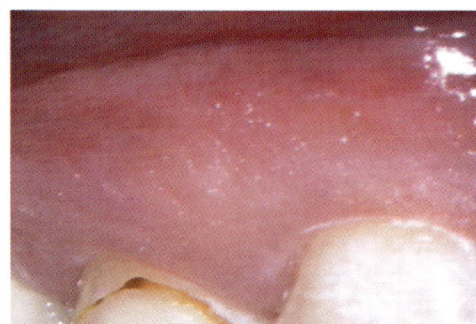

Fig. 6: One month post-op

Gingival Recontouring

When excess gingiva covers an area of the tooth that needs a restoration (i.e., subgingival caries in Class II, III, IV, or V situations), gingival recontouring is indicated.

Laser Parameters, Set 1: Pre-Conditioning

Waterlase MD laser system settings: MG-6 tip, 0.25W, 1% Water, 1% Air, 50 Hz for 2 minutes
Other Er,Cr:YSGG laser system settings: G-6 tip, 0.25W, 7% Water, 11% Air for 4 minutes

Direct the laser towards the tissue to be removed. It is used primarily to warm-up the patient to the laser energy, and also to make an outline of the tissue to be ablated. Occasionally, this may also be enough power to perform the procedure, and no further power settings will be necessary. The pre-conditioning of soft tissue surgery is feasible only on smaller areas that are involved in surgery.

Laser Parameters, Set 2: Ablation

Waterlase MD laser system settings: MG-6 tip, 0.50-1.50W, 7% Water, 11% Air, 30 Hz or 1.00-2.00W, 7% Water, 11% Air, 30 Hz, S mode
Other Er,Cr:YSGG laser system settings: G-6 tip, 0.50-1.25W, 7% Water, 11% Air

If the desired cutting speed cannot be obtained with 0.50W, increase the power in 0.25W increments every 30 seconds until the procedure can be finished efficiently and without causing pain to the patient.

Normally the highest power setting will be 1.50W for the Waterlase MD and 1.25W for other Er,Cr:YSGG laser systems.

Laser Parameters, Set 3: Hemostasis and Margin Refinement

Waterlase MD laser settings: MG-6 tip, 2.25W, 1% Water, 11% Air, 50 Hz, S mode
Other Er,Cr:YSGG laser system settings: C-6 tip, 0.50W, 2-6% Water, 11% Air

Move the tip quickly in a back-and-forth motion above the margin of the gingival crest for hemostasis and refinement of the gingival margin.

Case 1: Gingival Recontouring Before a Class V Prep

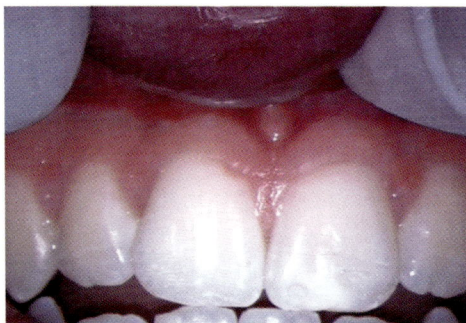

Fig. 1: Hyperplastic gingiva covers a Class V lesion the mesio-labial area of #8.

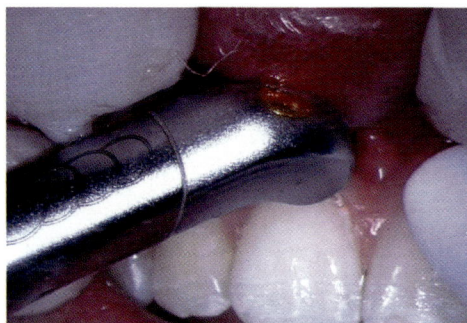

Fig. 2: The tip is focused and aimed at the hyperplastic gingiva to perform gingival recontouring.

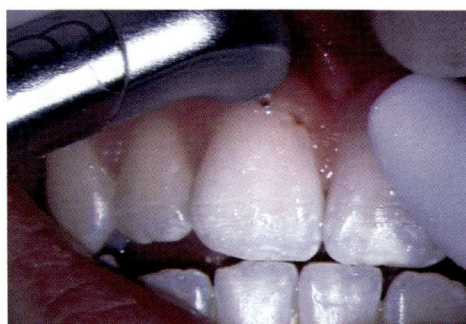

Fig. 3: The Class V caries is better revealed with the completion of gingival recontouring.

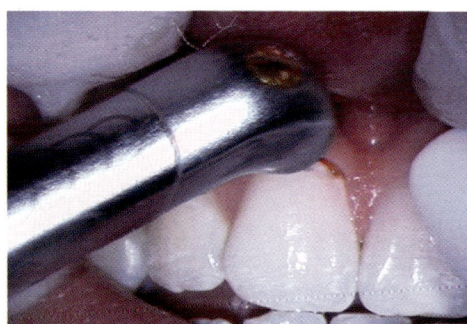

Fig. 4: The tip is focused and aimed at Class V lesion to start cavity preparation.

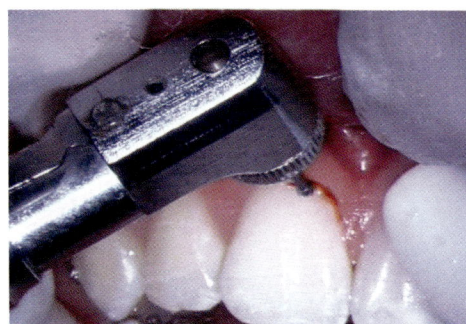

Fig. 5: A slow-speed round bur is used to remove and check caries.

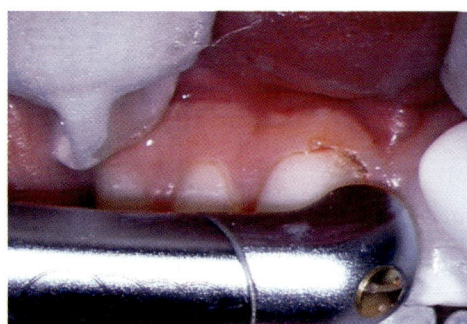

Fig. 6: The tip is focused and aimed to debride, clean and complete preparation.

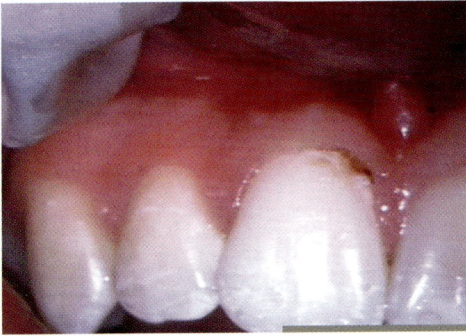

Fig. 7: Post-op. Gingival recontouring and
Class V cavity preparation are complete.

Crown and Veneer Preparation

Introduction

One can easily see why it is not always possible to prepare crowns and veneers with the exclusive use of the Er,Cr:YSGG laser system. In general, using the Er,Cr:YSGG laser system to prepare a veneer or crown can take significantly longer than using a rotary instrument. Longer procedures can lead to intra-operative muscle spasms and post-operatively, in the worst cases, can trigger TMJ dysfunction. Depending on the location of the tooth that requires crown placement, access to the tooth for purposes of using the laser may be a concern. In addition, the presence of metal restorations as a foundation of the crown may make it impossible for the laser to complete the preparation.

However, the laser system provides important advantages over the exclusive use of rotary instruments. The laser provides the ability to avoid micro fractures from the drill, which is well established in literature, as well as the ability to avoid using injectable anesthetics.

I prefer laser-assisted veneer and crown preparation, which combines the advantages of both the laser and the drill. This method uses the analgesic effect of the laser and retains the speed of the drill. The Er,Cr:YSGG offers advantages in removing the smear layer. The laser can be used to trough the gingiva of the crown prep instead of using cord before taking impression. The impression obtained after laser debridement can show debris-free margin. Post-operatively, because of the conditioning of marginal areas, patients normally have less sensitivity with the temporary crown.

Veneer preparations and some crown preparations on anterior teeth can be successfully performed without injectable anesthetics, using techniques similar to my Turtle Technique and a diamond bur. Anesthesia is almost always required in order to operate on posterior teeth. In either case, a high-speed diamond bur is needed to finish the prep and refine the margin.

An important consideration is that in some cases this is the only viable alternative for patients who require crown preparations, but are medically compromised or have negative responses to injectable anesthetic. Laser-assisted crown preparation makes it possible for these patients to obtain a crown restoration.

Er,Cr:YSGG Laser System Troughing in Crown Impression

Laser Parameters, Set 1: Troughing

Waterlase MD laser system settings: MG-6 tip, 1.50-1.75W, 7% Water, 11% Air, 30 Hz
Other Er,Cr:YSGG laser system settings: G-6 tip, 1.25-1.50W, 7% Water, 11% Air

> The tip is placed almost parallel to the long axis of the tooth, aimed at troughing a space between the tooth and the gingival crest. In a fast back-and-forth motion encompassing a 1.5-2.5mm segment of gingiva space at a time, trough the tissue between the tooth and the gingival crest. A controlled rapid speed will minimize the creation of any irregular spaces, and any irregular spaces that are created can be corrected by moving the tip back and forth over the rough areas.

Laser Parameters, Set 2: Hemostasis and Retaining the Trough

Waterlase MD laser system settings: MC-6 tip, 2.25W, 1-3% Water, 11% Air, 50 Hz
Other Er,Cr:YSGG laser system settings: C-6 tip, 1.00W, 1-3% Water, 11% Air

> Aim the tip at points that are bleeding, varying the pressure from focused to lightly touching. Move the tip quickly from one bleeding spot to another in a fast sweeping motion. This also helps to refine the trough.

Case 1: Crown Troughing – Alternative to Packing Cord

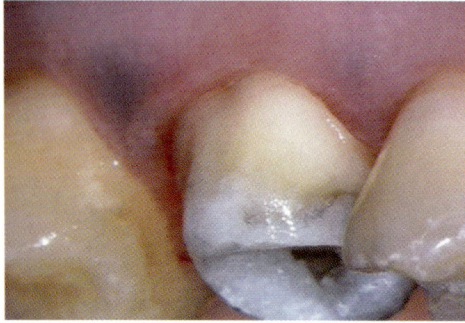

Fig. 1: Pre-op. After crown preparation, crown troughing is chosen over cord packing to prepare the crown for impression.

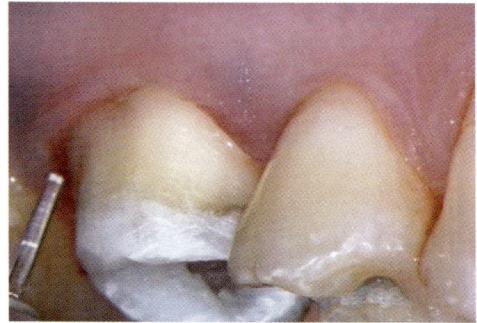

Fig. 2: A MG-6 (or MZ-6, or MC-6) is used.

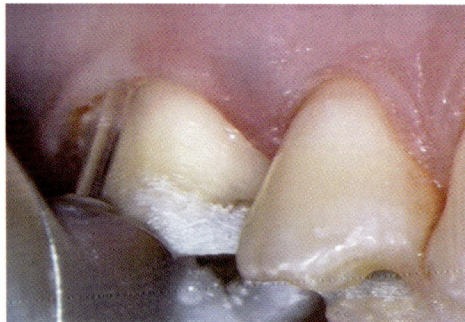

Fig. 3: The tip is placed in the space between gingiva and tooth margin. The setting is 1.50W, 15% Water, 11% Air, 30 Hz.

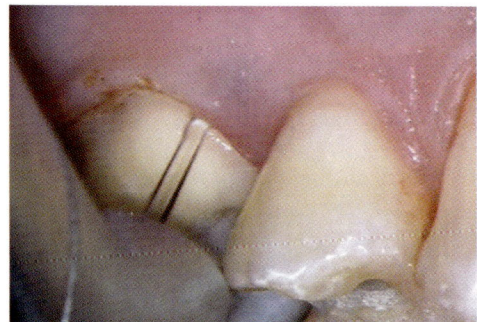

Fig. 4: One segment at a time, a trough is made between gingiva and tooth.

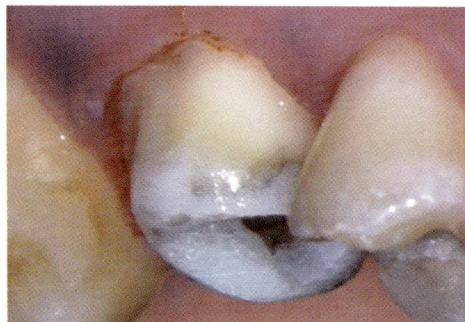

Fig. 5: Crown troughing is completed with no reduction of marginal gingiva.

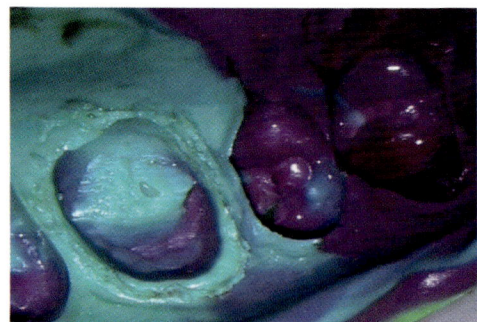

Fig. 6: A clean and accurate impression is shown.

Er,Cr:YSGG Laser System-Assisted Veneer Preparation (Anterior Tooth)

Laser Parameters, Set 1: Pre-Conditioning

Waterlase MD laser system settings: MC-12 tip, 0.50W, 0% Water, 0% Air, 50 Hz
(focused mode, approximately 1-2mm from the target)
Other Er,Cr:YSGG laser system settings: C-12 tip, 0.25W, 0% Water, 0% Air
(defocused at 3-5mm from the target)

The tip is angled perpendicular to the long axis of the tooth at the cervical area. For pre-conditioning, keep the tip aimed towards the approximate outline of the pulp, and move slowly around the outline of the pulp for 120 seconds.

Laser Parameters, Set 2: Ablation of Enamel

Waterlase MD laser system settings: MG-6, 3.00-3.50W, 60% Water, 80% Air, 15 Hz
Other Er,Cr:YSGG laser system settings: 3.50-4.00W, 60% Water, 65% Air

The tip is slightly angled, aiming at the enamel. Keeping the tip in focused mode, laser energy is used to ablate enamel evenly from the incisal edge to the gingival margin. Continue the enamel ablation again from the incisal edge to the gingiva until a relatively even thickness of enamel is established (approximately 1mm in thickness). This is followed by a high-speed diamond bur used to smooth and further reduce the labial surface by another 0.5mm.

Laser Parameters, Set 3: Removal of Smear Layer and Debris

Waterlase MD laser system settings: 2.00W, 60% Water, 80% Air, 30 Hz
Other Er,Cr:YSGG laser system settings: 2.00W, 30% Water, 30% Air

Reduce the laser settings and remove the smear layer and debris from the preparation.

Laser Parameters, Set 4: Completion of Prep

Waterlase MD laser system settings: MG-6, 2.00W, 60% Water, 80% Air, 40 Hz
Other Er,Cr:YSGG laser system settings: G-6 tip, 1.25W, 15% Water, 15% Air

Apply laser energy to the veneer surface in a disciplined up-and-down motion to remove smear and debris and to smooth the prep before restoration.

Case 1: Gingival Recontour, Laser-assisted Veneer Prep, MD Regular HP with MG-6 Tip

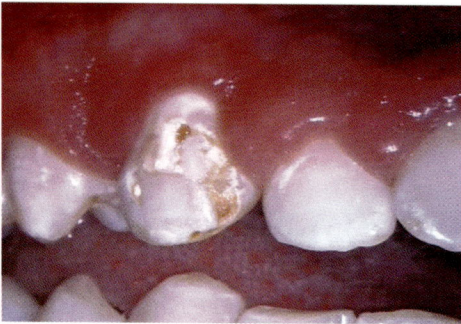

Fig. 1: Pre-op. #6 shows caries in the labial surface and needs a MIDFL composite veneer. The presence of hyperplastic gingival tissue also requires gingival recontouring of #6 and #7.

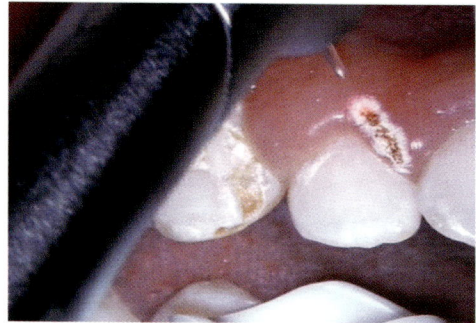

Fig. 2: Marking of the soft tissue to be removed on #7 is performed by a MG-6 (or MZ-6) tip. The setting is 0.50W, 0% Water, 11% Air, 30 Hz.

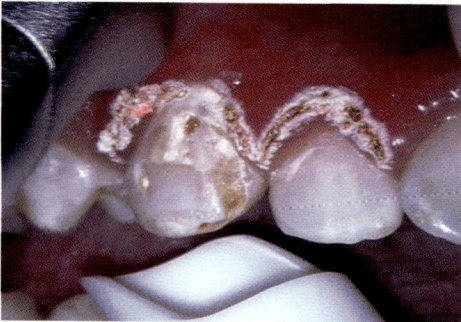

Fig. 3: Also perform "blue-print" marking on #6.

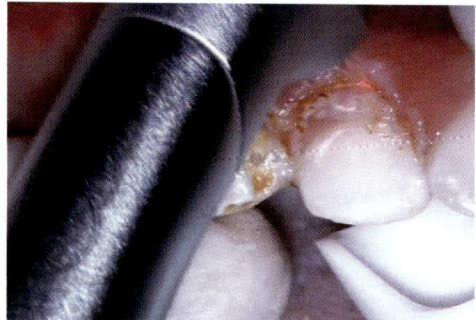

Fig. 4: Gingival recontouring is performed on #7 using the MG-6 (or MZ-6) tip. The setting is 1.75W, 7% Water, 11% Air, 30 Hz.

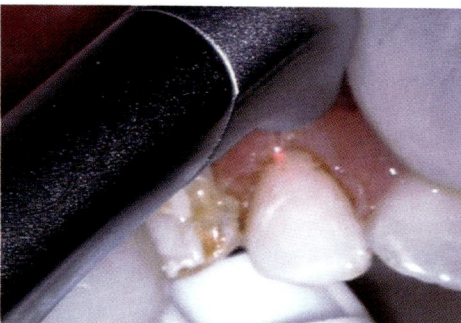

Fig. 5: Recontouring on #7 is refined with the setting of 1.75W, 7% Water, 11% Air, 30 Hz, S mode.

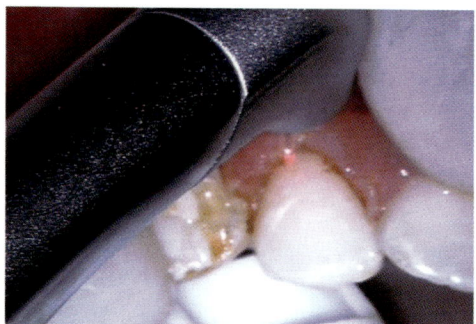

Fig. 6: Recontouring of labial gingiva of #6.

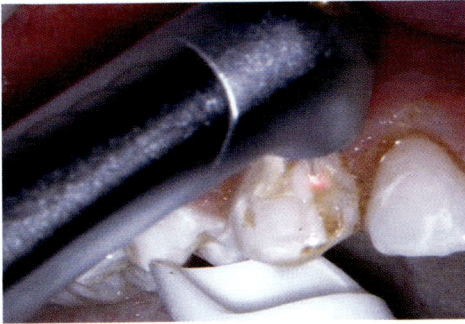

Fig. 7: Begin caries removal and veneer prep by using the MG-6 (or MZ-6) tip at 2.00W, 60% Water, 80% Air, 30 Hz.

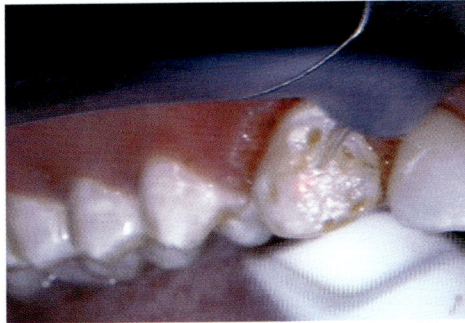

Fig. 8: The power is gradually increased by 0.25W at a time, until enamel is reduced at an efficient rate.

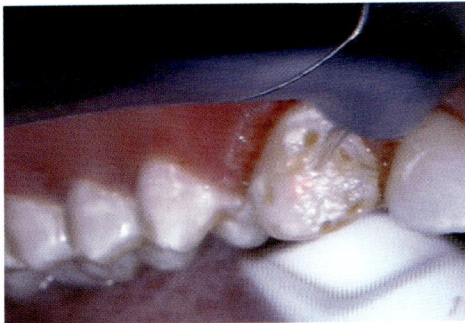

Fig. 9: After two minutes of relatively lower power, 3.00W, 60% Water, 80% Air, 15 Hz is used to finish removing decay and gross enamel and dentin reduction.

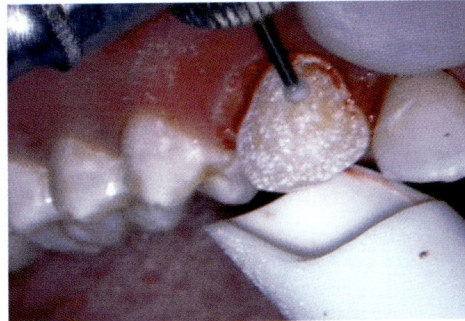

Fig. 10: A slow-speed round bur is used to remove and check caries.

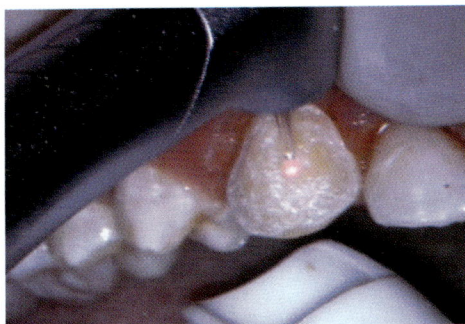

Fig. 11: Laser is used to remove smear, debris and finish the veneer prep. The setting is 2.00W, 60% Water, 80% Air, 30 Hz.

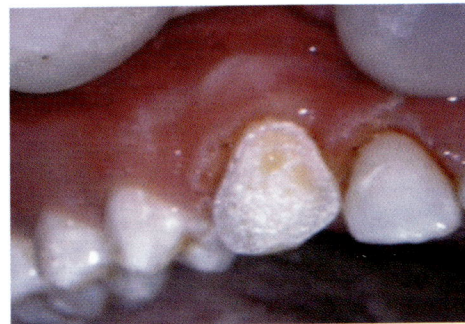

Fig. 12: Immediate post-op after gingival recontouring of #6 and #7 and veneer prep of #6.

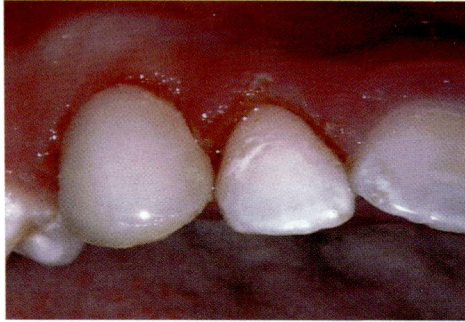

Fig. 13: Post-op after placement of composite veneer on #6.

Case 2: Laser-assisted Veneer Prep, M2 with G-6 Tip

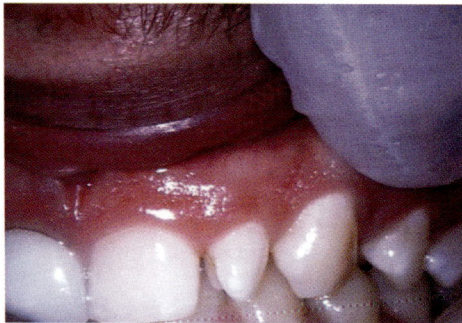

Fig. 1: Pre-op. #10 is a peg lateral that is treatment planned for a composite veneer restoration.

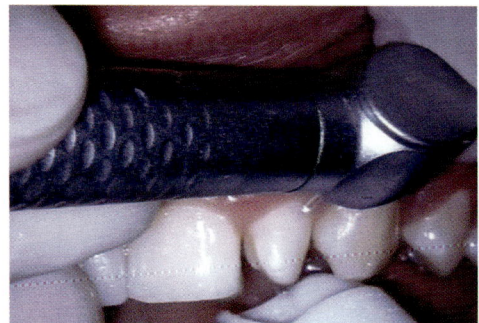

Fig. 2: A G-6 (or Z-6) tip is used to pre-condition the tooth. The setting is 1.25W, 15% Water, 15% Air.

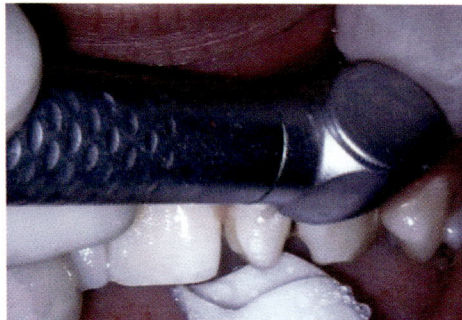

Fig. 3: The power is raised to 2.00W, 30% Water, 30% Air. More pre-conditioning and some ablation of enamel is noted.

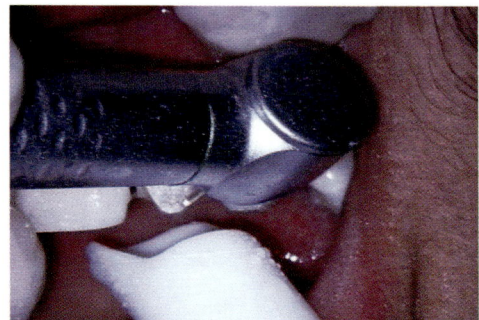

Fig. 4: The power is raised to 4.00W, 60% Water, 65% Air, to grossly reduce enamel.

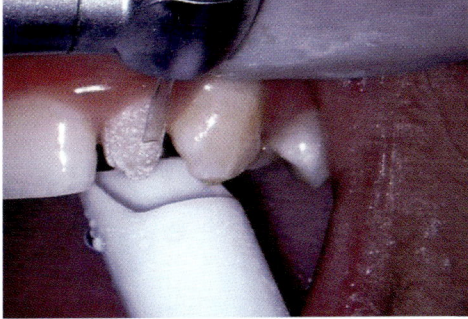

Fig. 5: A C-3 tip is used at 4.00W, 60% Water, 65% Air to continue reduction of the labial surface. It also reduces the roughness produced by the G-6 tip.

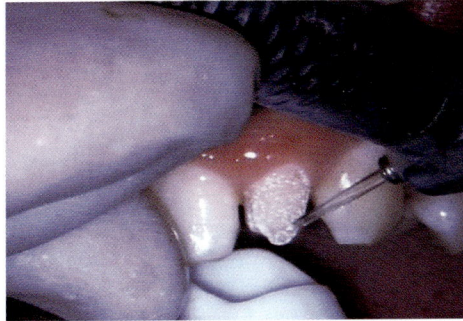

Fig. 6: The incisal bevel is prepared. The power is reduced to 2.00W, 30% Water, 30% Air to finish the prep.

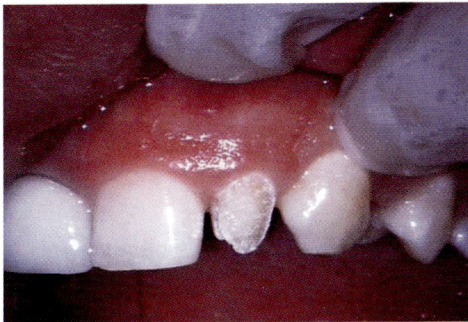

Fig. 7: Post–op.

Er,Cr:YSGG Laser System-Assisted Crown Preparation (Anterior Tooth)

Laser Parameters, Set 1: Pre-Conditioning

Waterlase MD laser system settings: MC-12 tip, 0.50W, 0% Water, 0% Air, 50 Hz (focused mode)
Other Er,Cr:YSGG laser system settings: C-12 tip, 0.25W, 0% Water, 0% Air (defocused to 3-5mm)

The tip is angled perpendicular to the long axis of the tooth at the cervical area. For pre-conditioning, keep the tip aimed towards the approximate outline of the pulp and move slowly around the outline of the pulp for 120 seconds.

Laser Parameters, Set 2: Enamel Ablation

Waterlase MD laser system settings: MG-6 tip, 4.50W, 60% Water, 80% Air, 15 Hz
Other Er,Cr:YSGG laser system settings: G-6 tip, 5.00-6.00W, 75% Water, 90% Air

Angle the tip perpendicular to the labial surface and at 1mm from the incisal edge. The ablation continues in a line parallel to the incisal edge until the incisal 1.5-2mm of tooth is removed.

Aim the tip at the mesial area, about 0.5mm from the mesial surface, to create a vertical cut down to 1mm from the gingival margin. A similar cut is made on the distal side. The mesial and distal walls are removed with laser energy cutting the base of these to smooth and finish margins at gingival crest with a shoulder at buccal, mesial, and distal area. The lingual margin is finished with a rounded tapered diamond to prepare a chamfer margin.

The tip is angled slightly and aimed at the buccal surface to reduce enamel evenly from occlusal to gingival margin, leaving about 1mm of enamel above the gingival crest. Similar reduction is done to the lingual surface. This is followed by using a narrow flat-ended diamond bur in a high-speed handpiece.

Laser Parameters, Set 3: Dentin Preparation

Waterlase MD laser system settings: 2.00W, 60% Water, 80% Air, 30 Hz
Other Er,Cr:YSGG laser system settings: 2.00W, 30% Water, 30% Air

Reduce laser settings and direct laser energy over all ablated sections of the tooth to remove the smear debris. A high-speed diamond is used to finish the margin. The prep is then finally completed with the laser to remove smear and debris.

Case 1: Preparation of Anterior Tooth (Incisor)

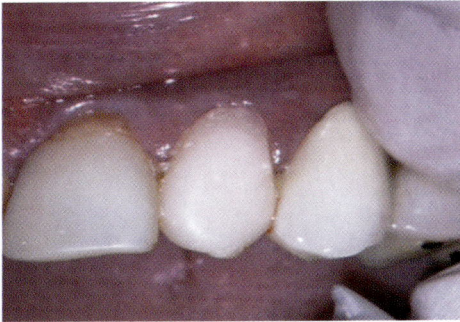

Fig. 1: Pre-op. Maxillary left lateral incisor is treatment planned to have a porcelain fused to metal crown after root canal therapy.

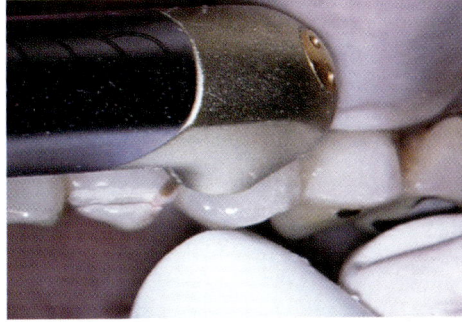

Fig. 2: An incisal cut is made with the laser, using a MZ-5 tip. About 2-3mm of enamel segment at the incisal edge is removed. The setting is 4.50W, 60% Water, 80% Air, 15 Hz.

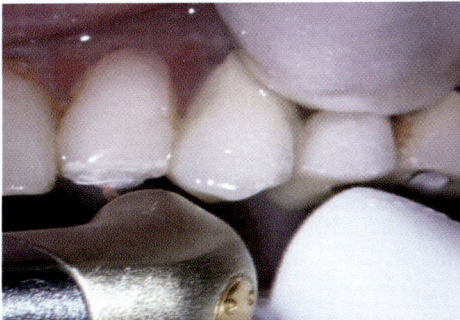

Fig. 3: Laser is used to smooth the rough finish by the initial incisal cut.

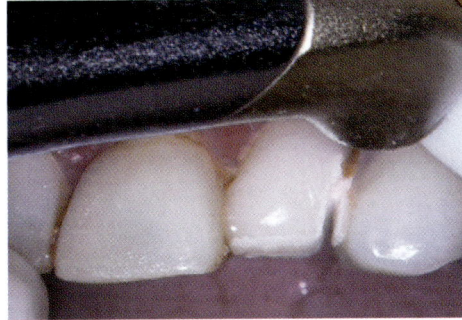

Fig. 4: A distal cut is made by the laser, leaving a thin layer of enamel. This enamel wall is removed by cutting the gingival base with the laser, leaving a rough shoulder margin. The same setting is used throughout the gross reduction at incisal, distal, and mesial cut.

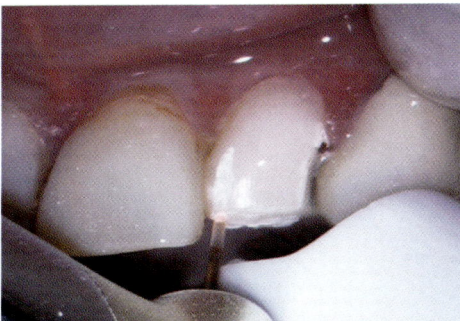

Fig. 5: A mesial cut is made by the laser, leaving a thin layer of enamel.

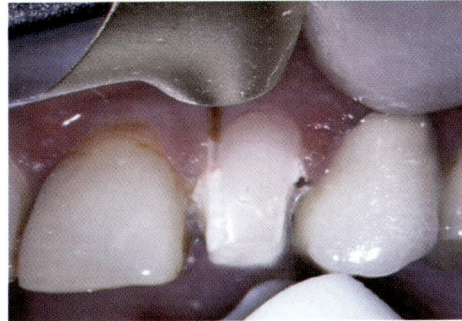

Fig. 6: The mesial enamel wall is removed by laser cutting the gingival base, leaving a rough shoulder margin.

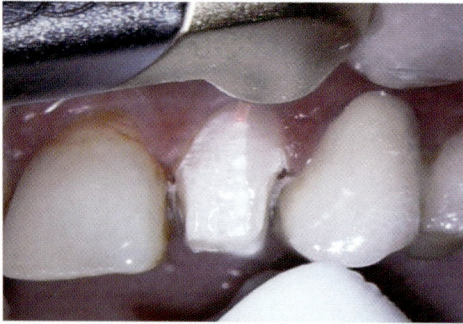

Fig. 7: The labial surface is evenly reduced in thickness similar to a veneer preparation. A rough shoulder margin is made.

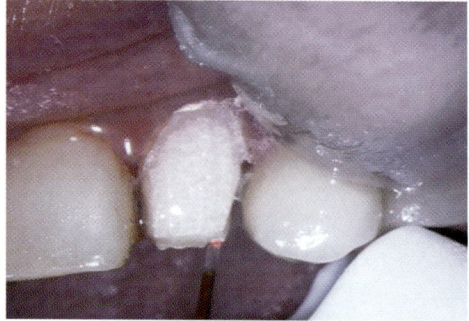

Fig. 8: The lingual surface is evenly reduced in thickness similar to the labial reduction. A rough chamfer margin is made.

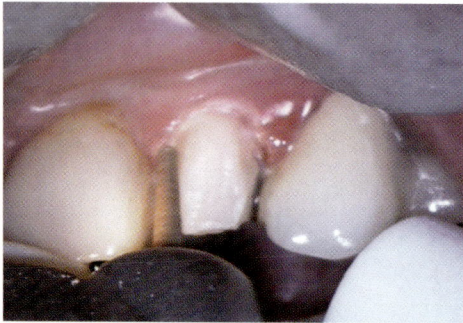

Fig. 9: The crown preparation is smoothed using an electric handpiece high-speed diamond drill to the final form.

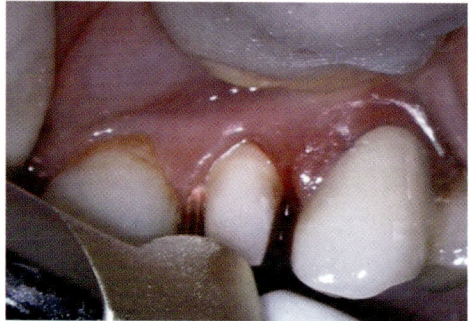

Fig. 10: Laser is used to remove smear and debris on the final prep. The setting is 0.25-0.50W, 60% Water, 80% Air, 30 Hz.

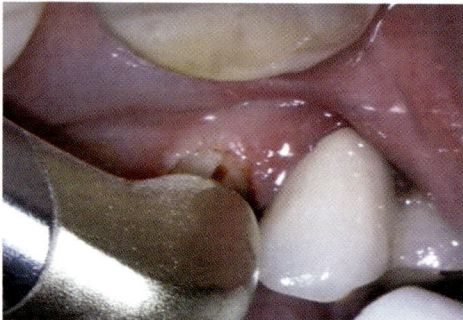

Fig. 11: Troughing is performed by the laser. The setting is 1.00-1.50W, 9-15% Water, 11% Air, 30 Hz. No retraction cord is used. Hemostasis setting is 2.00W, 1% Water, 11% Air, 50 Hz, S mode.

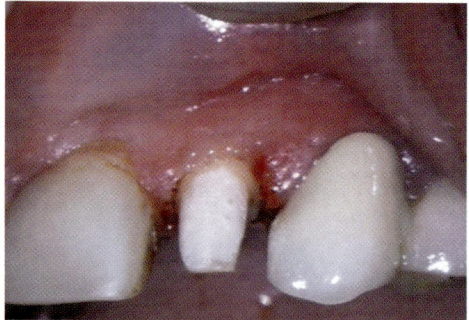

Fig. 12: Post-op. Both crown prep and troughing are complete.

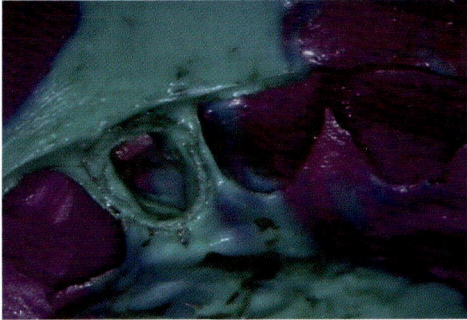

Fig. 13 The impression shows a clean and accurate duplication of the crown prep.

Anterior tooth: Supplementary Drawings

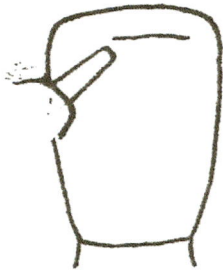

Fig. 1: The tip is aimed to ablate and remove the incisal reduction (labial view).

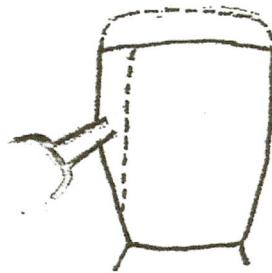

Fig. 2: The tip is aimed to ablate and remove one proximal wall (labial view).

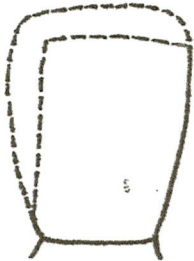

Fig. 3: Removal of one proximal wall is complete (labial view).

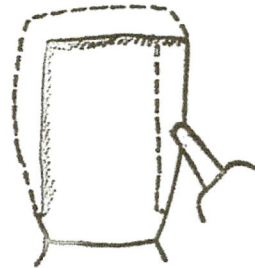

Fig. 4: The tip is aimed to ablate and remove the other proximal wall (labial view).

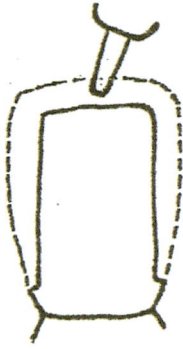

Fig. 5: The tip is aimed to reduce the labial surface (labial view).

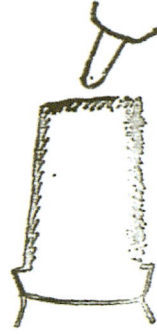

Fig. 6: The tip is aimed to reduce the lingual surface (labial view).

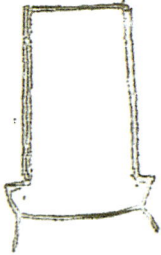

Fig. 7: The crown preparation is complete (labial view).

Er,Cr:YSGG Laser System-Assisted Crown Preparation (Posterior Tooth)

Laser Parameters, Set 1: Pre-Conditioning

Waterlase MD laser system settings: MC-12 tip, 0.50W, 0% Water, 0% Air, 50 Hz
(focused mode)
Other Er,Cr:YSGG laser system settings: C-12 tip, 0.25W, 0% Water, 0% Air
(defocused to 3-5mm)

The tip is angled perpendicular to the long axis of the tooth at the cervical area. For pre-conditioning, keep the tip aimed towards the approximate outline of the pulp and move slowly around the outline of the pulp for 120 seconds.

Laser Parameters, Set 2: Occlusal Reduction

Waterlase MD laser system settings: MG-6 tip, 4.50W, 60% Water, 80% Air, 15 Hz
Other Er,Cr:YSGG laser system settings: G-6 tip, 6.00W, 75% Water, 90% Air

Start a channel approximately 1mm below the occlusal surface to aim at sectioning off the occlusal layer. This reduction follows the occlusal anatomy.

Laser Parameters, Set 3: Proximal Surface Reduction

Waterlase MD laser system settings: MG-6 tip, 4.50W, 60% Water, 80% Air, 15 Hz
Other Er,Cr:YSGG laser system settings: G-6 tip, 6.00W, 75% Water, 90% Air

Start a channel at the mesial surface about ½ to 1mm from contact. The preparation extends to 1mm short of the gingival margin. A similar channel is prepared at the distal area.

Laser Parameters, Set 4: Facial and Lingual Surface Reduction

Waterlase MD laser system settings: MG-6 tip, 4.50W, 60% Water, 80% Air, 15 Hz
Other Er,Cr:YSGG laser system settings: G-6 tip, 6.00W, 75% Water, 90% Air

Both facial and lingual surface reductions are performed by using a similar technique as the one used in Set 3, proximal surface reduction. By the end of this procedure, a rough reduction of the crown on occlusal, mesial, distal, facial and lingual surfaces is established.

Laser Parameters, Set 5: High-Speed Drill

A high-speed diamond bur is used to smooth the different surfaces and the margin of the crown preparation.

Laser Parameters, Set 6: Tidy the Crown Prep

Waterlase MD laser system settings: 2.00W, 60% Water, 80% Air, 30 Hz
Other Er,Cr:YSGG laser system settings: 2.00W, 30% Water, 30% Air

This procedure is used to clean the crown prep and provide more laser anesthesia. The procedure is followed by using high-speed diamond burs to smooth the prep and complete the shoulder margin at the facial, mesial, and distal margin. The lingual margin is finished with a chamfer margin.

Laser Parameters, Set 7: Removal of Smear Layer and Debris

Waterlase MD laser system settings: 0.25-1.00W, 60% Water, 80% Air, 30 Hz
Other Er,Cr:YSGG laser system settings: 0.25-0.75W, 15% Water, 15% Air

Reduce laser settings and direct laser energy over all ablated sections of the tooth to remove the smear debris and finish the crown preparation.

Preparation of Bicuspid: Supplementary Drawings

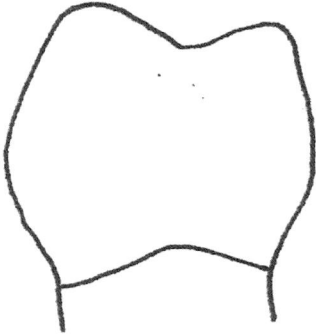

Fig. 1: Preparation: Proximal view.

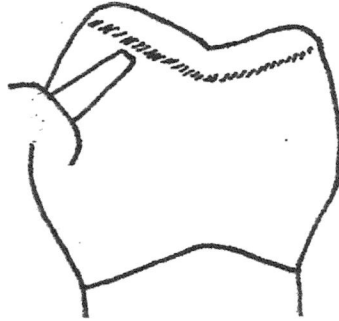

Fig. 2: The tip is aimed to ablate and remove the occlusal reduction (proximal view).

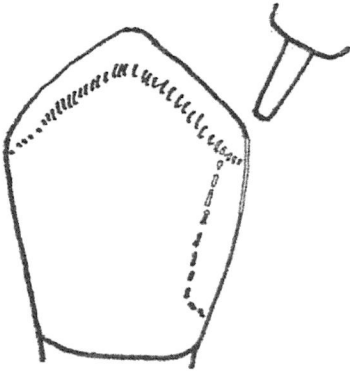

Fig. 3: The tip is aimed to ablate and remove one proximal wall (buccal view).

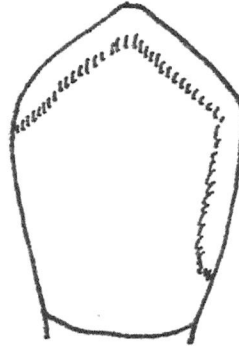

Fig. 4: Removing one proximal wall is complete (buccal view).

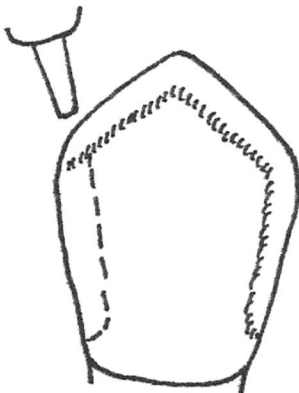

Fig. 5: The tip is aimed to ablate and remove the other proximal wall (buccal view).

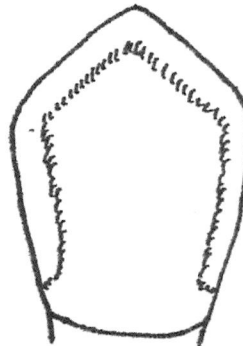

Fig. 6: Removing the other proximal wall is complete (buccal view).

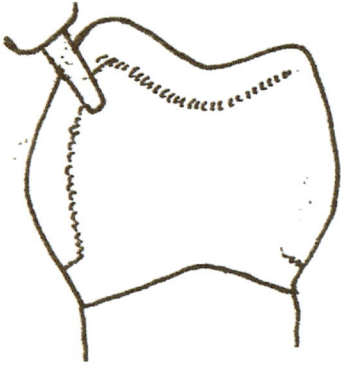

Fig. 7: The tip is aimed to reduce the buccal surface (proximal view).

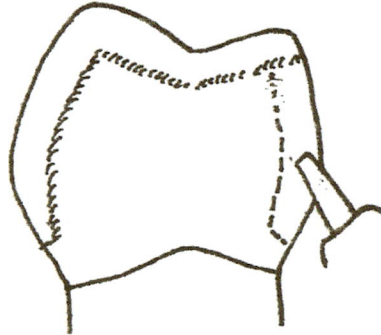

Fig. 8: The tip is aimed to reduce the lingual surface (proximal view).

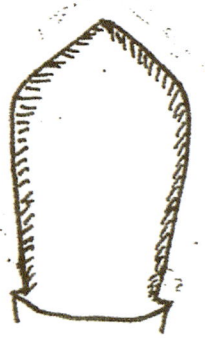

Fig. 9: The crown preparation is complete (buccal view).

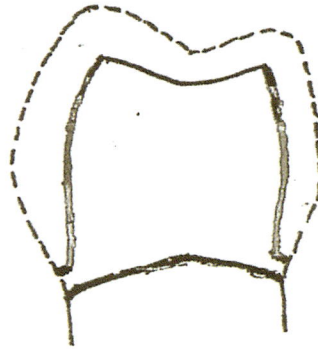

Fig. 10: The crown preparation is complete (proximal view).

Endodontic Procedures

Introduction

Nickel-titanium crown-down rotary instrumentation for root canal treatment is currently regarded as state-of-the-art endodontic therapy. However, the irrigation agent used in the conventional root canal therapy (such as NaOCl and EDTA) for debridement and cleaning has limited capabilities. Conventional root canal therapy can only penetrate 100 microns into the dentinal tubules, whereas bacteria penetrates up to 1000 microns. Obviously there is much room for improvement in the realm of cleaning and bactericidal treatment of root canals. The use of lasers provides an effective treatment to eliminate bacteria in endodontic therapy, as laser energy at different wavelengths is capable of penetrating up to 1000 microns to eliminate bacteria.

The American Association of Endodontists (AAE) has recognized the benefits of laser application in endodontics: the bactericidal capability of lasers and laser energy's ability to aid in removing the smear layer and debris along the canal wall. In addition, the AAE recognizes that lasers may aid in sealing the root canal. However, the AAE has a few concerns about the use of the laser in endodontic therapy, citing the potential detrimental thermal effect on the root and periodontal tissues. The AAE also has concerns about how laser energy can be delivered efficiently in complicated curvatures of some root canal systems. Hopefully this chapter will provide more information on how the laser is used in endodontic therapy, in order to begin dispelling such concerns.

The Er,Cr:YSGG laser system uses laser energy to treat the root canal without generating heat, thus providing minimal thermal side effects to the root canal and periodontal tissues. The Er,Cr:YSGG laser system also utilizes laser fiber tips that are narrow and very flexible, such that they can negotiate curved canals and deliver laser energy in many complicated root canal systems. The uniqueness of the Er,Cr:YSGG laser system's hard and soft tissue applications enables laser energy to treat the pulpal tissue, as well as the dentinal wall. In addition to its capabilities in pulpotomy, pulpectomy, debridement, cleaning and disinfection, the Er,Cr:YSGG laser system can be used for the enlargement and shaping of the root canal. This makes the Er,Cr:YSGG laser endodontic system a viable alternative to other root canal systems.

The Er,Cr:YSGG laser system also provides the doctor with the ability to perform surgery with reduced mechanical trauma and decreased lateral tissue damage. In apicoectomy procedures in particular, Er,Cr:YSGG laser system applications provide the same advantages as in other laser surgery procedures. These benefits include good hemostasis, on-site bactericidal effects, decreased post-operative swelling, scarring, pain, and superior post-operative patient conditions.

To summarize, there are many advantages to using the Er,Cr:YSGG laser system in endodontics:

1. Laser energy does not cause microfractures in tooth structures during the access opening and cleaning of root canals.
2. Laser energy removes pulpal tissue efficiently and effectively.
3. Laser energy removes dentin from root canal walls (including diseased tissue) efficiently and effectively.
4. Laser energy provides on-site bactericidal treatment.
5. Laser energy removes smear layer and debris.
6. Laser energy penetrates deep in the dentinal walls in the accessory canals, and the tubule system to reduce bacteria pathogens, to provide better obturation and sealing of the root canal system.
7. Laser energy reduces the need for antibiotics.
8. Laser energy reduces post-operative pain, discomfort and swelling.
9. Laser energy reduces the need for intra-canal irrigation by irrigants such as NaOCl, and eliminates the 30-minute of effective treatment time that is usually required for bactericidal effects by these irrigants.
10. Laser energy reduces the need for post-operative treatment.
11. The advantages of other types of surgeries are shown in apicoectomy procedures. Principles of laser therapy in soft tissue, bone tissue and tooth tissue are applied in apicoectomy procedures, using a laser wavelength in a refined space. The laser uses energized water molecules in performing the functions without the concern of lateral damage. It shows the extraordinary advantages of using the Er,Cr:YSGG laser system in dentistry.

When assessing the following specific root canal therapy procedures, please consider the following diagrams:

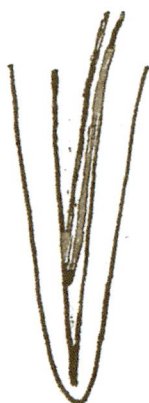

Fig. 1: The Endo fiber tip is placed in the root canal 1-2mm from the root end, aiming at the canal wall (cross-section view).

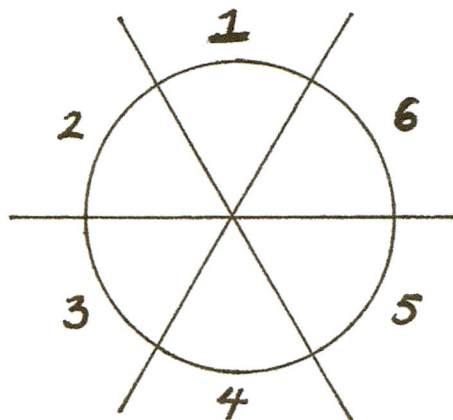

Fig. 2: The root canal is roughly divided into six segments (incisal view). Each sequence of laser firing will debride, clean and enlarge that segment of the root canal.

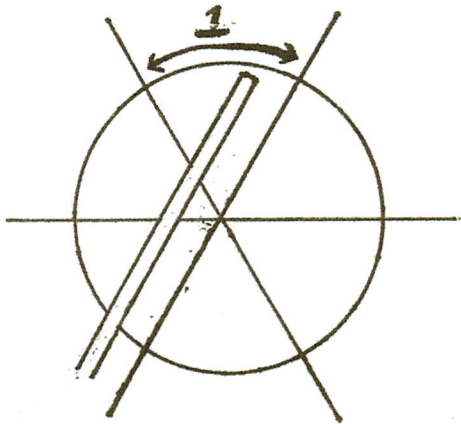

Fig. 3: Aim the tip at the first segment of the canal wall (incisal view).

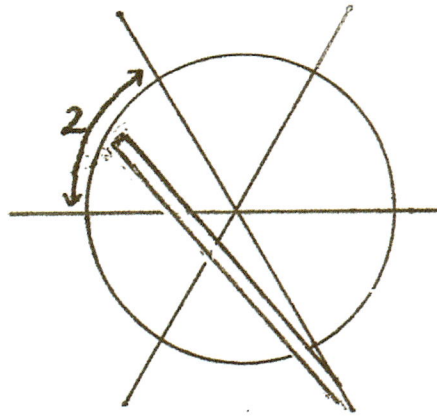

Fig. 4: Aim the tip at the second segment of the canal wall. Proceed for sections 3-6.

Anterior Teeth (Single Canal Root Canal Therapy)

Laser Parameters, Set 1: Access Opening in Enamel

Waterlase MD laser system settings: MG-6 tip, 3.50-4.50W, 60% Water, 80% Air, 15 Hz
Other Er,Cr:YSGG laser system settings: G-6 tip, 4.00-6.00W, 75% Water, 90% Air

Since the tooth is anesthetized, use a high-power enamel ablation setting to start the access opening. Prepare a sufficiently large access opening in the enamel above the pulp chamber.

Laser Parameters, Set 2: Dentin Ablation and Pulp Exposure

Waterlase MD laser system settings: 2.00-3.00W, 60% Water, 80% Air, 15 Hz
Other Er,Cr:YSGG laser system settings: 3.50W, 60% Water, 65% Air

Reduce the power once the dentin is reached. The fiber tip should be aimed towards the pulp. This should be estimated from a lateral and then incisal view to ensure the accuracy of position of the laser fiber tip to avoid over-ablation of tooth structure or perforation of the side of the pulp chamber.

The tip should slowly descend into the crown until it drops into the pulp chamber. Carefully inspect the site to ensure that the pulp is fully exposed. (Note: A high-speed bur can be used to refine the access opening into the pulp. This is done with a careful light shaving motion of the bur.)

Laser Parameters, Set 3: Pulpotomy

Waterlase MD laser system settings: MG-6 tip, 2.75W, 11% Water, 11% Air, 30 Hz, H mode
Other Er,Cr:YSGG laser system settings: G-6 tip, 2.50W, 7% Water, 11% Air

Reduce the power and use the laser to carefully expose the pulp and perform a pulpotomy.

A #10 or #15 K-file is then used to establish the working length of the canal. This is confirmed by either a periapical x-ray or an apex locator. The procedure is followed by the nickel-titanium crown-down rotary instrumentation to enlarge the canal space to about 250μm (about the same size as a #25 K file). One technique involves using Gates Glidden #1, #2, #3 into 1/5 to 1/4 the distance of the canal, followed by a series of nickel-titanium crown-down files of 0.1 taper, 0.08 taper, 0.06 taper, cleaning to about half the distance up to the canal, then continue the preparation with a series of 0.04 rotary files to the working length.

Laser Parameters, Set 4: Canal Wall Ablation

Waterlase MD laser system settings: MZ-2 tip, 1.25W, 24% Water, 34% Air, 20 Hz
Other Er,Cr:YSGG laser system settings: Z-2 tip, 1.25W, 24% Water, 34% Air

The laser procedure will follow the crown down preparation. A 25mm length Z-2 tip is placed in the canal to the root end, and then retrieved 2-3mm. The tip is angled to aim at the dentinal wall. Start laser ablation and continue to aim the tip at the canal wall. With a slow motion, from side-to-side and with a very slow up-and-down motion, the tip is moved in a coronal direction. The goal is to clean one portion of the canal wall at a time.

Continue the slow side-to-side and slight up-and-down motions in a disciplined and controlled ablation of calculus and plaque on the dentinal wall from the apical to coronal regions. Each sequence of laser firing should be approximately 15-30 seconds and should cover approximately 1/6 of the area of the canal wall (see previous diagram).

A total of six sequences of laser firing should cover the canal wall for laser debridement, cleaning and enlargement of the canal space.

Laser Parameters, Set 5: Continue Canal Wall Ablation

Waterlase MD laser system settings: MZ-3 tip, 1.25W, 24% Water, 34% Air, 20 Hz
Other Er,Cr:YSGG laser system settings: Z-3 tip, 1.25W, 24% Water, 34% Air

Replace tip with a Z-3/MZ-3 tip and continue the laser treatment using the same settings and approach. (Note: The Z-3 tip is less flexible than the Z-2.) Again, a total of six sequences of laser firing follow along the canal wall.

Laser Parameters, Set 6: Continue Canal Wall Ablation

Waterlase MD laser system settings: MZ-4 tip, 1.25W, 24% Water, 34% Air, 20 Hz
Other Er,Cr:YSGG laser system settings: Z-4 tip, 1.25W, 24% Water, 34% Air

Replace tip with a Z-4/MZ-4 tip to finish the laser preparation. Again, follow the same technique and use the same number of sequences.

After laser instrumentation, the canal space should be able to accommodate a #35 K-file down to the working length. The shape of the canal space should be similar to the conventionally prepared funnel-shape. Any obturation system can be used to complete the root canal therapy.

(Note: In-between the Z-2, Z-3 and Z-4 laser firing sequences, a K-file should be used to check the patency of the canal. If there is ledging, #20 and #25 K-files are used to recapitulate the canal.) Make sure finish the root canal preparations with laser debridement and proper cleaning.

Case 1: Anterior Tooth Endo, MD Regular HP, with MG-6, and End-Firing Endo Tips

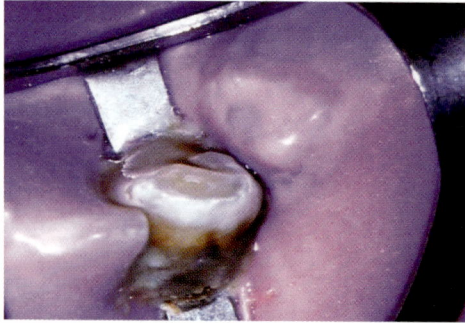

Fig.1: Pre-op photo

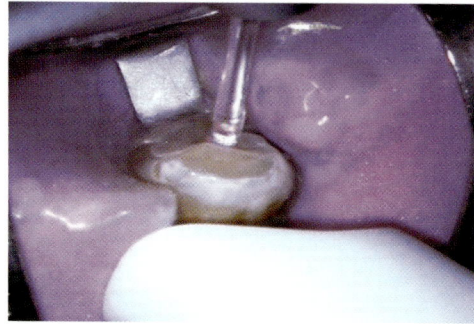

Fig. 2: A MG-6 tip is used for access opening. The setting is 4.50W, 60% Water, 80% Air, 15 Hz.

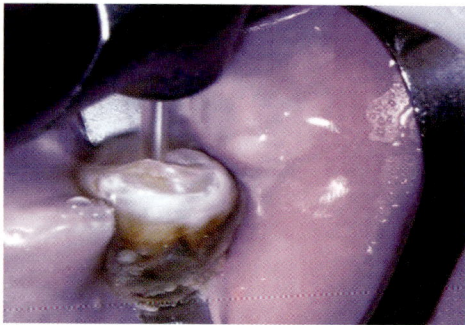

Fig. 3: As the ablation progresses into the dentin, the tip is focused closer to the pulp. The setting is reduced to 3.00W, 60% Water 80% Air, 15 Hz.

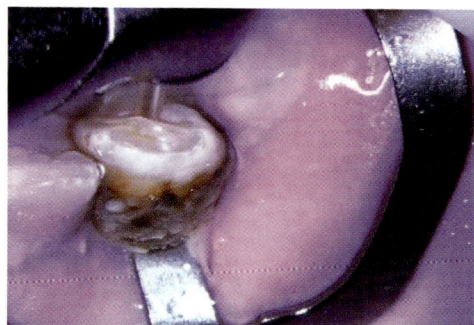

Fig. 4: The tip is in the pulp performing pulpotomy. The setting is 2.00W, 7% Water 11% Air, 30 Hz.

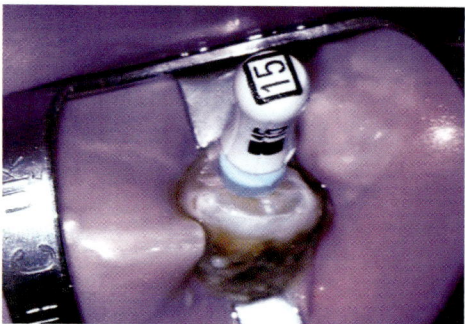

Fig. 5: Working length is measured by inserting a #15 K-file to root end.

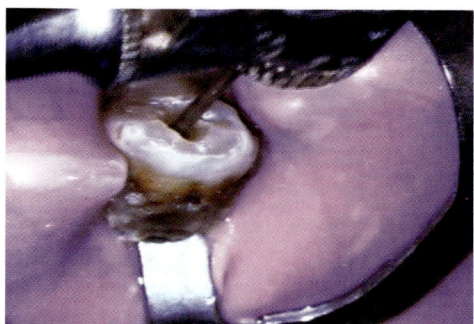

Fig. 6: The canal opening is enlarged by a short series of Gates-Glidden.

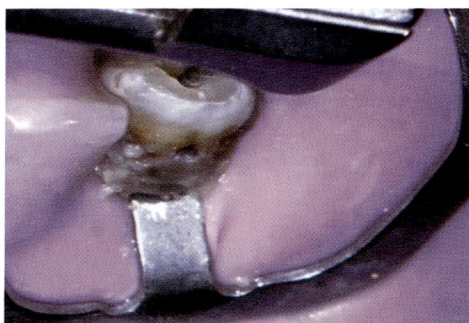

Fig. 7: The root canal is enlarged by a short series of nickel-titanium rotary files to 250 µm.

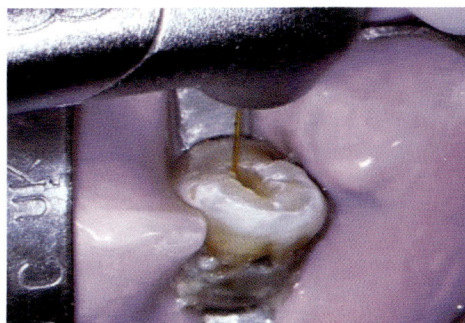

Fig.8: A MZ-2 tip placed at 2mm short of apex aimed at one side of the canal wall. Laser energy is applied to the wall as the tip retrieves from the canal. The setting is 1.25W, 24% Water, 34% Air, 30 Hz.

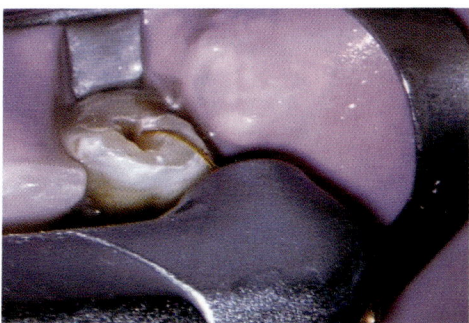

Fig. 9: The MZ-2 tip is cleaning another segment of the root canal wall.

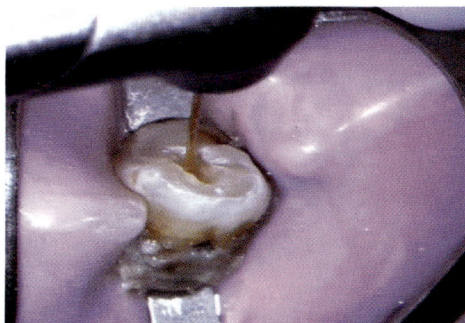

Fig. 10: A MZ-3 tip is used to clean, debride and enlarge the root canal using same setting and similar technique as with the MZ-2.

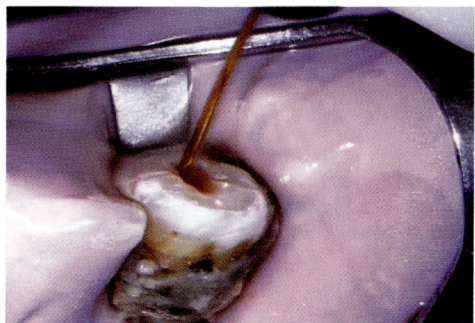

Fig.11: A MZ-4 tip is used to finish the root canal preparation.

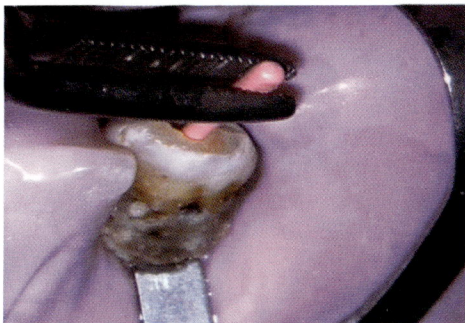

Fig.12: A gutta-percha master cone is fitted to the working length.

Case 2: Anterior Tooth Endo, M2 and End-Firing Endo Tips

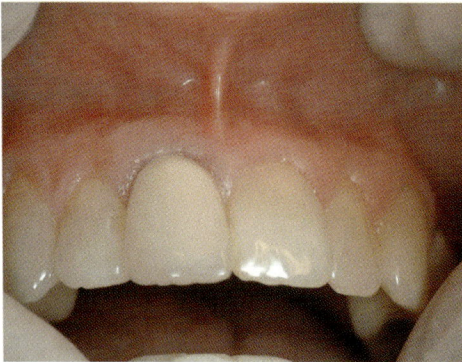

Fig. 1: Pre-op. #9 is diagnosed to have a reversible pulpitis and requires a root canal therapy.

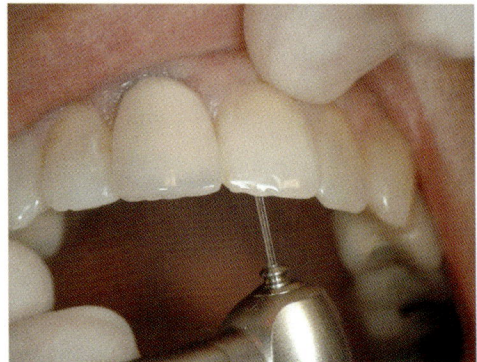

Fig. 2: Access opening is performed without a rubber dam so that laser energy can be applied more accurately to access opening and to avoid perforation. A G-6 (9mm) tip is used with a setting of 5.50W, 25% Water, 90% Air.

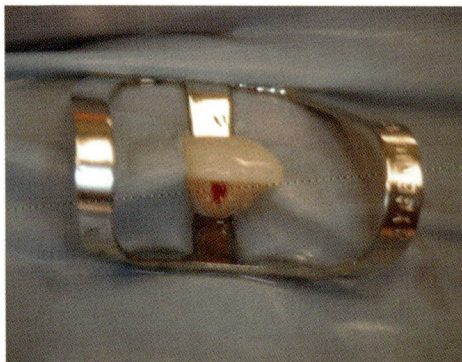

Fig. 3: Lingual view to show that pulp has been exposed.

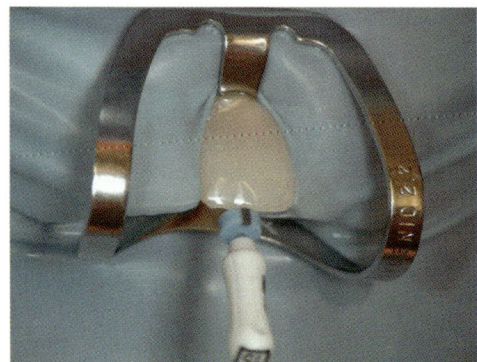

Fig. 4: Working length is measured by a #15 K-file. This is followed by enlargement of the root canal by a K-file of up to 250μm diameter.

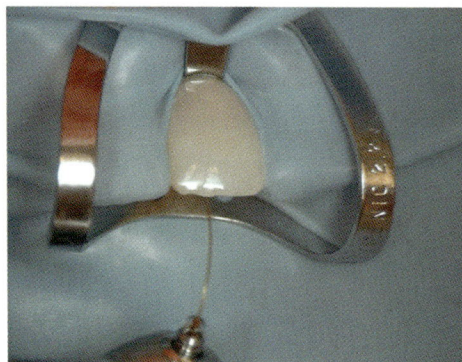

Fig. 5: A Z-2 (25mm) tip is placed at 1mm short of apex. The tip end is placed to aim at the side of the canal. Laser energy is applied as the fiber tip is retrieved from the root end position in a sweeping motion that cleans a segment of the canal wall. The setting is 1.25W, 24% Water, 34% Air. Six sequences of

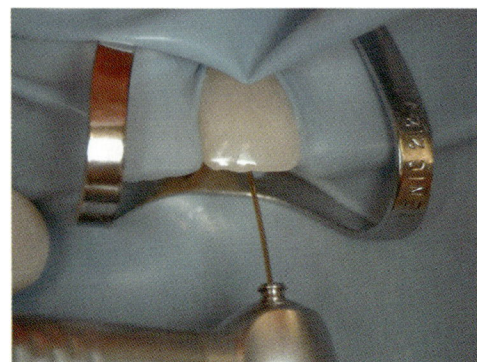

Fig. 6: A Z-3 (25mm) tip is used with a similar technique and setting as with the Z-2 tip. Again, six sequences of treatment are used to further debride, clean and enlarge the canal.

treatment follow using the Z-2 tip.

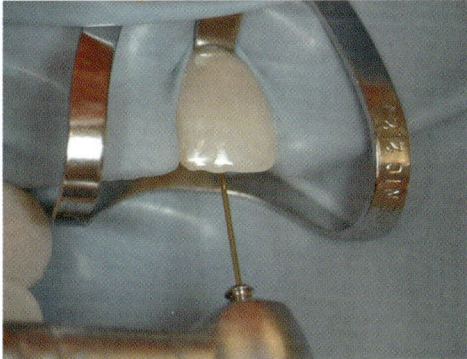

Fig. 7: A Z-4 (25mm) tip is used with a similar technique and setting as with the Z-2 tip. Again, six sequences of treatment are used to finish debriding, cleaning and enlarging the canal.

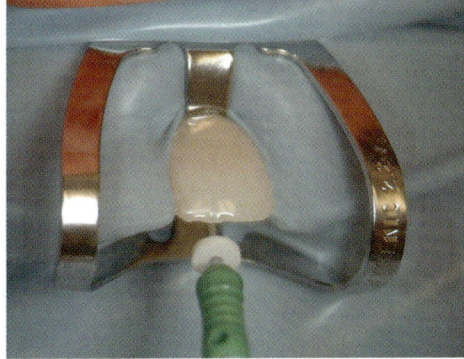

Fig. 8: A #35 K-file is used to check patency and to check that a funnel-shaped canal is being prepared.

Case 3: Anterior Tooth Endo, M2 and End-Firing Endo Tips

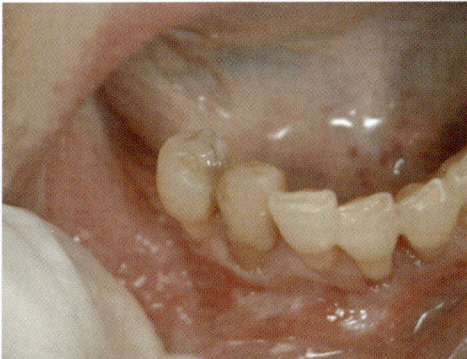

Fig. 1: Pre-op. #27 is diagnosed to have an irreversible pulpitis, root canal therapy is indicated.

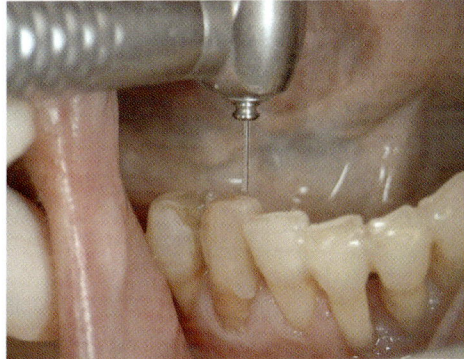

Fig. 2: Access opening is performed without the rubber dam to give a more accurate assessment of the canal and to avoid perforation. A G-6 tip is used. The setting is 4.00W, 60% Water, 60% Air.

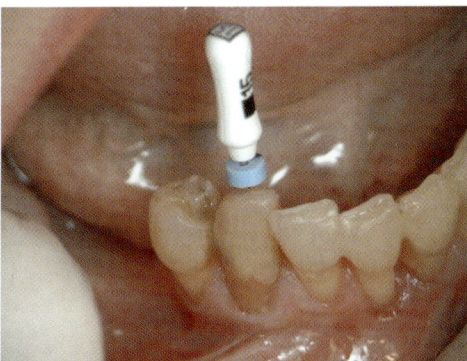

Fig. 3: Working length is measured with a #15 K-file.

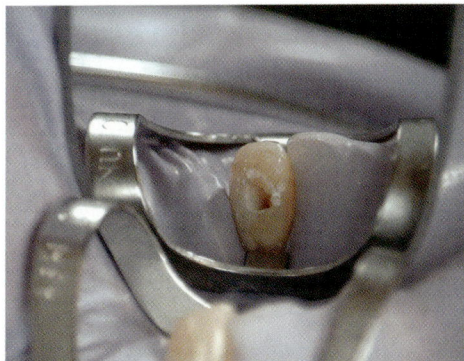

Fig. 4: Lingual view of #27 with rubber dam and clamp in place.

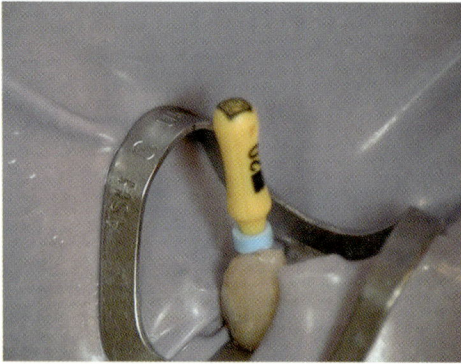

Fig. 5: The root canal is enlarged further by a #20 K-file.

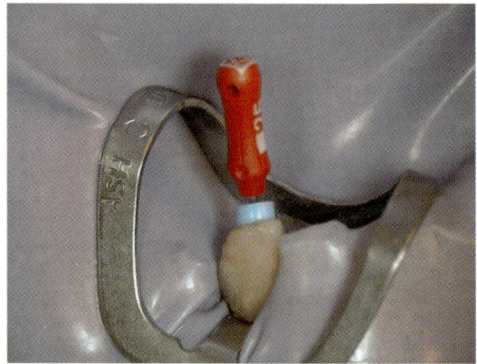

Fig. 6: The root canal is enlarged to a 250μm diameter by a #25 K-file.

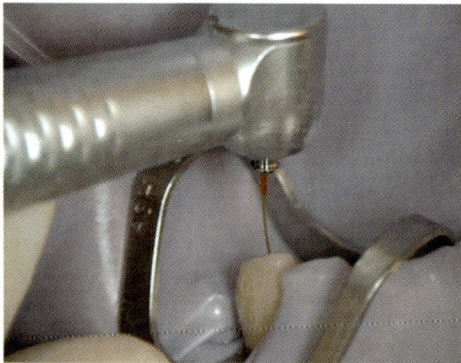

Fig. 7: A Z-2 (25mm) tip is placed at 1mm short of root end, aiming at the canal wall. Laser energy is applied as the tip slowly retrieves from the canal, cleaning one segment of the canal wall at a time. Six sequences of treatment are used to debride, clean and enlarge the root canal. The setting is 1.25W, 24% Water, 34% Air.

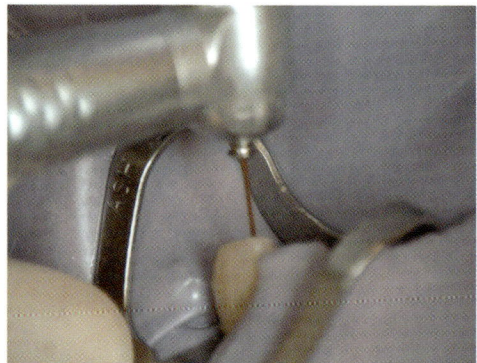

Fig. 8: A Z-3 (25mm) tip is used with similar technique and setting as with the Z-2 tip. Additional debridement, cleaning and enlargement occurs.

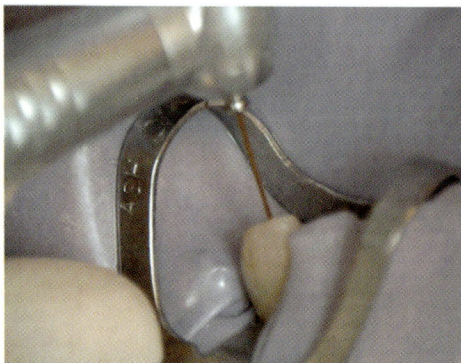

Fig. 9: A Z-4 (25mm) tip is used to complete debridement, cleaning and enlargement of the root canal.

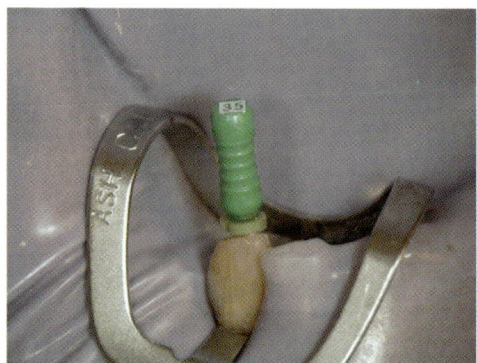

Fig. 10: A #35 K-file can fit to working length showing a funnel shaped finished root canal preparation.

Bicuspid Teeth
(Single or Two-Canal Root Canal Therapy)

The procedure for accessing bicuspid teeth is in all respects the same as for single rooted anterior teeth, except that in accessing the dentin, care should be taken to avoid access openings leading into the interproximal surfaces of the tooth. Use a round bur to refine the preparation of the access opening into the buccal and lingual canals, as necessary.

Treatment of a bicuspid with a single, relatively straight canal is identical to that described above for single-rooted anterior teeth. For teeth with more than one canal or with curved canals, the canal space should be prepared with the crown-down technique in its entirety.

Follow the conventional treatment by performing treatment as described for single-rooted teeth.

Case 1: Bicuspid Endo, MD Regular HP with End-Firing Endo Tips

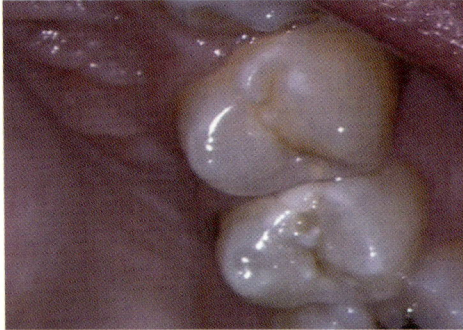

Fig.1: Pre-op, a maxillary left second premolar requires root canal therapy due to an irreversible pulpitis.

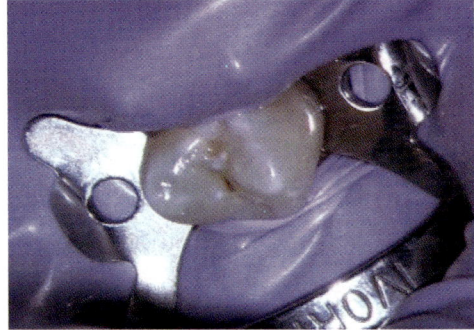

Fig. 2: After giving a local anesthetic, a rubber dam clamp and rubber dam are placed on the site.

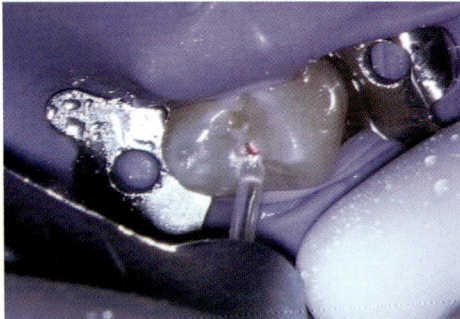

Fig. 3: A MG-6 tip is used to access opening into the root canal. The setting is 4.50W, 60% Water, 80% Air, 15 Hz.

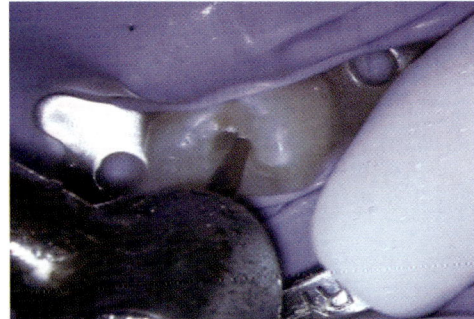

Fig. 4: The opening of the canal is assisted by using a high-speed round bur.

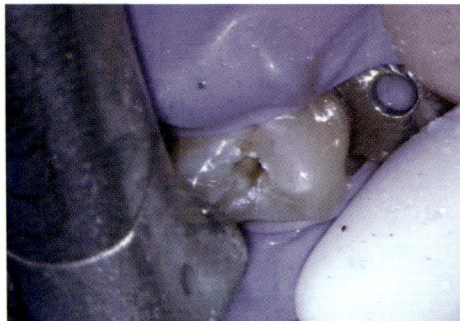

Fig. 5: A pulpotomy is performed. The setting is 2.00W, 7% Water, 11% Air, 30 Hz.

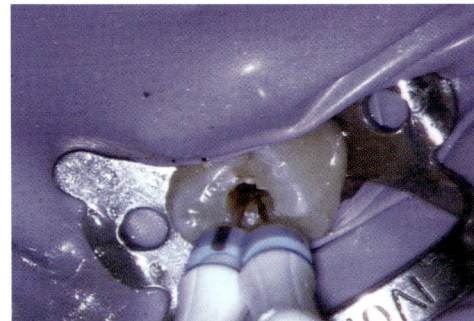

Fig. 6: Two #15 K-files are in place to measure the working lengths of both the buccal and lingual canals.

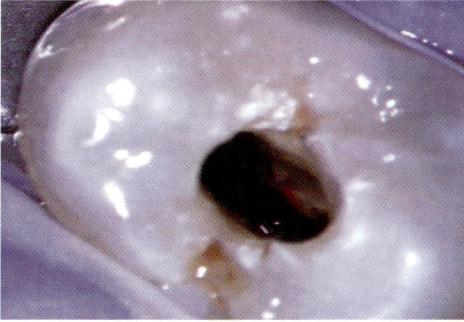

Fig. 7: A close-up look at the pulp chamber.

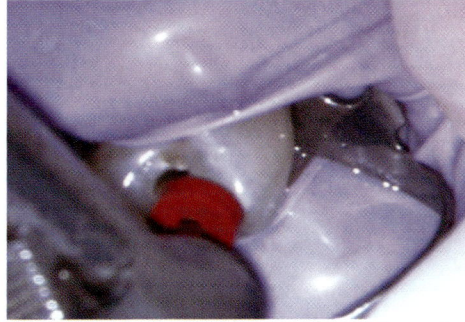

Fig. 8: The root canals are enlarged by a short series of Gates-Glidden and nickel-titanium crown-down instrumentation to 250μm.

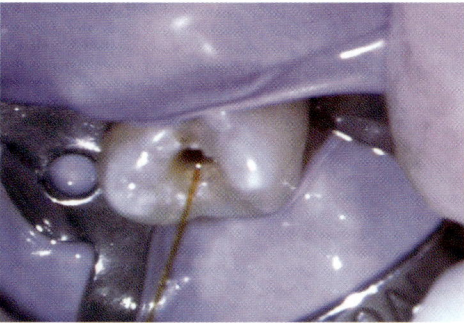

Fig. 9: A MZ-2 tip is used to clean, debride and enlarge both canals. The setting is 1.25W, 24% Water, 34% Air, 30 Hz.

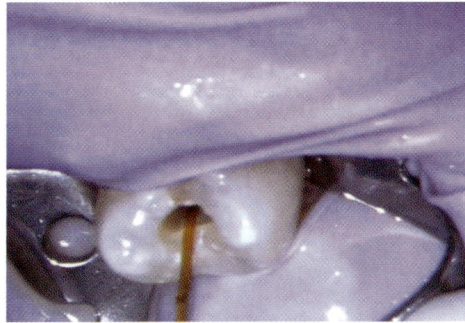

Fig. 10: A MZ-3 tip is used to continue cleaning, debridement and enlargement of the canals.

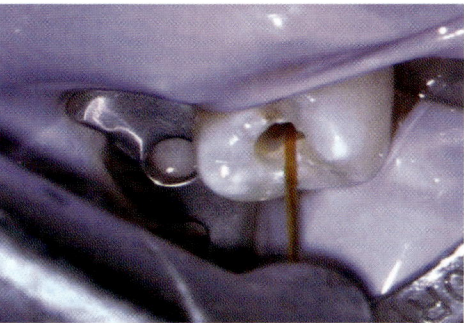

Fig. 11: A MZ-4 tip is used to complete the preparation.

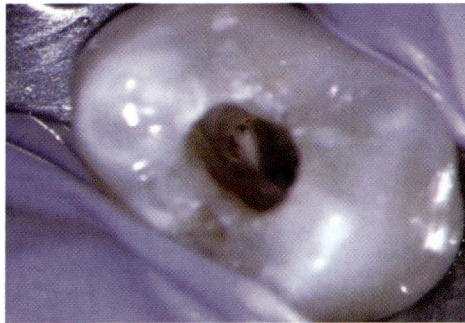

Fig. 12: A close-up look of the pulp chamber after completion of the root canal therapy.

Molars (3$^+$ Roots)

In the treatment of molars with more than three roots, several procedures are performed in similar fashion to the procedures described in earlier chapters: access opening, root canal path finding, working length measurements and enlargement of canals.

In laser preparation, only MZ-2 and MZ-3 tips are used, and power settings should not exceed 1.00W in curved root canals.

For the lingual canal of maxillary first molars and the distal canal of mandibular first molars, the MZ-2 tip can be placed at 2mm from the root end. After the canal has been cleaned and enlarged, the MZ-3 tip can be used about 2mm from the root end. For the remaining canals of both the maxillary and mandibular molars, the MZ-2 tip should initially start 3mm from the root end, and the MZ-3 should start up to 4mm from the root end. Laser treatment of molars requires a more time-consuming process because of the complexity and curvature of the canals. Each tip only has four sequences of usage within the root canals rather than six as described above. This helps to reduce the risk of melting dentin and losing the patency of the canals.

Case 1: Molar Endo, MD Regular HP with End-Firing Endo Tips

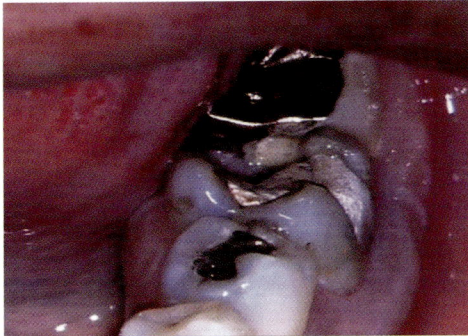

Fig. 1: Pre-op. Mandibular left first molar needs RCT due to an irreversible pulpitis from deep caries.

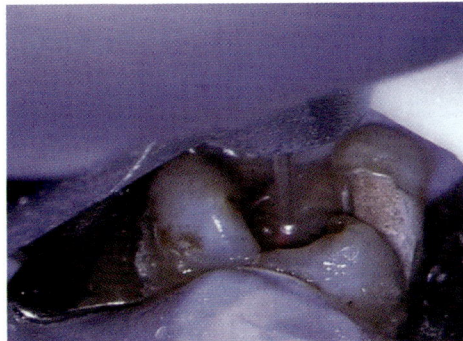

Fig. 2: After local anesthetic is administered, a rubber dam clamp and rubber dam are placed. The old amalgam is removed by a high-speed bur, followed by using a MG-6 for further access opening. The setting is 4.50W, 60% Water, 80% Air, 15 Hz.

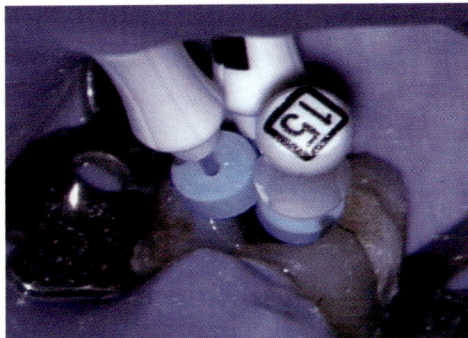

Fig. 3: Working lengths of the canals are measured by using #15 K-files.

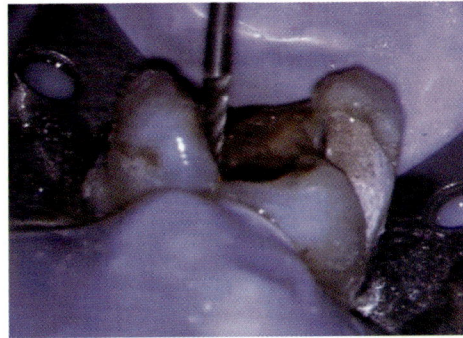

Fig. 4: The canals are enlarged to 200-250μm by using Gates-Glidden and nickel-titanium crown-down instrumentation.

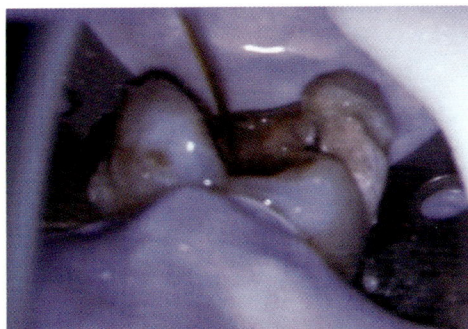

Fig. 5: A MZ-2 tip is used to clean and debride the canals. The setting is 1.00W, 24% Water, 34% Air, 30 Hz.

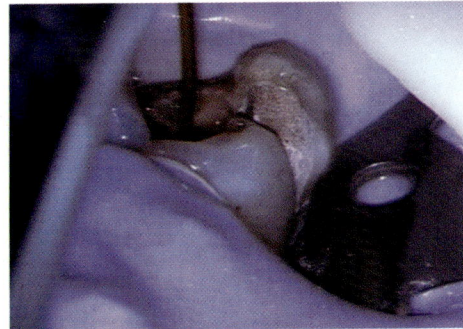

Fig. 6: A MZ-3 tip is used to complete cleaning and debridement in the canals. The setting is 1.00W, 24% Water, 34% Air, 30 Hz.

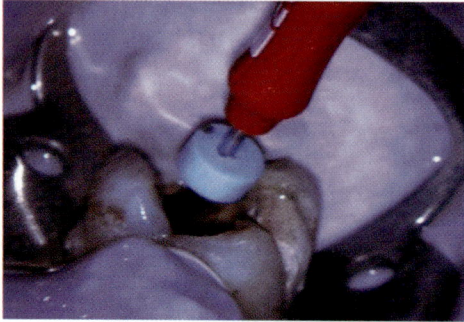

Fig. 7: Patency is checked with a #25 K-file.

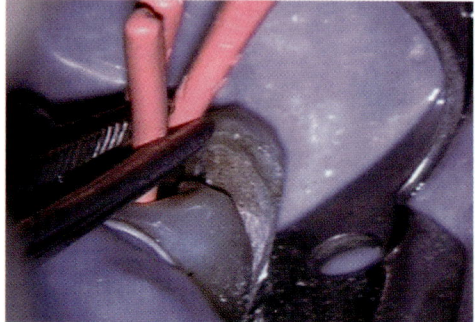

Fig. 8: Gutta percha master cones are placed.

Case 2: Molar Endo, M2 with End-Firing Endo Tips

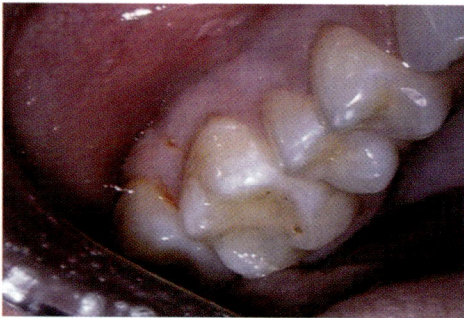

Fig. 1: Pre-op. The maxillary right first molar is treatment planned for root canal therapy because the diagnosis is an irreversible pulpitis.

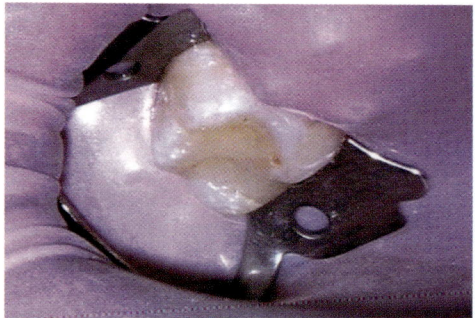

Fig. 2: After local anesthesia is administered, a rubber dam clamp and rubber dam are placed.

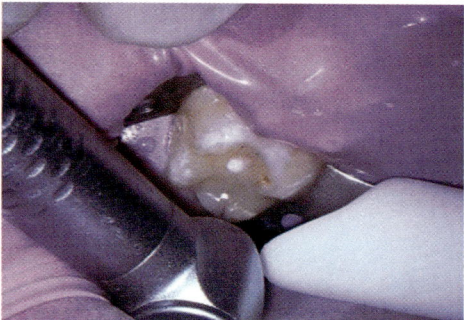

Fig. 3: A G-6 (9mm) tip is used for access opening. The setting is 5.50W, 75% Water, 90% Air.

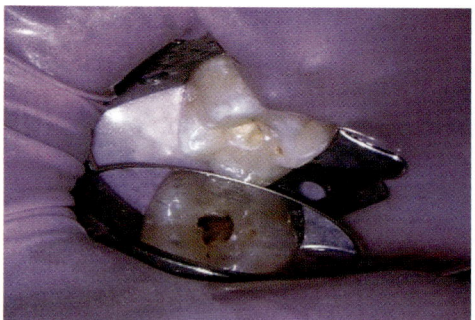

Fig. 4: An initial access opening has been prepared by the laser.

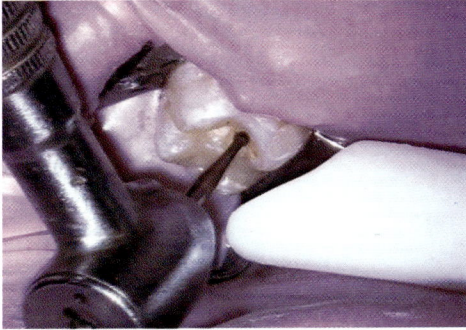

Fig. 5: A high speed round bur is used to finish the access opening in the pulp chamber and the root canal openings.

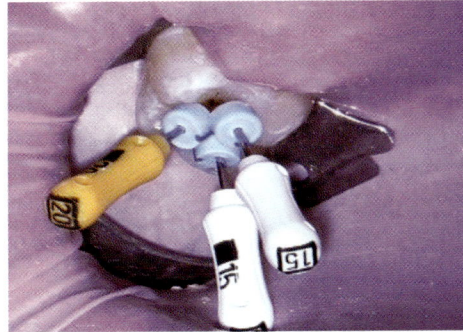

Fig. 6: K-files are in place to measure the working length of the three root canals.

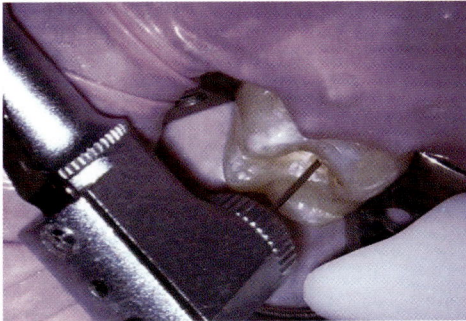

Fig. 7: Gates-Glidden is used to enlarge the root canal openings.

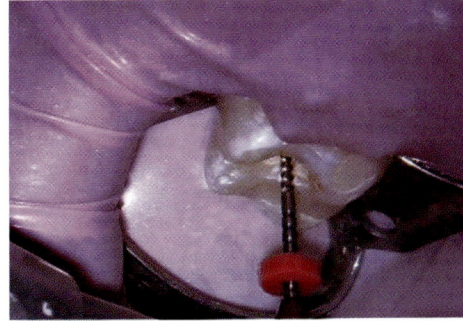

Fig. 8: A short series of crown-down nickel-titanium rotary files is used to enlarge the root canals to working length.

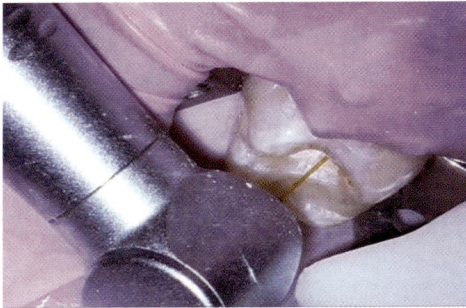

Fig. 9: A Z-2 tip is placed 2 mm from the root end of the palatal root. Laser energy is applied to a segment of the canal wall as the tip retrieves from the root end. The setting is 1.00W, 24% Water, 34% Air.

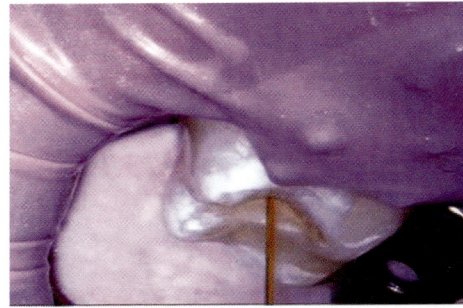

Fig. 10: A Z-3 tip is used to continue to clean, debride and enlarge the root canal. The setting is 1.00W, 24% Water, 34% Air.

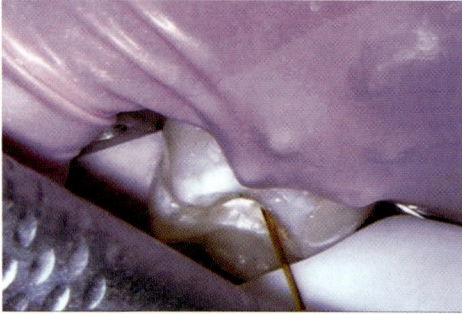

Fig. 11: A Z-4 tip is used to finish cleaning, debridement and enlargement of the root The setting is 1.00W, 24% Water, 34% Air.

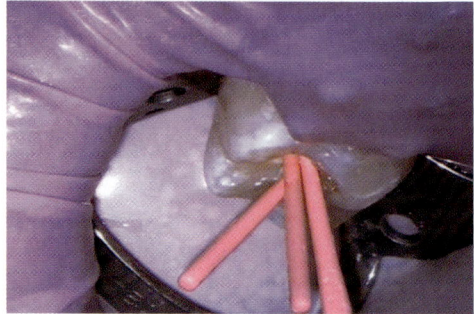

Fig. 12: Master cone gutta percha points are tried in the root canals.

Er,Cr:YSGG Laser System Root Canal Therapy
(Without Local Anesthesia)

Only selective cases of root canal therapy can be successfully performed without local anesthesia. It may be preferred to perform Er,Cr:YSGG laser system root canal therapy without local anesthesia with certain types of patients:

1. Medically compromised patients for whom local anesthesia creates a risk;
2. Patients who are severely needle phobic;
3. Patients who have a partially or totally necrosed pulp; and
4. Patients whose root canal pulp is large enough to allow Z-2 as a path finding instrument (typically, anterior teeth and some bicuspids).

Laser Parameters, Set 1: Pre-Conditioning

Waterlase MD laser system: MG-6 tip, 2.00W, 60% Water, 80% Air, 30 Hz, 120 seconds
Waterlase MD laser system alternate technique #1: MC-12 tip, 0.50W, 0% Water, 0% Air, 50 Hz, 120 seconds
Waterlase MD laser system alternate technique #2: MG-6 or MZ-6 tip, 0.25W, 0% Water, 0% Air, 50 Hz, 120 seconds
Other Er,Cr:YSGG laser system settings: G-6 tip, 1.25W, 15% Water, 15% Air

Keeping the fiber tip in focused mode at all times (1.5-2mm), direct the fiber tip perpendicular towards the fissure, down the long axis of the tooth. When ablating, the motion used is semi-circular and back-and-forth, but primarily aiming at the area where the lesion is located. Move slowly along the length of the lesion. Fire the laser at starting settings for 120 seconds.

Waterlase MD alternate technique: The MC-12 tip is placed focused 1-2mm from the cervical area of the tooth. The tip is moved slowly aiming at the cervical third of the tooth in the shape of the pulp. Time spent for the laser analgesia is 120 seconds.

Laser Parameters, Set 2: Enamel Ablation

Waterlase MD laser system settings: 3.50-4.50W, 60% Water, 80% Air, 15 Hz
Other Er,Cr:YSGG laser system settings: 4.00W, 60% Water, 65% Air

Ablation of the enamel should take place at this power setting. In my experience, more than 80% of bicuspid and deciduous molar enamel ablation can take place using 4.00W.

For most anterior teeth and bicuspids, 4.00W is enough for ablation of enamel. If necessary, after 30 seconds, increase power by 0.50W.

Laser Parameters, Set 3: Dentin Ablation

Waterlase MD laser system settings: 3.00W, 60% Water, 80% Air, 15 Hz
Other Er,Cr:YSGG laser system settings: 2.00-2.50W, 60% Water, 65% Air

Once the dentin is reached, the power is reduced to the above settings to continue with ablation. Use the next settings when the depth of the access opening gets close to the pulp.

Laser Parameters, Set 4: Pulp Exposure

Waterlase MD laser system settings: 3.00W, 60% Water, 80% Air, 30 Hz
Other Er,Cr:YSGG laser system settings: 2.00W, 60% Water, 65% Air

When exposing the pulp, the settings used should never be higher than those listed above, or there will be a high chance of causing discomfort to the patient. The lower power settings allow for better control in creating the depth of the opening and exposing the pulp.

Laser Parameters, Set 5: Laser Analgesia Applied Directly to Nerve

Waterlase MD laser system settings: MZ-2 tip, 0.25-0.75W, 15% Water, 15% Air, 30 Hz
Other Er,Cr:YSGG laser system settings: Z-2 tip, 0.25-0.75W, 15% Water, 15% Air

Change the tip and laser settings for direct nerve laser anesthesia. Using a slow up-and-down pumping motion, the tip is slowly immersed into the root canal for 60-120 seconds. The immersion continues in the canal until the fiber reaches about one-half to two-thirds of the way into the canal.

A #10 or #15 K file is used at this point to measure the working length. (Note: If the Z-2 directed nerve anesthesia is performed well, the patient will not feel discomfort when the K-file is placed in the canal).

At this point, the same technique as used for single-rooted anterior teeth should be used. On completing the preparation, any obturation system can be used to finish the root canal therapy.

Laser Parameters, Set 6: Pulpotomy

Waterlase MD laser system settings: 2.00-2.25W, 7% Water, 11% Air, 30 Hz
Other Er,Cr:YSGG laser system settings: 1.25W, 7% Water, 11% Air

Once in the pulp chamber, change settings and perform the pulpotomy. After a partial pulpotomy is successfully completed without causing pain, a #2 round bur is used to enlarge the access opening and prepare the pulp chamber. Use the laser to treat the remainder of the pulp to complete the pulpotomy.

Case 1: Laser Endo with No Injection Anesthesia, MD Regular HP with End-Firing Endo Tips

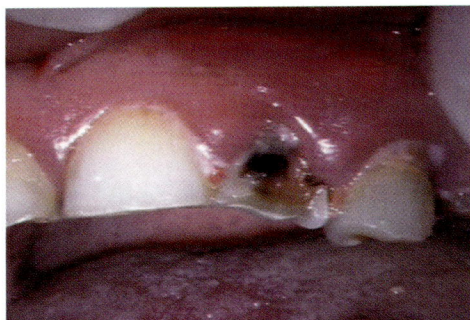

Fig. 1: Pre-op. The maxillary left lateral incisor is treatment planned for root canal therapy, post and core build-up and a PFM crown.

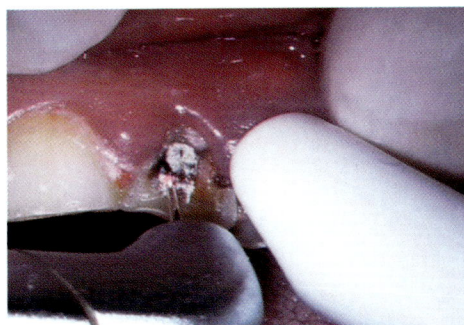

Fig. 2: A MG-6 tip is used to aim at the pulp with a low level laser power to pre-condition the pulp. The setting is 0.25W, 0% Water, 0% Air, 50 Hz.

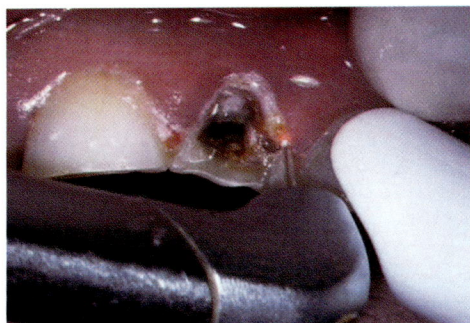

Fig. 3: Laser energy is used to pre-condition the gingiva and the CEJ at the labial surface.

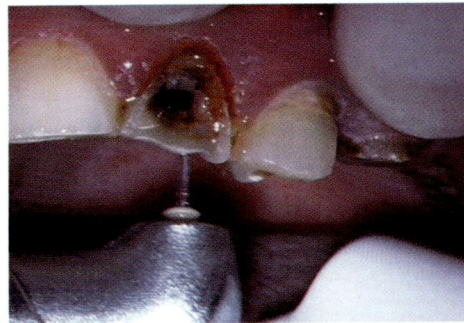

Fig. 4: Laser energy is used to pre-condition the gingiva and the CEJ at the lingual surface.

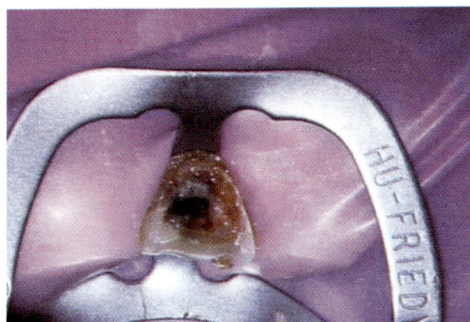

Fig. 5: A rubber dam clamp and rubber dam are placed at the lateral incisor.

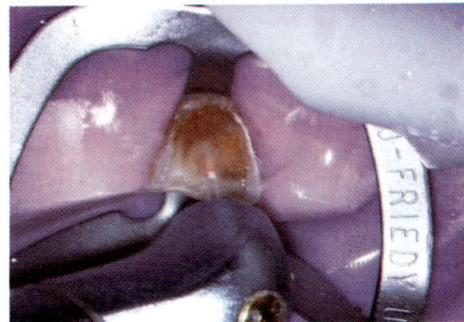

Fig. 6: The MG-6 tip is aimed at the pulp to access open the root canal. The setting is 3.00W, 60% Water, 80% Air, 15 Hz.

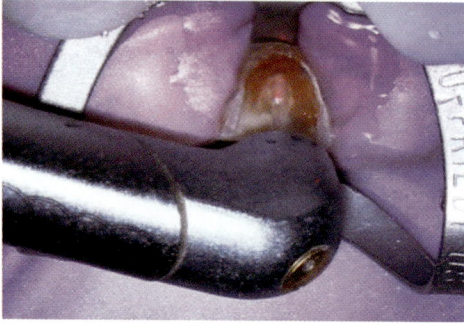

Fig. 7: The setting is changed to 3.00W, 60% Water, 80% Air, 30 Hz to expose the pulp.

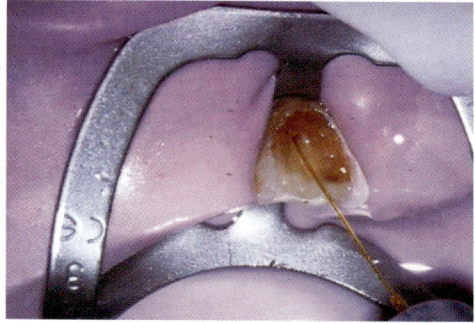

Fig. 8: After pulpotomy is performed with a MG-6 tip at 2.00W, 7% Water, 11% Air, 30 Hz, a MZ-2 tip is used to apply lower level laser in the root canal. The setting is 0.25W, 20% Water, 20% Air, 30 Hz.

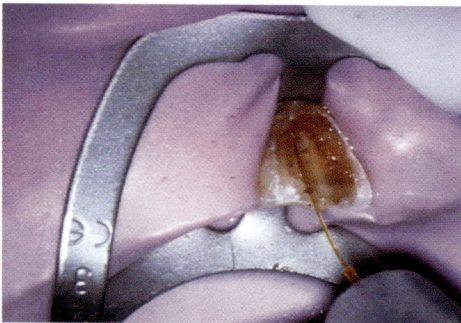

Fig. 9: About ½ to 1/3 of the root canal is reached with the MZ-2.

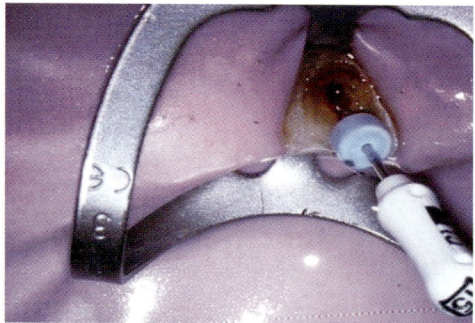

Fig. 10: A #15 K-file is used to measure the working length.

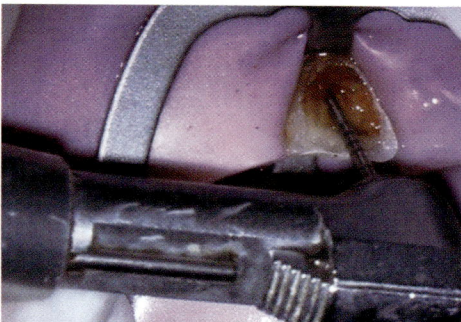

Fig. 11: Gates-Glidden drills are used to enlarge the root canal opening.

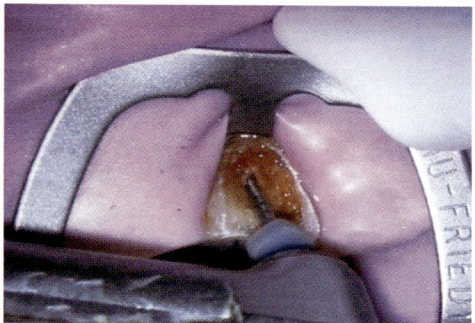

Fig. 12: A short series of crown-down nickel-titanium rotary files is used to enlarge the root canal to a 250μm diameter.

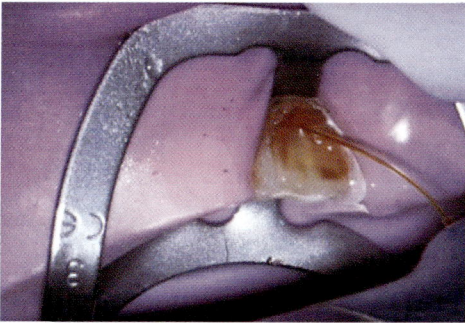

Fig. 13: The MZ-2 tip is used to clean, debride and enlarge the root canal. The setting is 1.25W, 24% Water, 34% Air, 30 Hz.

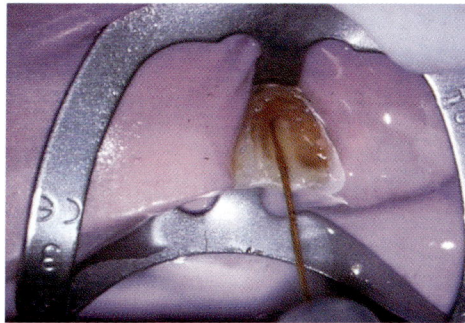

Fig. 14: A MZ-3 tip is used to continue cleaning, debridement and enlargement of the root canal.

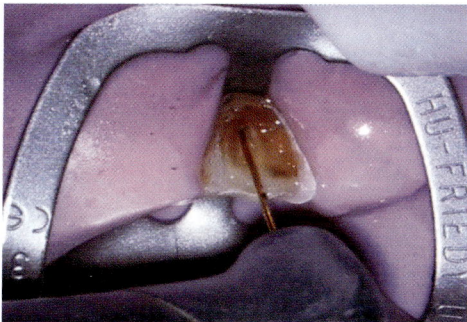

Fig. 15: A MZ-4 tips is used to finish cleaning, debridement and enlargement of the root canal.

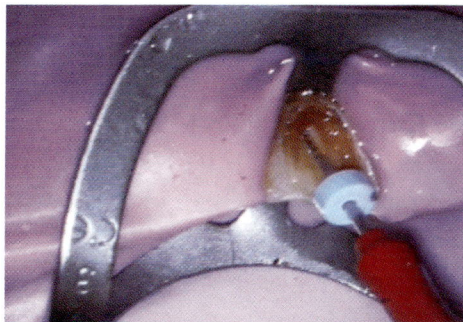

Fig. 16: A #25 K-file is used to check the patency of the canal.

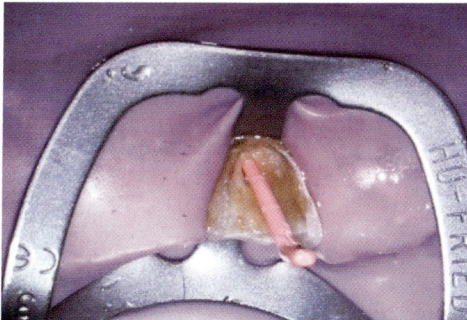

Fig. 17: A master cone gutta percha point is placed.

Er,Cr:YSGG Laser System Apicoectomy

Administer anesthesia carefully with the bevel of the needle facing the alveolar bone. Make sure the injection is given next to the bone and not in the mucogingival tissue. This will reduce bleeding during the surgery.

Laser Parameters, Set 1: Incision and Flap

Waterlase MD laser system settings: MT-4 tip, 1.75-2.50W, 7% Water, 11% Air, 30 Hz
Other Er,Cr:YSGG laser system settings: T-4 tip, 1.00-1.50W, 7% Water, 11% Air

> For flap design in apicoectomy, use your preferred technique. I prefer using a semilunar flap incision 4-5mm from the apex and in the mucogingival area. Other flap designs include a trapezoid or a rectangle. The apex of the tooth can be approximated from the working length by using a ruler. If there is a very large periapical lesion that may have extensive bone loss up to the middle of the root, a full thickness flap is preferred.

Laser Parameters, Set 2: Osteotomy

Waterlase MD laser system settings: MG-6 tip, 2.50-4.50W, 60% Water, 80% Air, 20 Hz
Other Er,Cr:YSGG laser system settings: G-6 tip, 2.50-4.50W, 30% Water, 30% Air

> Aim at the approximate position of the root end and remove bone carefully to expose the root end. In some cases a bony defect already exists, and lower power should be used to retrieve the root end.

Laser Parameters, Set 3: Remove Granulation Tissue

Waterlase MD laser system settings: 1.50-2.50W, 7% Water, 11% Air, 30 Hz
Other Er,Cr:YSGG laser system settings: 1.25-2.00W, 7% Water, 11% Air

> After the outline of the root end is exposed, change the settings as outlined above to remove some granulation tissue around this area. This will enable you to evaluate the anatomy of the root end.

Laser Parameters, Set 4: Remove Root End

Waterlase MD laser system settings: 2.00-3.00W, 60% Water, 80% Air, 30 Hz
Other Er,Cr:YSGG laser system settings: 1.75-2.75W, 30% Water, 30% Air

> Amputate 3mm off of the root end by making a cut perpendicular to the long axis of the tooth. This is done with a 15-25 degree angle to better expose the root canal sealant material. For a smaller diameter root end, use a MT tip to clean the root end cavity. Use power settings of 1.00-1.50W, 60% Water, 80% Air, 30 Hz. Remove the root end from the treatment site.

Laser Parameters, Set 5: Removal of Remaining Granulation Tissue and Gutta Percha

Waterlase MD laser system settings: 1.50-2.50W, 7% Water, 11% Air, 30 Hz
Other Er,Cr:YSGG laser system settings: 1.25-2.00W, 7% Water, 11% Air

Complete the process of removing granulation tissue from the root end lesion. Any tenacious granulation tissue can be removed with periodontal surgical curettes, especially in the lingual area of the root. Use an endodontic surgical Cavitron to remove 2-3mm of gutta percha from the root end.

Laser Parameters, Set 6: Debride and Clean the Root End

Waterlase MD laser system settings: 2.00-2.25W, 60% Water, 80% Air, 30 Hz
Other Er,Cr:YSGG laser system settings: 1.50-2.00W, 30% Water, 30% Air

Lower laser energy is used to clean and debride the cavity at the root end and the exterior surface of the root end. This is followed by placement of MTA (mineral trioxide aggregate) as a retrograde filling material. The surgical site must be kept clean and dry to allow MTA to set, and it should feel hard to the touch before closing the flap and placing sutures to finish.

Laser Parameters, Set 7: Hemostasis

Waterlase MD laser system settings: MG-6 tip 1.25W, 0% Water, 11% Air, 30 Hz or
MC-12 tip, 1.50 W, 0% Water, 11% Air, 30 Hz
Other Er,Cr:YSGG laser system settings: G-6 tip, 1.00 W, 0% Water, 11% Air

The tip is defocused from 3-5mm from the surgical site. Low-level laser energy is used to blanket the surgical site for the purpose of hemostasis, bactericidal effects, and any anti-inflammatory action, to promote faster healing and faster regeneration.

Case 1: Apicoectomy, Maxillary Central Incisor, MD Regular HP with MG-6 Tip

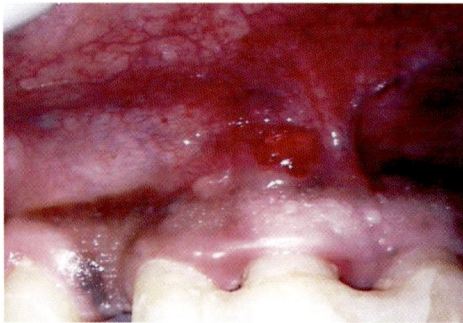

Fig. 1: Pre-op. The maxillary right central incisor shows a fistula at the labial surface. The tooth had root canal therapy in the past and is showing failure. Apicoectomy is treatment planned.

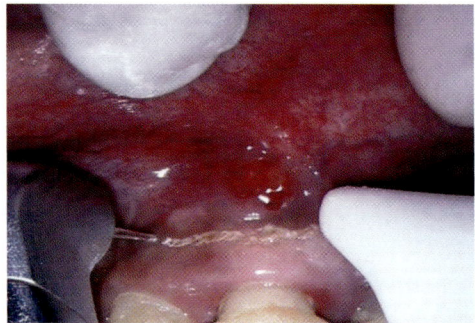

Fig. 2: A MT-4 tip is used to make a semilunar incision for flap. The setting is 2.00W, 7% Water, 11% Air, 30 Hz.

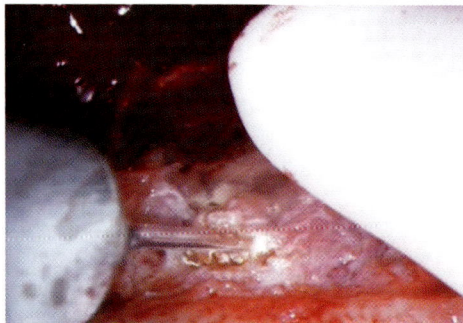

Fig. 3: A MG-tip is used to ablate bone to expose the root end. The setting is 4.00W, 60% Water, 80% Air, 20 Hz.

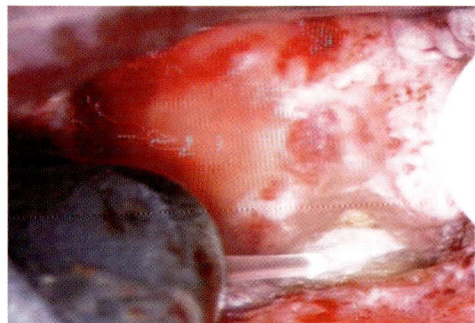

Fig. 4: Apicoectomy is performed by using laser. The setting is 2.50W, 60% Water, 80% Air, 20 Hz.

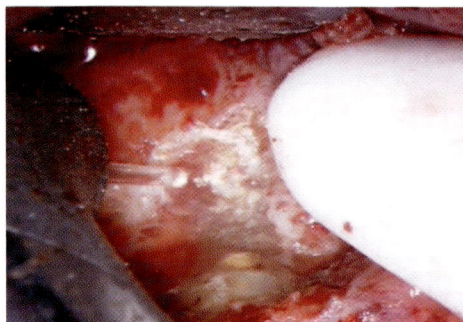

Fig. 5: Gutta percha is revealed after apicoectomy. Laser is used to remove granulation tissue in bone and around root end. The setting is 2.00W, 7% Water, 11% Air.

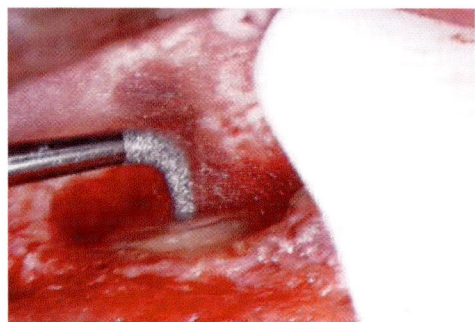

Fig. 6: A surgical endodontic Cavitron tip is used to remove gutta percha 2-3 mm in the root end.

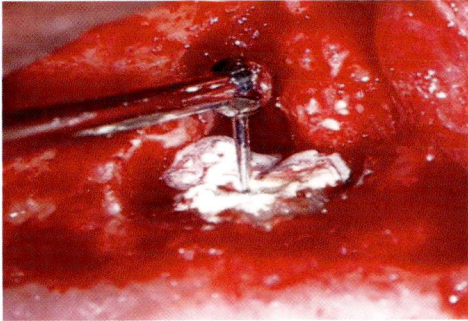

Fig. 7: MTA is placed at the root end as a retrofill restoration.

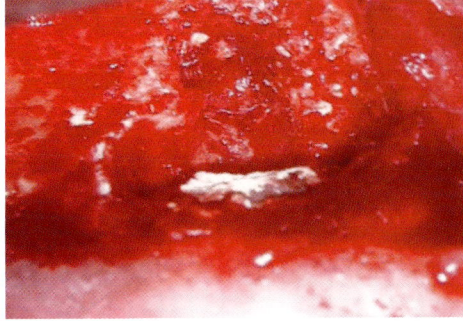

Fig. 8: After removing excess MTA, it is allowed to set hard before closure of the surgical site.

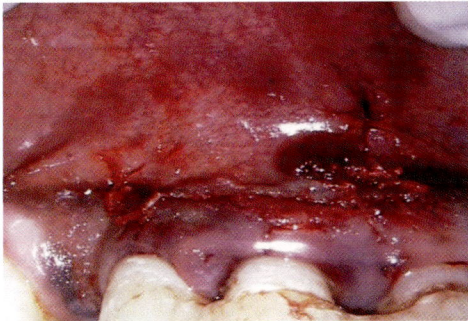

Fig. 9: A 4-0 vicryl suture is placed (mattress suture)

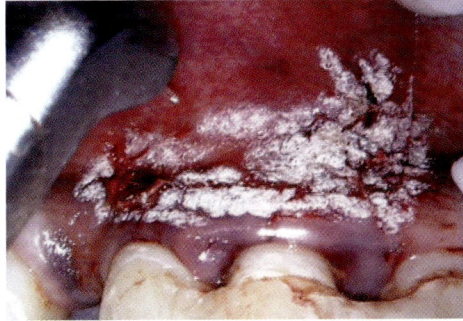

Fig. 10: Biologic band-aid is applied by laser. The setting is 1.00W, 0% Water, 11% Air. The MG-6 tip is refocused 5 mm.

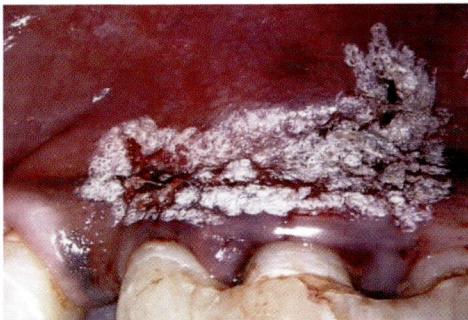

Fig. 11: Immediate post-op.

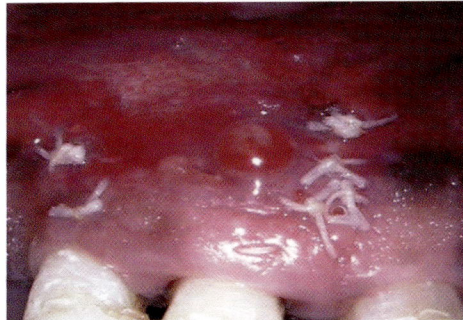

Fig. 12: Ten day post-op.

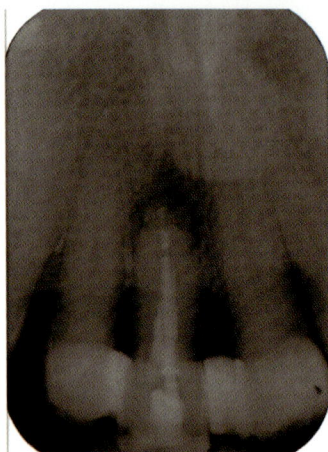

Fig. 13: Pre-operative x-ray

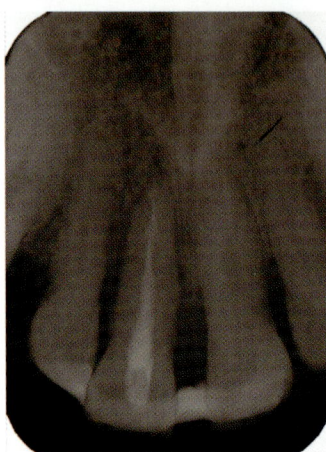

Fig. 14: Post-operative x-ray (18 months)

Case 2: Apicoectomy, Maxillary 1st Premolar, MD Regular HP with MG-6 Tip

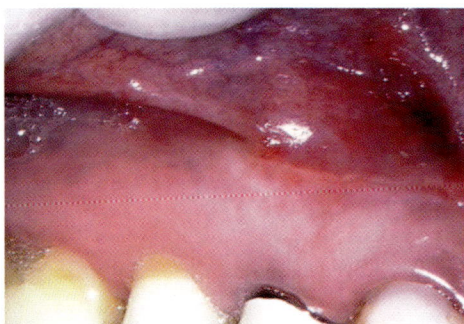

Fig. 1: Pre-op. Maxillary right first premolar shows a fistula and a periapical lesion. The tooth already had root canal therapy in the past. Apicoectomy is treatment planned.

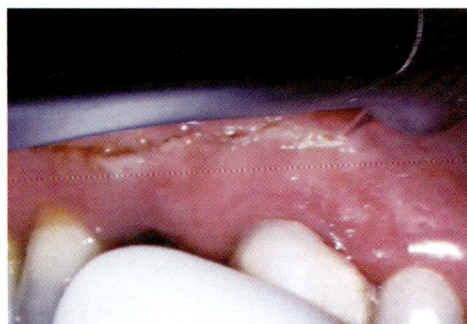

Fig. 2: A MT-4 tip is used to make a semilunar incision at the mucogingival tissue from mesial of #6 to distal of #4. The setting is 2.00W, 7% Water, 11% Air, 30 Hz.

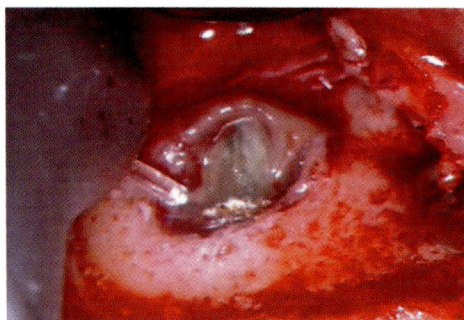

Fig. 3: A MG-6 tip is used to apply laser energy to open a window in the alveolus to expose the root end. The setting is 4.00W, 60% water, 80% air, 20 Hz, H mode.

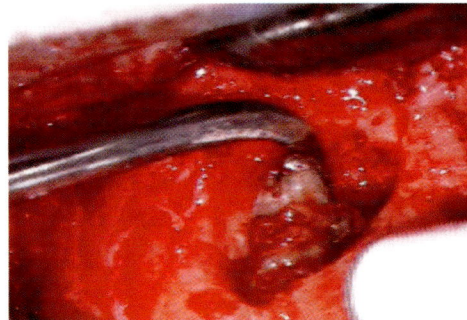

Fig. 4: Removal of gross amount granulation tissues by periodontal surgical curette.

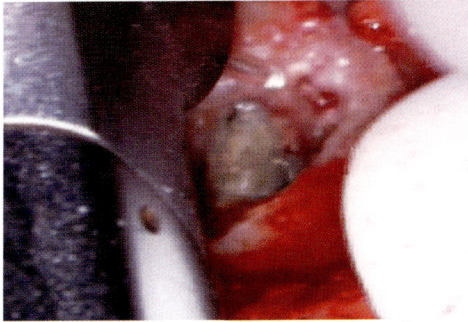

Fig. 5: Granulation around the infected root Is removed by laser energy. The setting is 2.00W, 7% Water, 11% Air, 30 Hz.

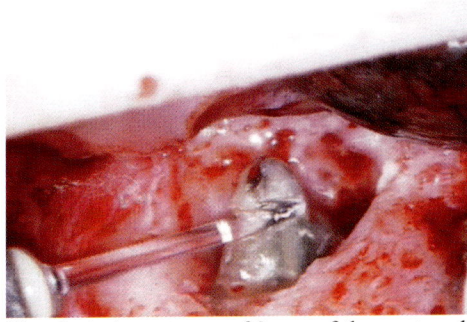

Fig. 6: Apicoectomy of 3mm of the root end is performed by using laser energy. The setting is 2.50W, 60% Water, 80% Air, 20 Hz.

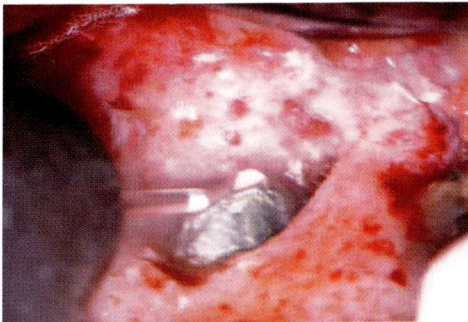

Fig. 7: Gutta percha and sealant is revealed after apicoectomy.

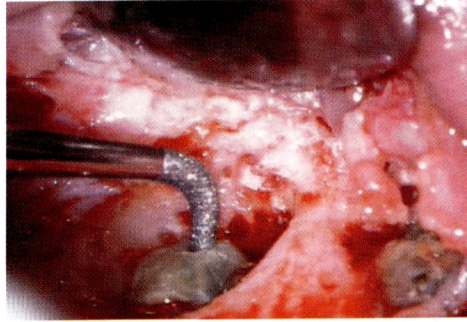

Fig. 8: An endodontic surgical Cavitron tip is used to remove 2-3mm of gutta percha from the root end.

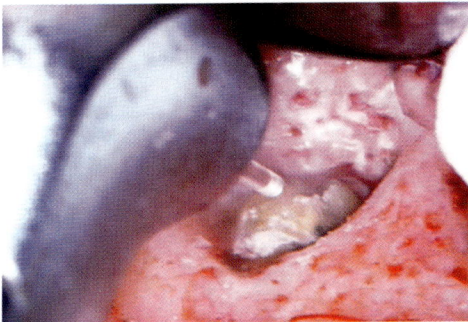

Fig. 9: Laser is used to clean and debride the root canal.

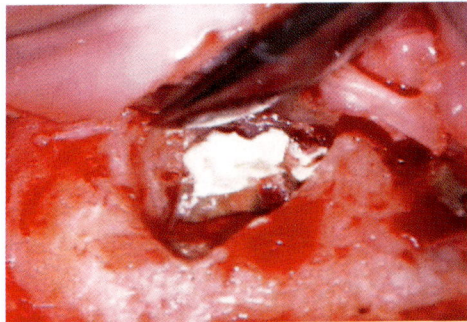

Fig. 10: MTA is placed as a retrofill restoration.

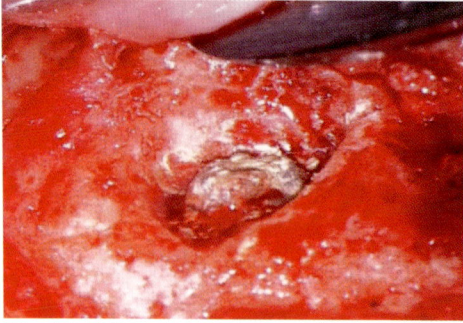

Fig. 11: After removing excess MTA, it is let to set hard before closure of the surgical site.

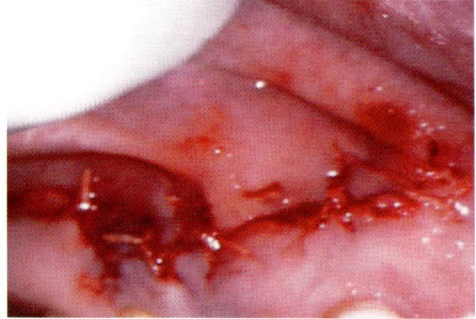

Fig. 12: A 4-0 vicryl suture is used to close the surgical site. (A mattress suture is placed)

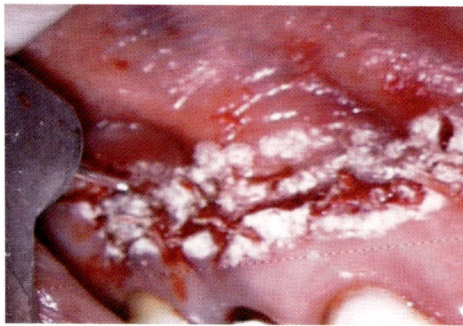

Fig. 13: Biologic band-aid is applied to the surgical site. The setting is 1.25W, 0% Water, 11% Air, 30 Hz. The MG-6 tip is defocused 5 mm while applying laser.

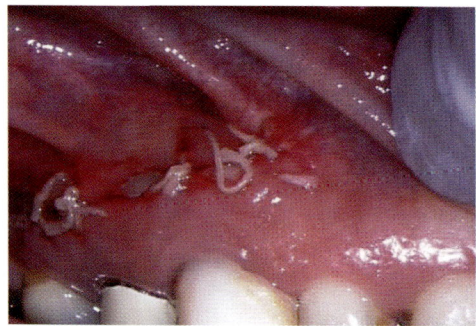

Fig. 14: One week post-op

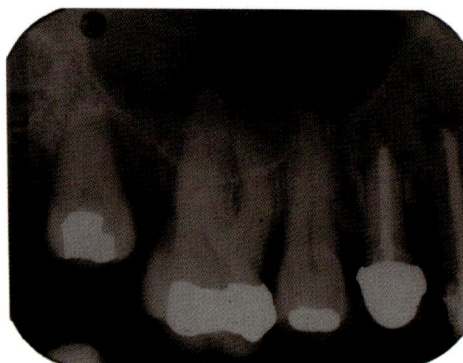

Fig. 13: Pre-operative x-ray

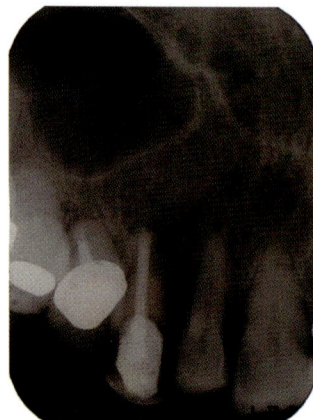

Fig. 14: Post-operative x-ray (12months)

Case 3: Apicoectomy, Maxillary 1st Premolar, M2 with G-6 Tip

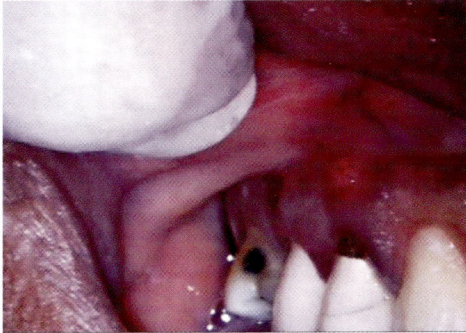

Fig. 1: Pre-op. The maxillary right 1st premolar shows a fistula at the buccal surface. Root canal therapy was done in the past. Apicoectomy is treatment planned.

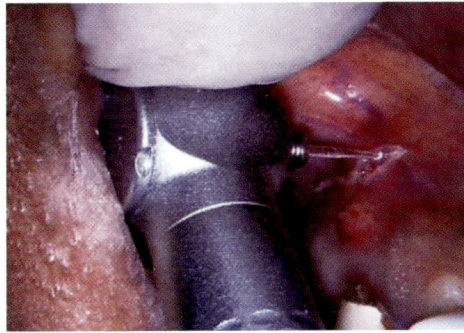

Fig. 2: A T-4 tip is used to make a semilunar flap. The setting is 1.50W, 7% Water, 11% Air. The incision is made to avoid cutting the fistula.

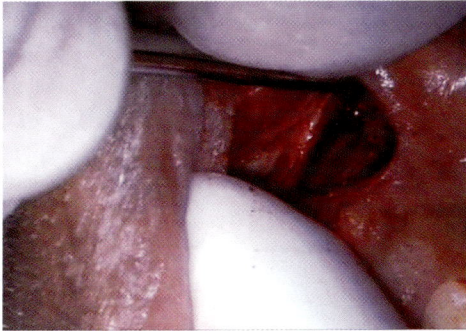

Fig. 3: Tissue is retracted to expose the alveolus.

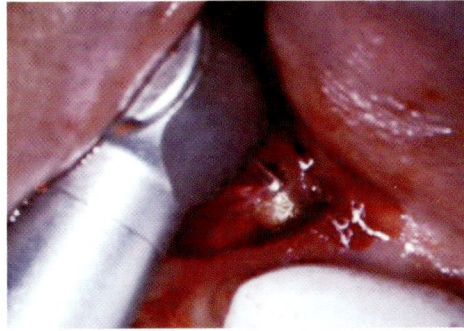

Fig. 4: A G-6 tip is used to ablate bone to expose the root end. The setting is 4.00W, 60% Water, 65% Air.

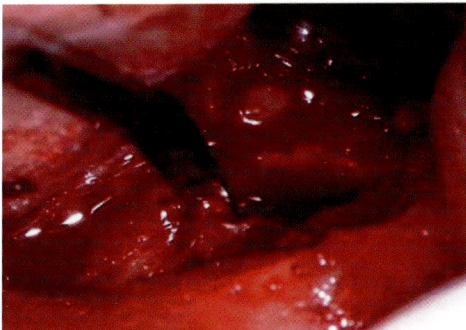

Fig. 5: A periodontal surgical curette is used to remove gross granulation tissue around the root end.

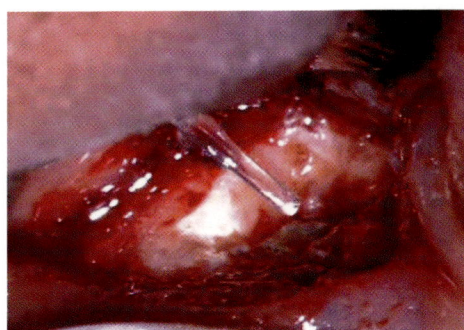

Fig. 6: Laser is used to remove tenacious granulation tissues around the root end and alveolus. The setting is 1.75W, 7% Water, 11% Air.

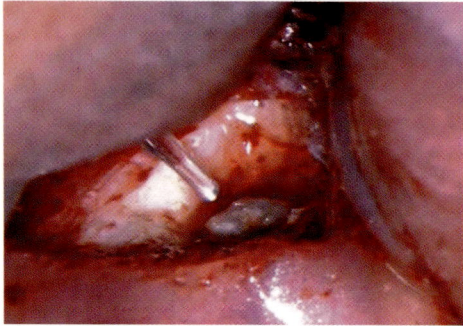

Fig. 7: Apicoectomy is performed by the laser. The setting is 2.50W, 40% Water, 40% Air.

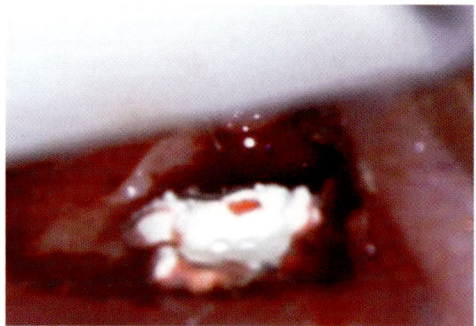

Fig. 8: MTA is used as a retrofill restoration.

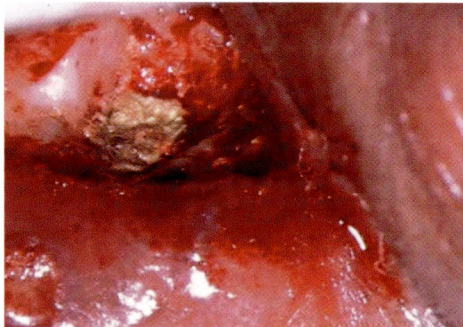

Fig. 9: After removing excess MTA, the material is let to set hard before closure of the surgical site.

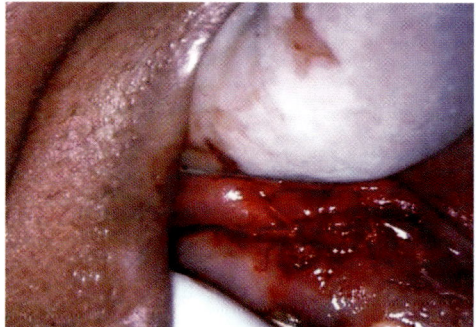

Fig. 10: A 4-0 vicryl suture is placed. (Mattress suture)

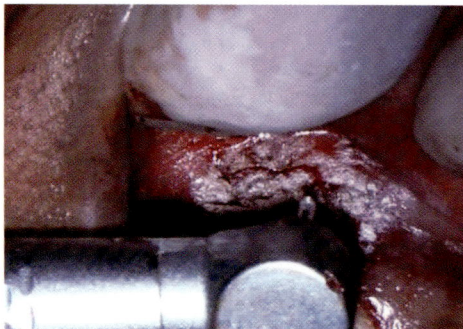

Fig. 11: Biologic band-aid is applied to the surgical site. The setting is 1.00W, 0% Water, 11% Air.

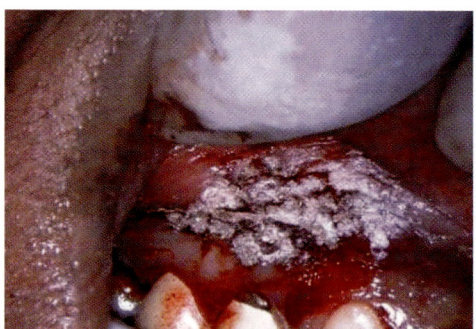

Fig. 12: Immediate post-op.

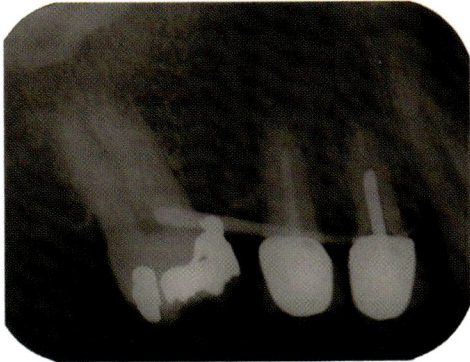

Fig. 13: Pre-operative x-ray

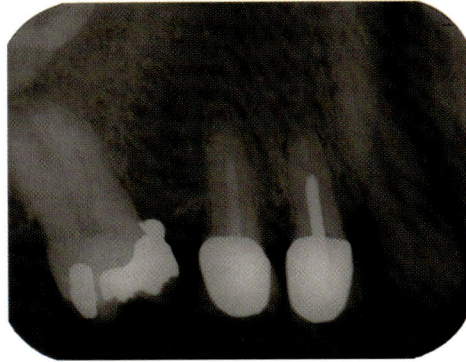

Fig. 14: Post-op x-ray (3 months).

Case 4: Apicoectomy of 2 Maxillary Anterior Tooth, MD Regular HP with MG-6 Tip

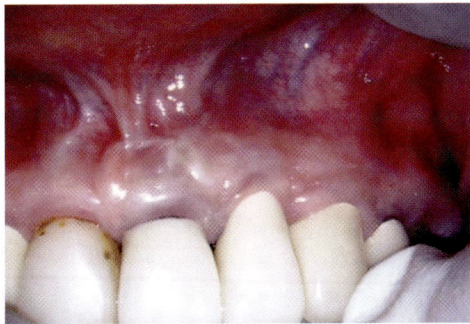

Fig. 1: Pre-op. Teeth #9 and #10 show fistulas and failure of previously performed apicoectomy.

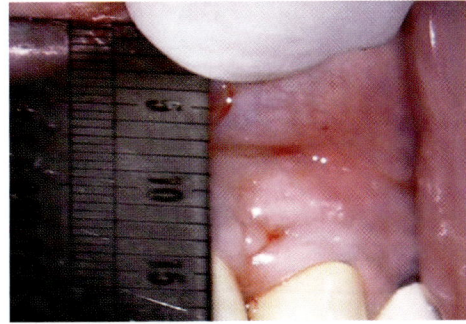

Fig. 2: Apical positions of #9 and #10 are approximated by using an endo ruler.

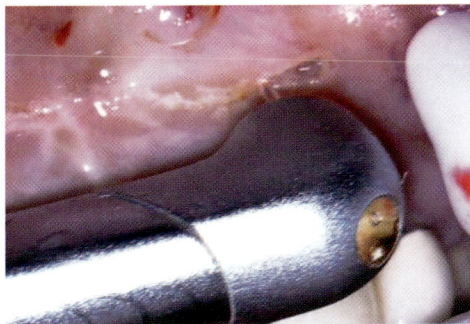

Fig. 3: After profound local anesthesia is administered, a semi-lunar flap is made by laser. A MT-4 tip is used. The setting is 1.50-1.75W, 7% Water, 11% Air, 30 Hz.

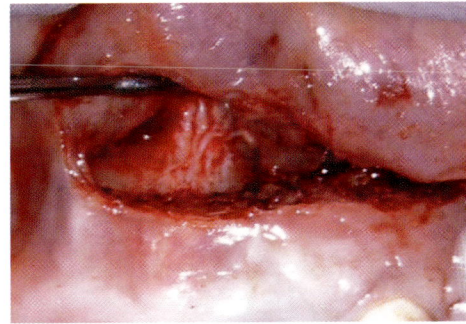

Fig. 4: A flap is made using a periosteal elevator.

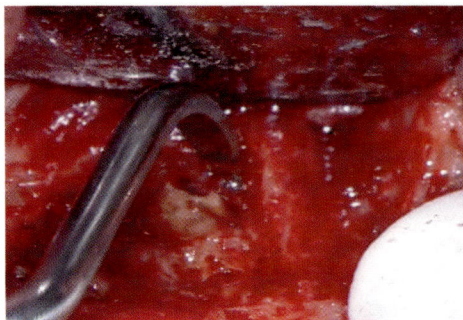

Fig. 5: A periodontal surgical curette is used to remove gross amount of granulation tissues in the apical areas of #9 and #10.

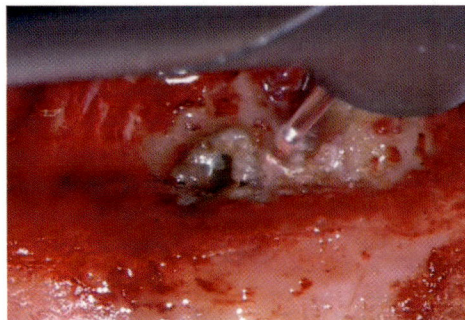

Fig. 6: Laser is used to remove the tenacious granulation tissue adhered to the root and alveolus in the surgical area. The tip used is MG-6 (or MZ-6). The setting is 2.00-2.50W, 11% Water, 11% air, 30 Hz. The same setting is used to remove fistula at the inner surface of the mucogingival tissue.

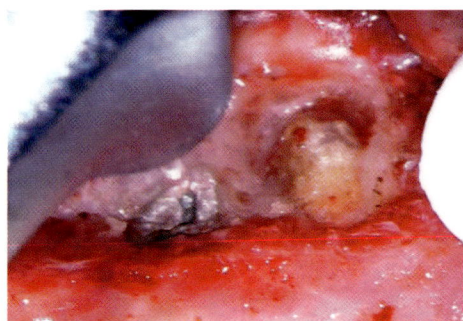

Fig. 7: Apical debridement and cleaning of #9 is done by a MG-6 (or MZ-6) using 2.00W, 60% Water, 80% Air, 30 Hz.

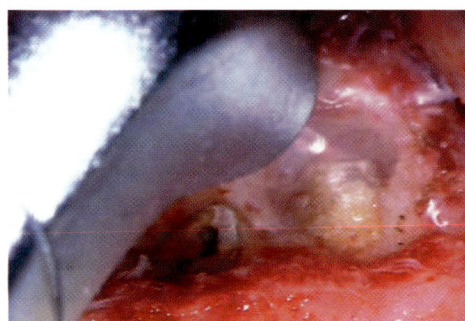

Fig. 8: Apicoectomy is performed on the #10 to remove an additional mm of root end. The setting is 2.50W, 60% Water, 80% Air, 30 Hz. This is followed by debridement and cleaning at 2.00W, 60% Water, 80% Air, 30 Hz.

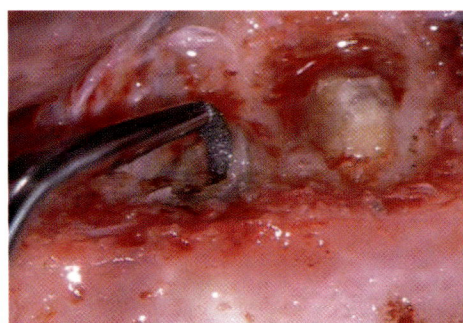

Fig. 9: Removal of the amalgam used in the previous apico surgery from #9 is done by a surgical cavitron.

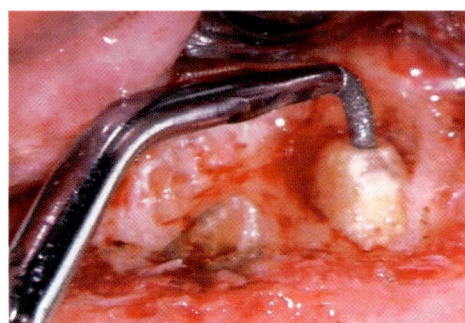

Fig. 10: Removal of gutta percha from the apical area of #10 is done by a surgical cavitron.

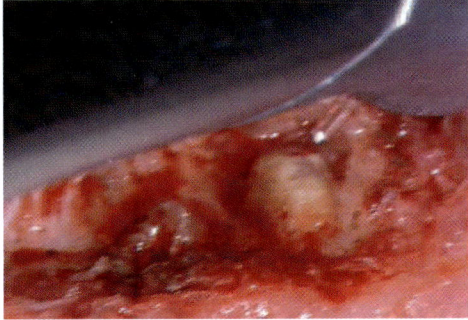

Fig. 11: This is followed by debridement and cleaning in the retrofill preparation area using 2.00W, 60% Water, 80% Air, 30 Hz.

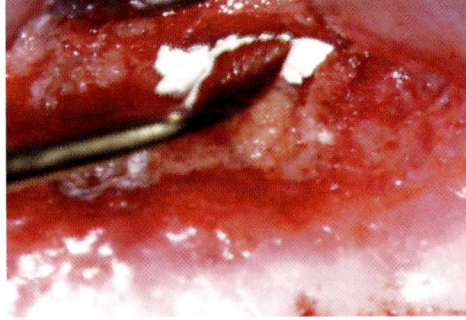

Fig. 12: MTA is placed as the retrofill material.

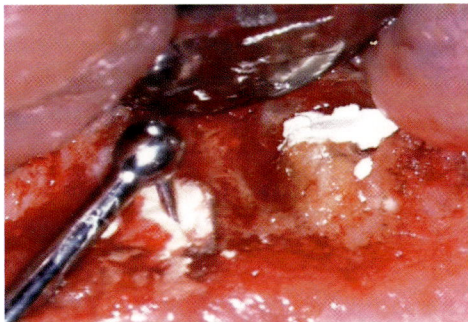

Fig. 13: Condensation of the MTA into the apical preps of #9 and #10.

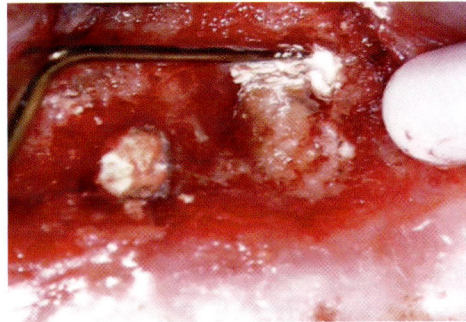

Fig. 14: Carving of MTA to remove excess material.

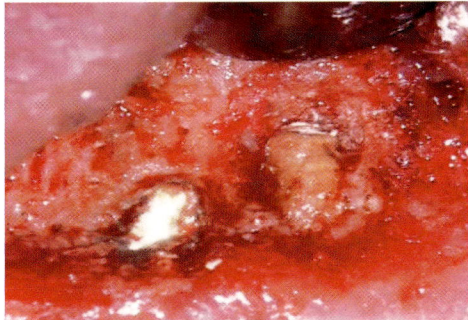

Fig. 15: MTA is allowed to set hard. Good hemostasis allows MTA to set properly before closure. This is crucial in getting a high percentage of success for apicoectomy.

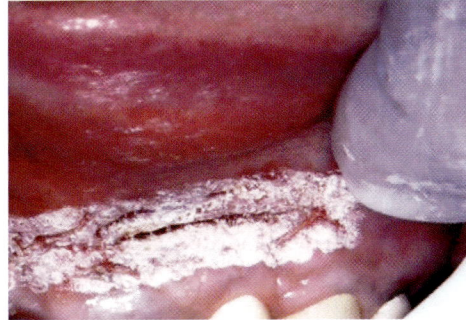

Fig. 16: After mattress suture is placed using a resorbable suture. Laser biologic band-aid is applied. A MZ-12 tip is used at 1.50W, 0% Water, 11% Air, 30 Hz at a 3-5 defocused distance.

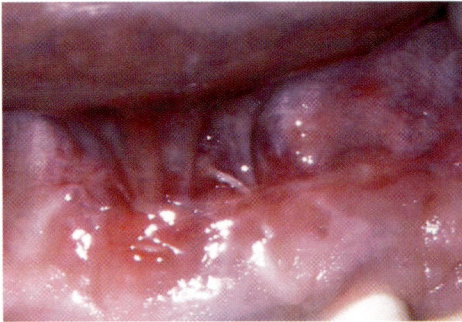
Fig. 17: One month post-op. No complication. Good healing.

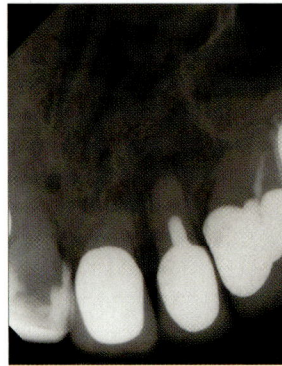
Fig. 18: Before x-ray

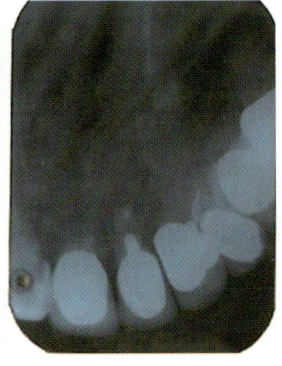
Fig. 19: After x-ray

Radial-Firing Tips

Clinical Procedures for Waterlase MD Root Canal Therapy Using Radial-Firing Tips

Laser Parameters, Set 1: Access Opening

MZ-5 tip (if using MD Gold Handpiece) or MG-6/MZ-6 (if using standard MD handpiece), 3.50-4.50W, 60% Water, 80% Air, 15 Hz

> The laser is used to prepare access opening. A high-speed round bur can be used to make the coronal and apical extensions to allow better access for instrumentation in the canal. The preparation continues until the pulp is exposed. Working length is measured with a #10 or #15 K-file and the use of a periapical x-ray apex locator.

> Enlargement of the root canal to 300μm diameter is performed by using nickel titanium crown-down instrumentation.

Laser Parameters, Set 2: Enlargement of the Canal to 300μm Diameter

RFT-2 tip, 1.25W, 24% Water, 34% Air, 50 Hz

> The RFT-2 is placed 1mm short of root end. Laser energy is applied as the tip is slowly retrieved from the root end in a straight line. The retrieval should take approximately one second per 1mm retrieved. The tip also maintains contact with the side surface of the canal wall during the entire apical to coronal movement. Two or more sequences of laser applications are used at different portions of the canal wall.

Laser Parameters, Set 3: Laser Cleaning and Enlargement

RFT-3 tip, 1.25W, 24% Water, 34% Air, 50 Hz

> The debridement, cleaning and enlargement of the root canal continues with the RFT-3 starting at the junction between the apical and middle third in the root canal (3-5mm from the root end). The apical to coronal sequence of firing should take approximately one second per 1mm. The laser procedure is repeated three more times on different portions on the root canal wall.

Laser Parameters, Set 4: Laser Disinfection

RFT-2 tip, 0.75W, 0% Water, 10% Air, 20 Hz

> The RFT-2 is placed 1mm short of the root end. Laser energy is applied as the tip moves from apex to the coronal area at approximately 1mm per second. Three to four laser applications are repeated with the tip in contact with different portions of the canal wall.

Laser Parameters, Set 5: Complete Laser Disinfection

RFT-3 tip, 0.75W, 0% Water, 10% Air, 20 Hz

> The RFT-3 is placed at the junction between apical and middle third. Laser energy is applied as the tip moves from apical to coronal area at 1mm per second. The laser procedure is repeated 4 to 5 times on different portions of the canal wall.

Laser Parameters, Set 6: Obturation

> After preparation of the root canal, the conventional funnel-shaped canal space is prepared. Any conventional obturation technique can be used to finish the root canal therapy.

Case 1: Anterior Tooth MD Gold HP Using Radial-Firing Endo Tips

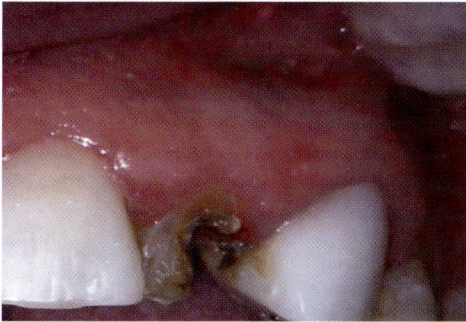

Fig. 1: Pre-op clinical view of #10.

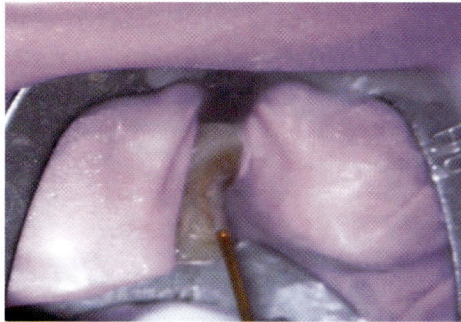

Fig. 2: Access opening is performed by laser. The fiber tip is MZ-5 in a MD Gold Handpiece. The setting is 3.00W, 60% Water, 80% Air, 15 Hz.

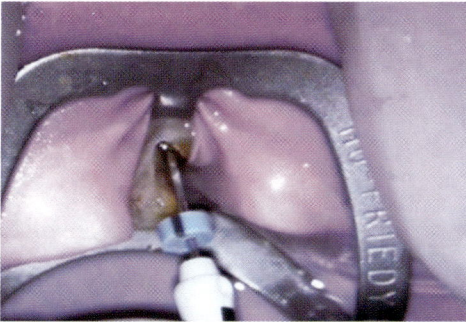

Fig. 3: Working length is measured by using a #15 K-file.

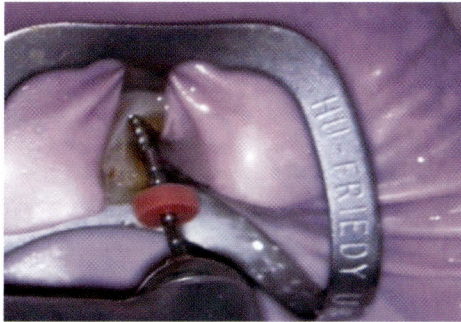

Fig. 4: The canal is enlarged to 300μm by using nickel-titanium crown-down rotary files.

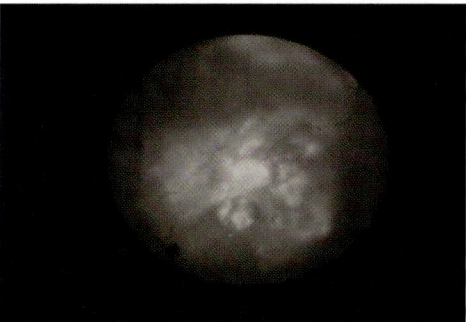

Fig. 5: Endoscope (x48) showing a smear and debris-covered dentinal wall.

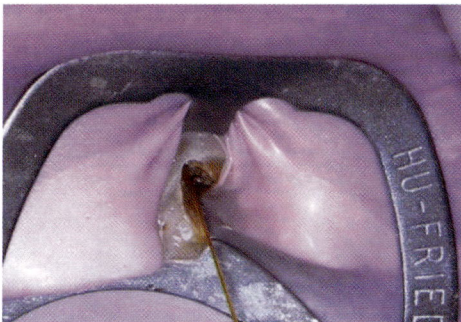

Fig. 6: RFT-2 is used to debride, clean and enlarge the canal. The setting is 1.25W, 24% Water, 34% Air, 50 Hz. Four sequences of RFT-2 firing are used to clean 1mm from root end to the coronal area.

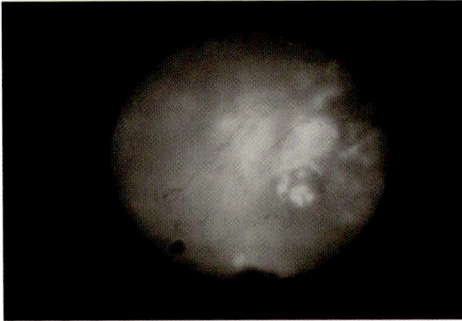

Fig. 7: Endoscope (x48) showing partially cleaned canal wall.

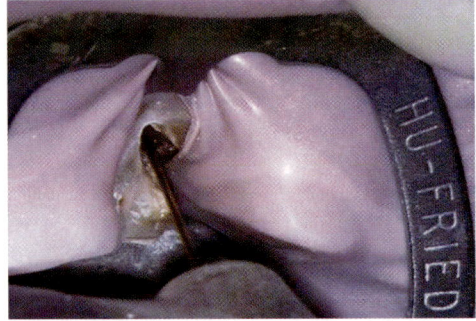

Fig. 8: RFT-3 is used to continue debridement, cleaning and enlargement of the canal. Same setting is used as in Fig. 6.

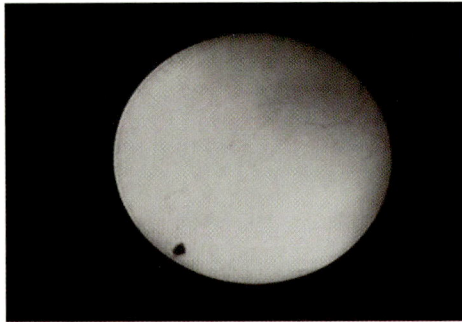

Fig. 9: Endoscope (x48) showing no smear, no debris and no charring.

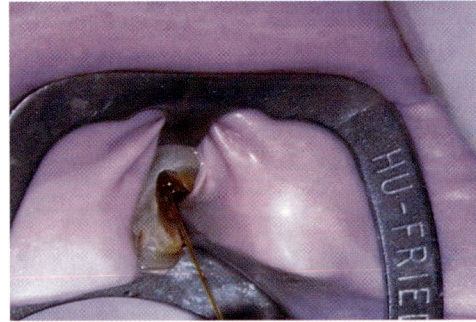

Fig. 10: RFT-2 is used for disinfection. The setting is 0.25W, 0% Water, 10% Air, 20 Hz.

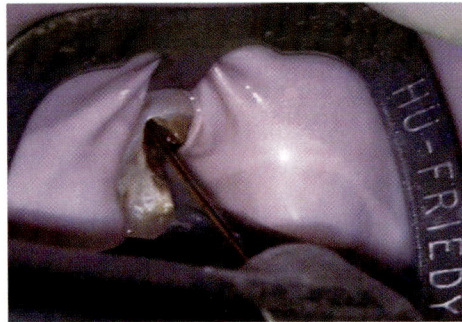

Fig. 11: RFT-3 is used to finish disinfection.

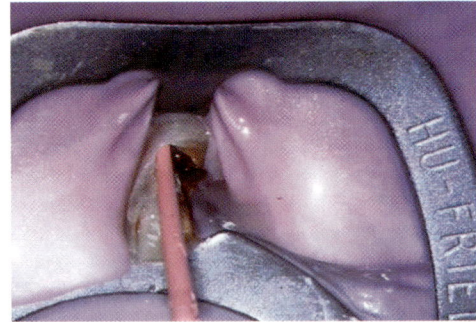

Fig. 12: A gutta percha master cone is tried in showing a funnel-shaped canal is prepared.

Case 2: Anterior Tooth, MD Gold HP Using Radial-Firing Endo Tips

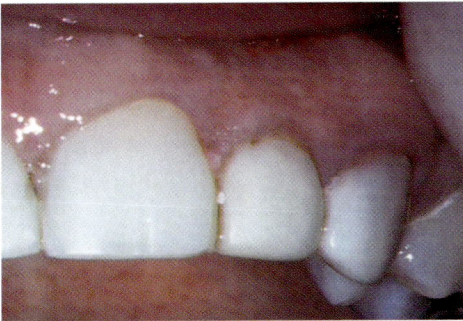

Fig. 1: Pre-op, #10 is diagnosed as having an irreversible pulpitis. A root canal therapy by using the radial firing endodontic tips is planned.

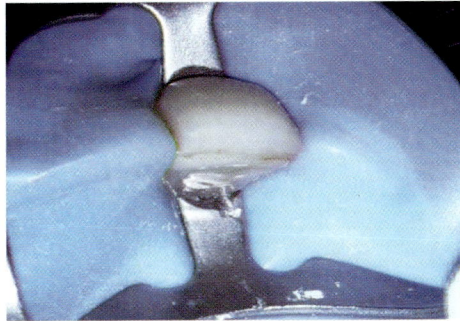

Fig. 2: Rubber dam and clamp is placed on #10.

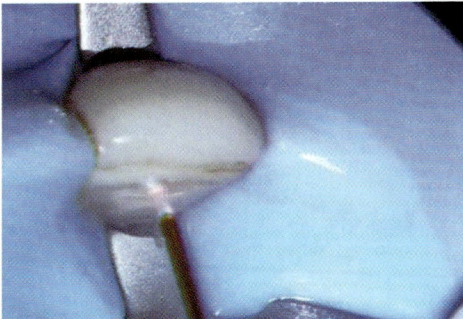

Fig. 3: MZ-5 tip in a MD gold handpiece is used for access opening. The setting is 4.50W, 60% Water, 80% Air, 15 Hz.

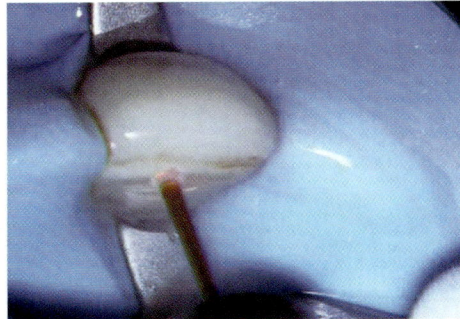

Fig. 4: Access opening continues into pulp chamber. The setting is reduced to 3.00W 60% Water, 80% Air, 15 Hz.

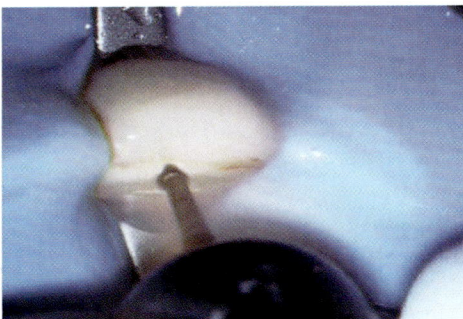

Fig. 5: A high speed round bur is used to improve and complete access opening.

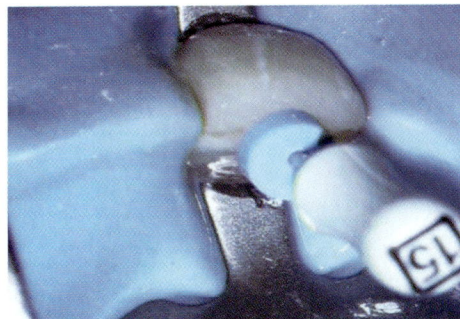

Fig. 6: Working length is measured by a #15 K-file.

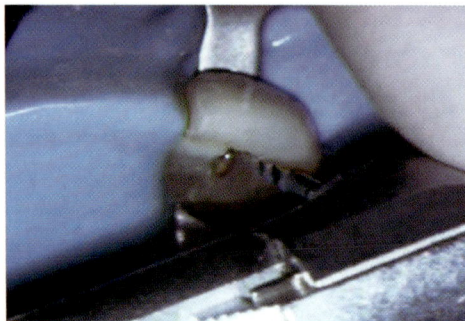

Fig. 7: The root canal is enlarged to 300μm diameter by nickel titanium crown down instrumentation.

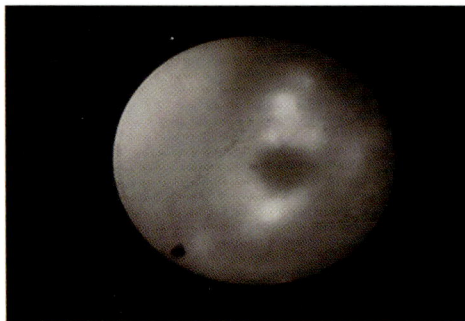

Fig. 8: A photo of the canal scoping with a magnification of 48x shows debris filled canal wall after rotary instrumentation.

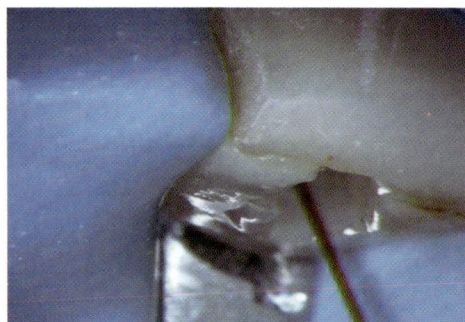

Fig. 9: A radial-firing tip 2 (RFT-2) is placed 1mm from apex and leaning against the mesial wall. Laser energy starts as the tip slowly retrieves from the apex. The setting is 1.25W, 24% Water, 34% Air, 50 Hz.

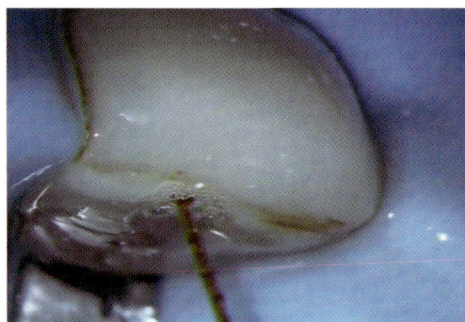

Fig. 10: RFT-2 is placed at the middle portion of the canal at 1mm from apex. The same laser setting is used as the fiber tip is moved slowly coronally.

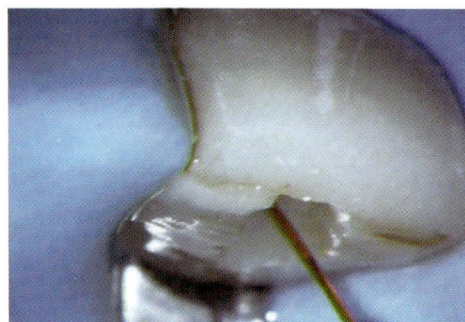

Fig. 11: The RFT-2 is used to treat the canal two more times at two new positions (distal and center opposing sides of wall).

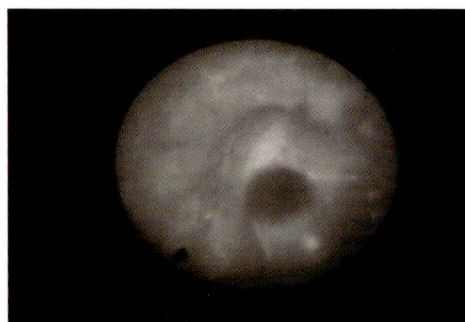

Fig. 12: A photo of the canal after four sequences of laser therapy by RFT-2.The cleanliness of the canal has improved.

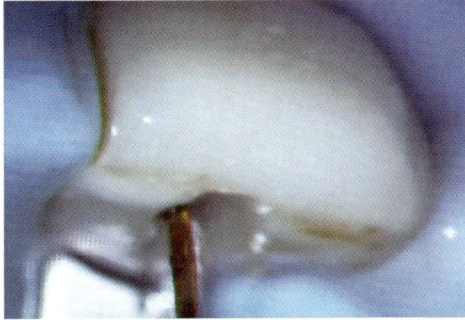

Fig. 13: A RFT-3 is placed at 5mm from the apex, leaning against the mesial wall. Laser energy is applied as the tip is slowly retrieved from the initial tip position. The setting is 1.25W, 24% Water, 34% Air, 50 Hz.

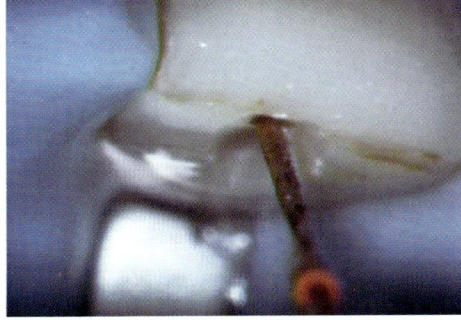

Fig. 14: The RFT-3 is placed 5mm from the apex, leaning against the center wall position. Again laser firing is applied as the tip is retrieved from the middle of the root canal.

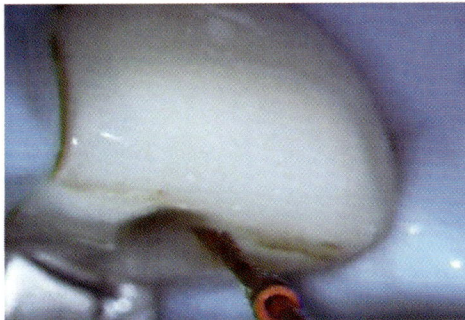

Fig. 15: The RFT-3 is placed at a new position of the root canal wall. A similar technique and setting is used to clean the canals at three different positions.

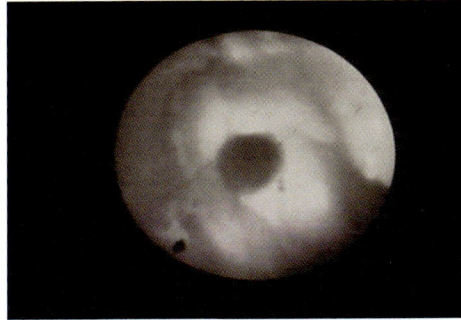

Fig. 16: A photo of the scoping of the root canal after initial treatments by RFT-2 and RFT-3.

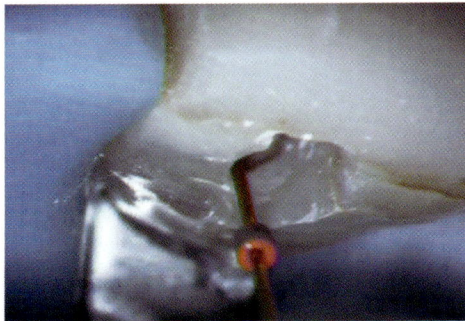

Fig. 17: The RFT-2 is placed 1mm from the apex. The laser is fired as the tip is slowly retrieved from the apex. Disinfection of the canal begins. The setting is 0.75W, 0% Water, 10% Air, 20 Hz. Conduct three to four more sequences of treatment with the RFT-2 at the same setting.

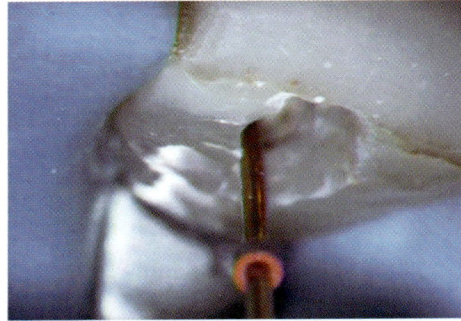

Fig.18: The RFT-3 is placed at 5mm from the apex. The laser is fired as the tip is retrieved coronally. Disinfection continues. The setting is 0.75W, 0% Water, 10% Air, 20 Hz. Four sequences of laser treatment with the RFT-3 are used to complete the endodontic disinfection.

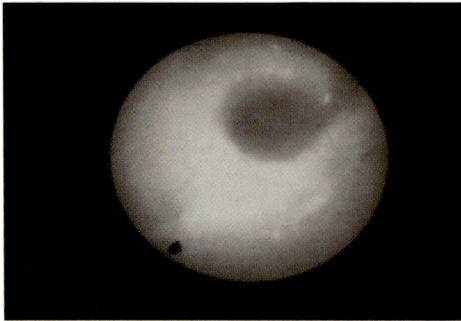

Fig. 19: A photo of the scoping of the canal shows smear and debris are removed. The canal is cleaned and debrided for obturation.

Case 3: Anterior Tooth, MD Gold HP Using Radial-Firing Endo Tips

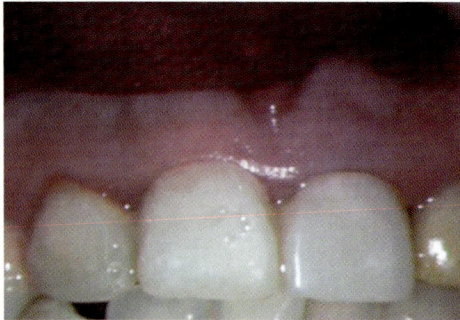

Fig. 1: Pre-op, #8 is fractured with pulp exposure. A core buildup with a composite crown is placed as a temporary. The tooth needs root canal therapy.

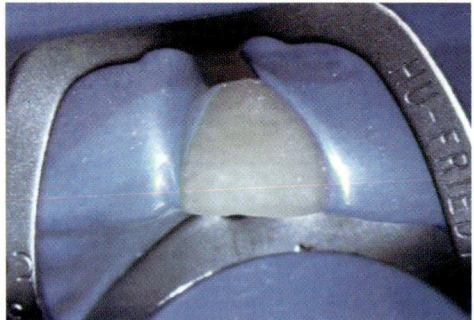

Fig. 2: A rubber dam clamp and rubber dam is placed.

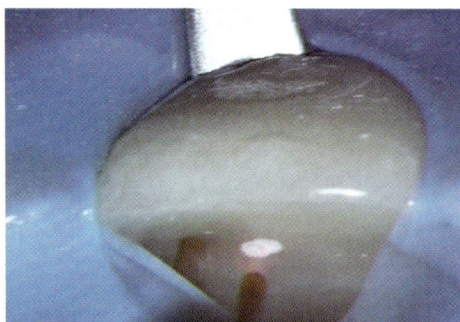

Fig. 3: Access opening starts with a MZ-5 tip in a MD Gold Handpiece. The setting is 4.50W, 60% Water, 80% Air, 15 Hz.

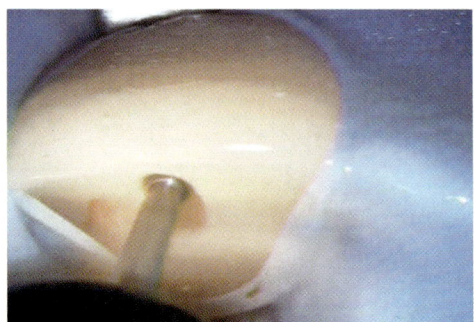

Fig. 4: Access opening is improved and completed with a high speed round bur.

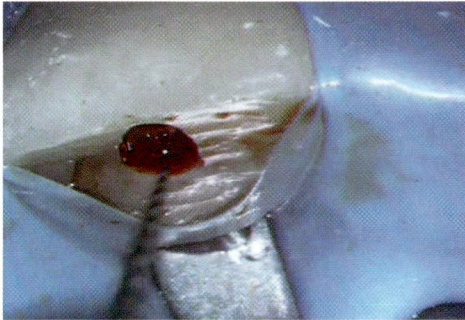

Fig. 5: Nickel-titanium crown-down instrumentation is used to enlarge the canal to 300μm diameter.

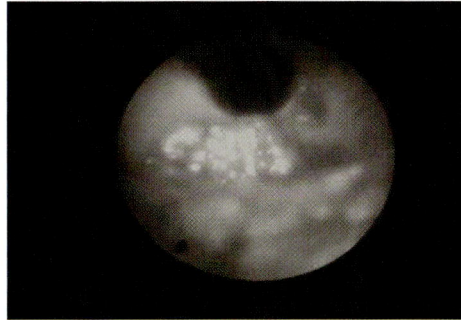

Fig. 6: A photo of the scoping of the canal shows a debris-filled canal wall from the rotary instrumentation.

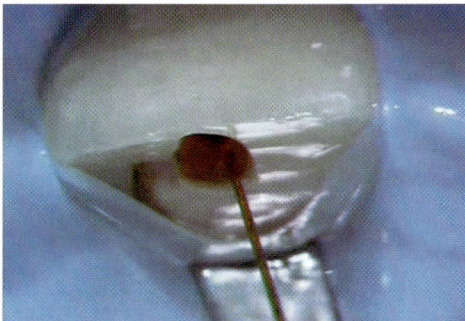

Fig. 7: A RFT-2 is placed 1mm from the apex for debridement, cleaning and enlargement. The setting is 1.25W, 24% Water, 34% Air. 50 Hz.

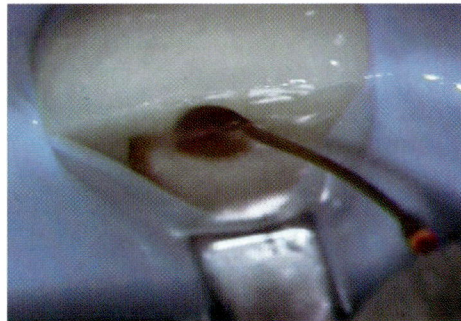

Fig. 8: The RFT-2 is fired 4-5 sequences with the same setting.

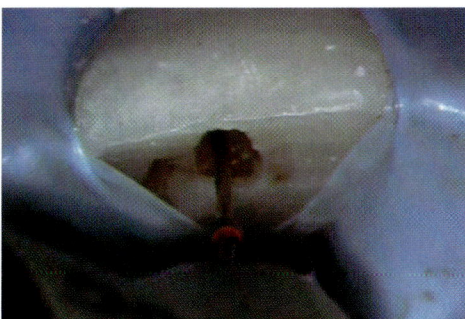

Fig. 9: A RFT-3 is placed 5mm from the apex for further debridement, cleaning and enlargement. Similar setting and technique are used as with RFT-3. Total of 5 sequences of treatment.

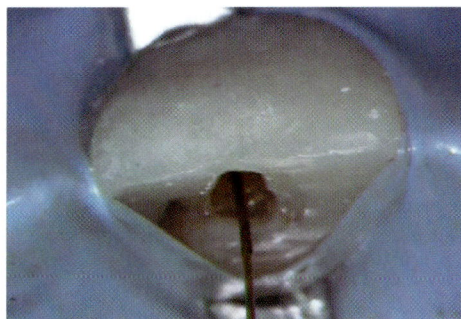

Fig. 10: The RFT-2 without water, is used for disinfection. 4-5 sequences of treatment at 0.75W 0% Water, 10% Air, 20 Hz.

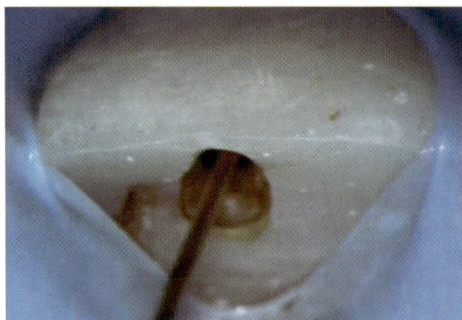

Fig. 11: The RFT-3, used without water, is utilized to complete disinfection of the canal for a sequence of five treatments at 0.75W, 0% Water, 10% Air, 20 Hz.

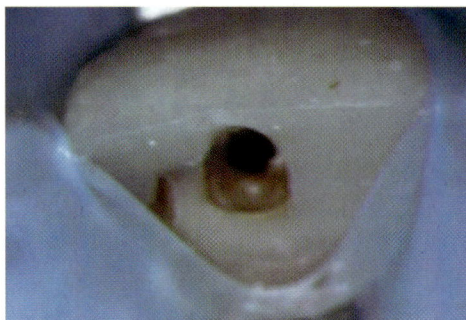

Fig 12: The preparation of the canal is complete.

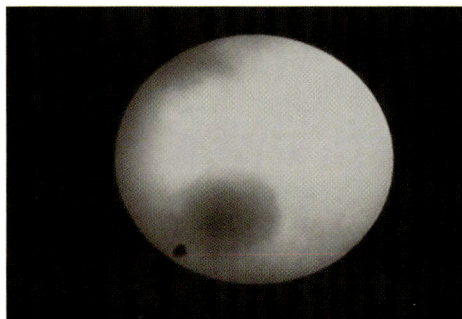

Fig. 13: A photo of the post-op. Scoping shows very clean, debris and smear free surface of the canal wall.

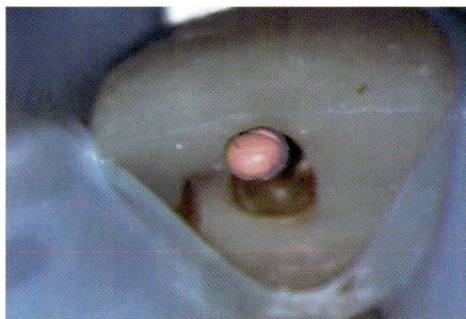

Fig 14: A gutta percha master cone is in place to the working length showing a funnel-shaped canal preparation.

Case 4: Molar Tooth, MD Gold HP Using Radial-Firing Endo Tips

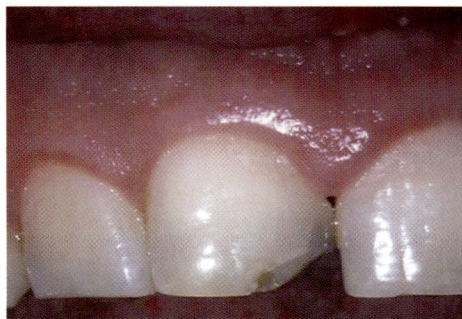

Fig. 1: Pre-op clinical view of #8.

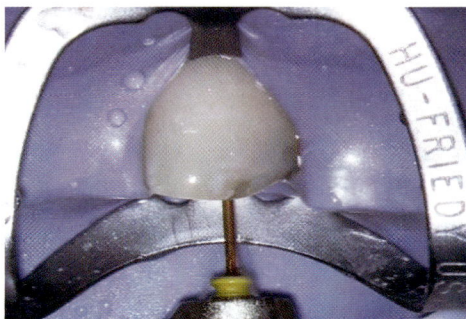

Fig. 2: Access opening is done with a laser using a MD Gold Handpiece and a MZ-5 tip. The setting is 4.00W, 60% Water, 80% Air, 15 Hz.

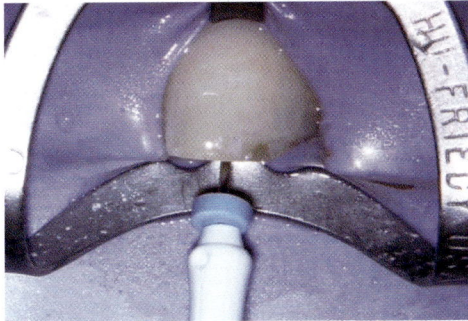

Fig. 3: A #15 K-file is used to measure the working length.

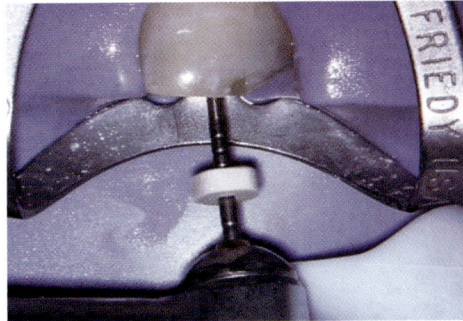

Fig. 4: The root canal is enlarged to 300μm by using crown-down nickel-titanium rotary files.

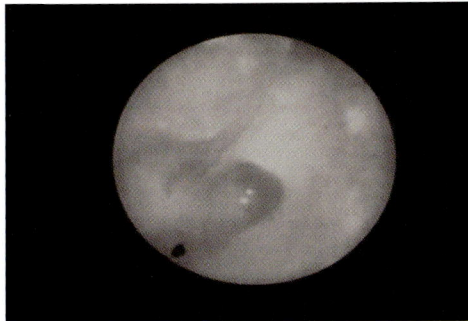

Fig. 5: Endoscope (x48) showing smear and debris-covered dentinal wall.

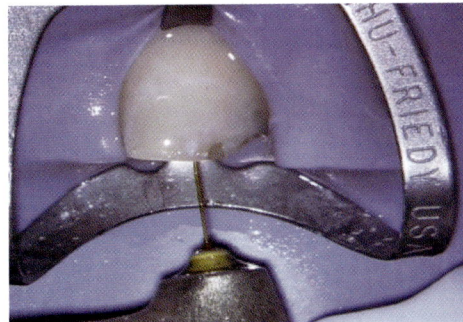

Fig. 6: A RFT-2 is used to debride, clean and enlarge the canal. The setting is 1.25W, 24% Water, 34% Air, 50 Hz. 4 sequences of laser application from 1 mm short of root end to the coronal area.

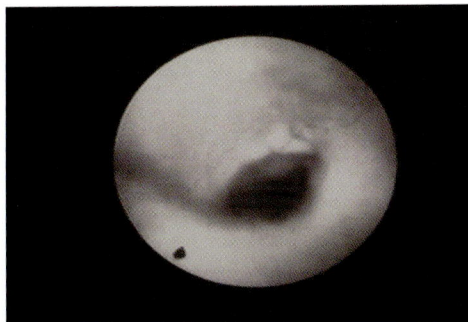

Fig. 7: Endoscope (x48) showing that the canal wall is much cleaner than after rotary instrumentation.

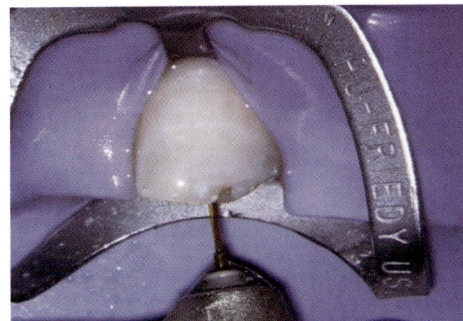

Fig. 8: A RFT-3 is used to continue debridement, cleaning and enlargement of the canal. Same setting is used as in Fig. 6.

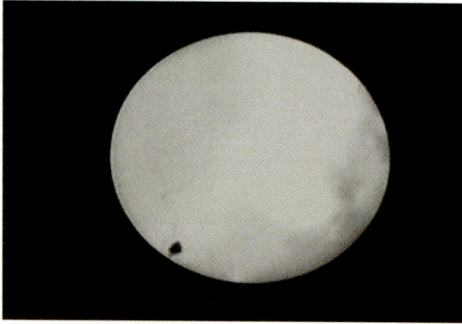

Fig. 9: Endoscope (x48) showing that the canal wall is very clean and shiny, without smear, debris and any melting.

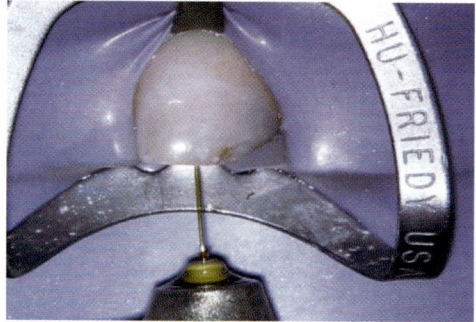

Fig. 10: A RFT-2 is used in disinfection. The setting is 0.75W, 0% Water, 10% Air, 20 Hz.

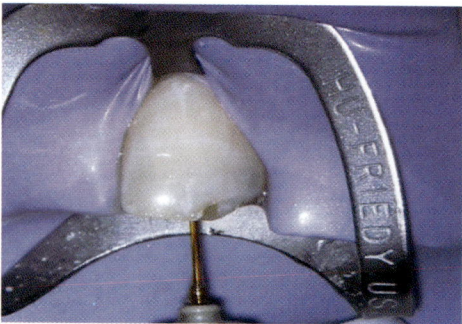

Fig. 11: A RFT-3 is used in disinfection. Same setting is used as in Fig. 10.

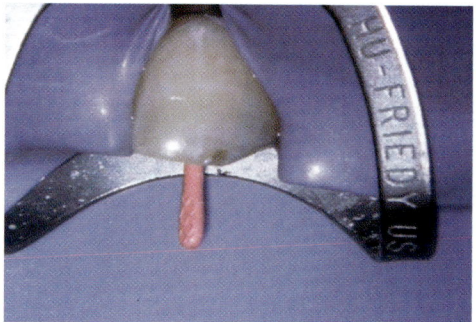

Fig. 12: A master cone gutta percha point is used to accomplish the traditional funnel shape preparation.

Case 5: Molar Tooth, MD Gold HP Using Radial-Firing Endo Tips

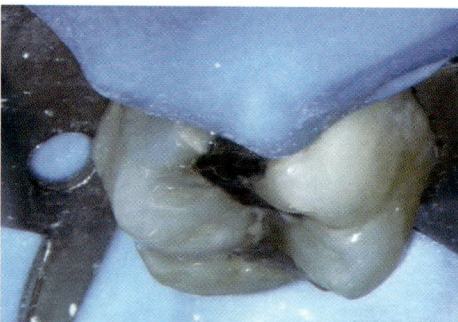

Fig. 1: Pre-op. #3 is diagnosed to have an irreversible pulpitis due to deep caries.

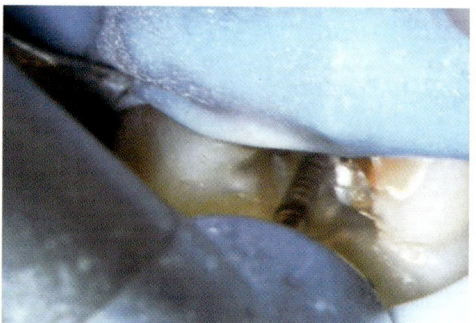

Fig. 2: Due to the presence of amalgam restoration, access opening is performed by a high speed 557 bur and a round bur.

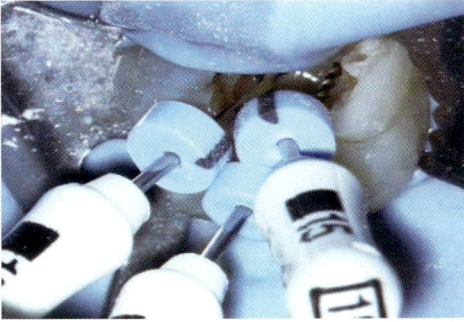

Fig. 3: Working lengths of the lingual, mesio-buccal, disto-buccal canals are measured.

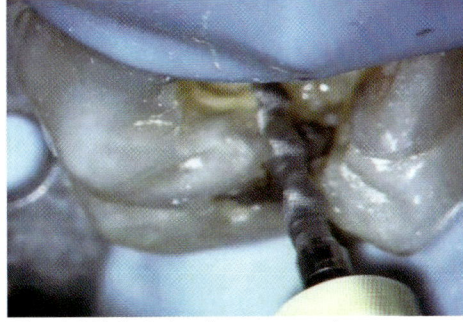

Fig. 4: Nickel-titanium crown-down rotary instrumentation is used to enlarge the lingual canal to 300µm diameter.

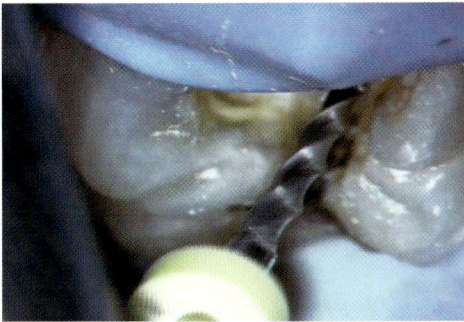

Fig. 5: Nickel-titanium crown-down rotary instrumentation is used to enlarge the mesio-buccal canal to 250µm.

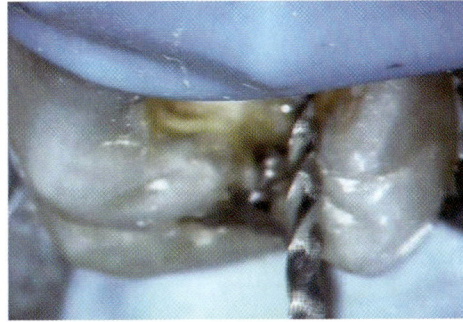

Fig. 6: Nickel-titanium crown-down rotary instrumentation is used to enlarge the disto-buccal canal to 250µm.

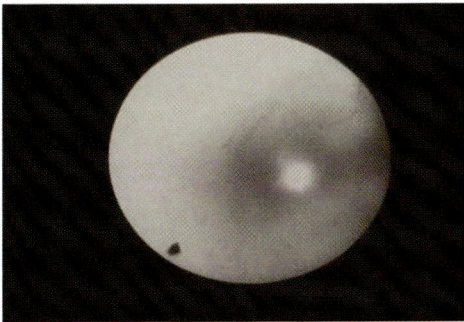

Fig. 7: A photo of the canal scoping at 48x magnification, showing debris covered canal wall in the lingual canal.

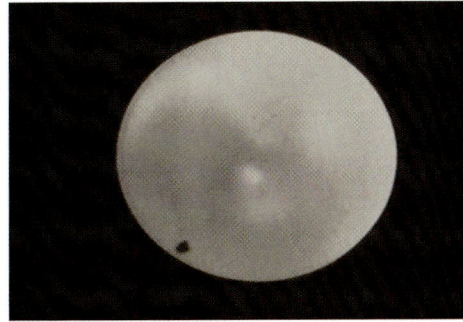

Fig. 8: A photo of the canal scoping showing debris covered canal wall in the mesio-buccal canal.

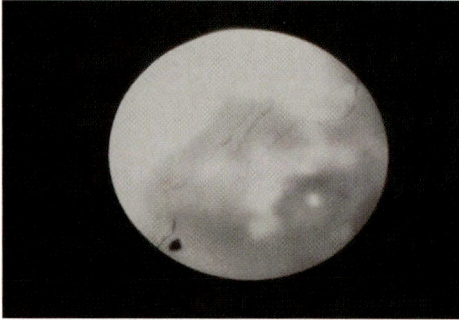

Fig. 9: A photo of the canal scoping showing debris covered canal wall in the disto-buccal canal.

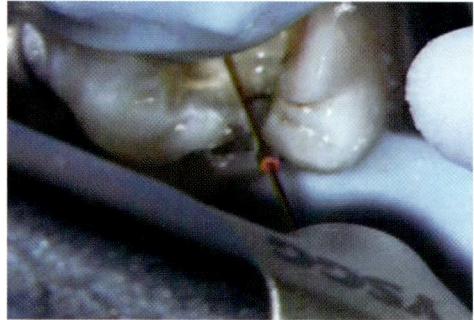

Fig. 10: A RFT-2 is used for debridement, cleaning and enlargement in the lingual, mesio-buccal and disto-buccal canals. The setting is 1.25W, 24% Water, 34% Air, 50 Hz.

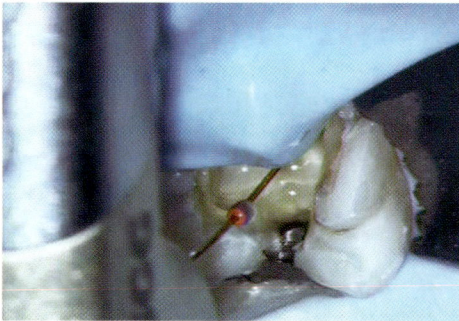

Fig. 11: A RFT-3 is used to continue debridement, cleaning and enlargement of all three canals. Similar setting as in Fig. 10 is used.

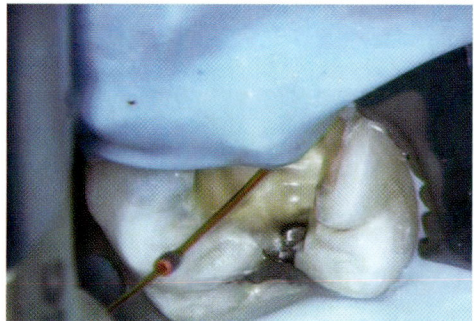

Fig. 12: This is followed by disinfection treatment with RFT-2 in all three canals. The setting is 0.75W, 0% Water, 10% Air, 20 Hz.

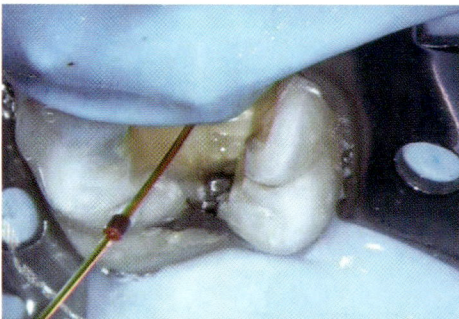

Fig. 13: The disinfection treatment is completed with RFT-3 in all three canals. The setting is 0.75W, 0% Water, 10% Air, 20 Hz.

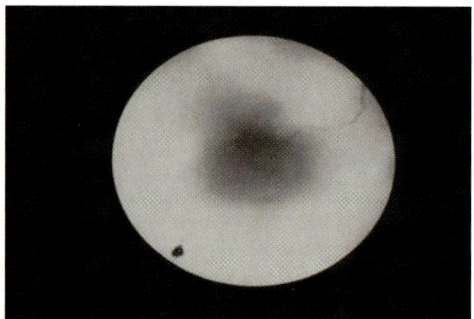

Fig. 14: A photo of the scoping of the lingual canal showing a smear and debris free canal wall.

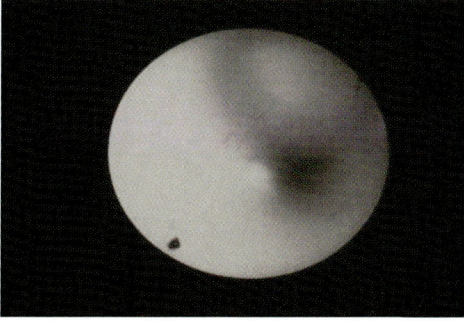

Fig. 15: A photo of the scoping of the mesio-buccal canal showing a smear and debris free canal wall.

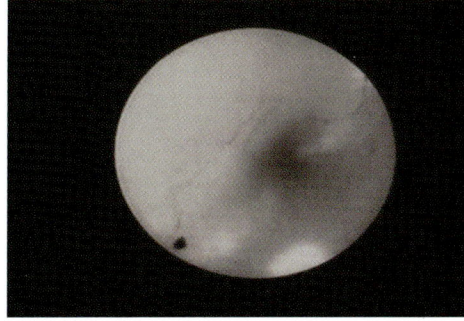

Fig. 16: A photo of the scoping of the disto-buccal canal showing a smear and debris free canal wall.

Endodontic X-rays Pre- and Post-Laser Treatment
Anterior Teeth:

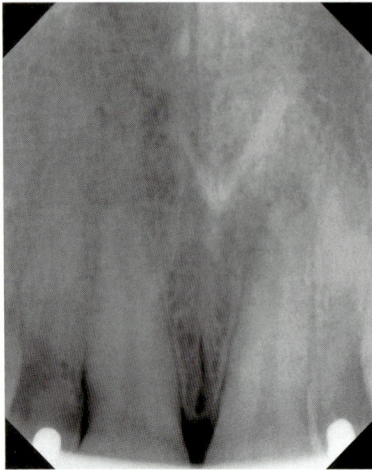

Fig. 1a: Pre-op x-ray, #9

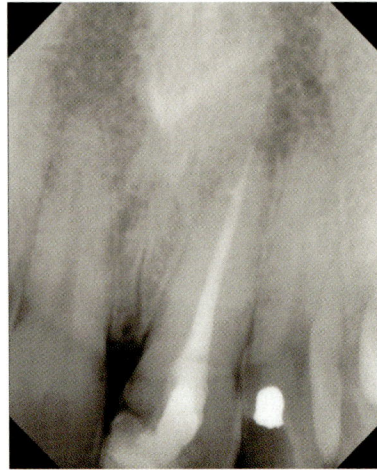

Fig. 1b: Post-op x-ray, #9

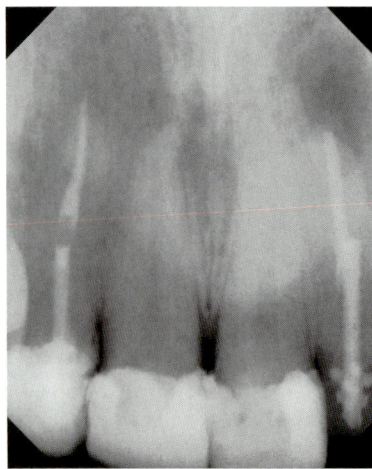

Fig. 2a: Pre-op x-ray, #8

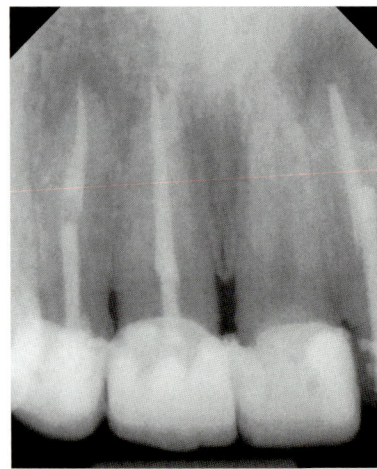

Fig. 2b: Post-op x-ray, #8

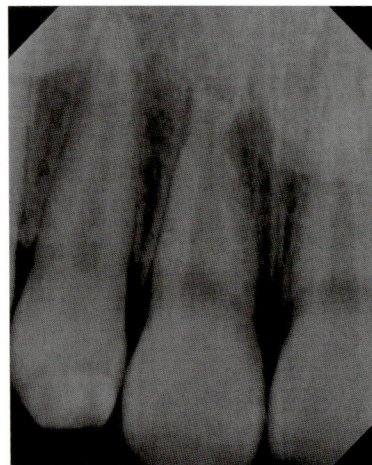

Fig. 3a: Pre-op x-ray, #8

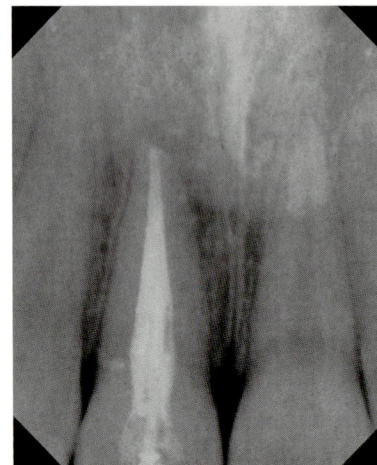

Fig. 3b: Post-op x-ray, #8

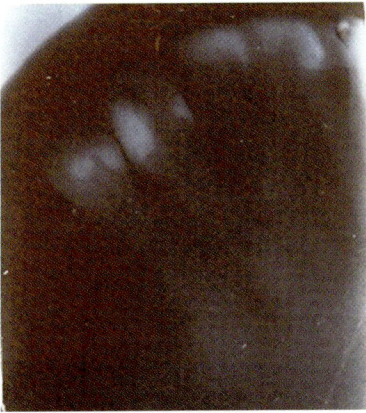
Fig. 4a: Pre-op x-ray, #27.

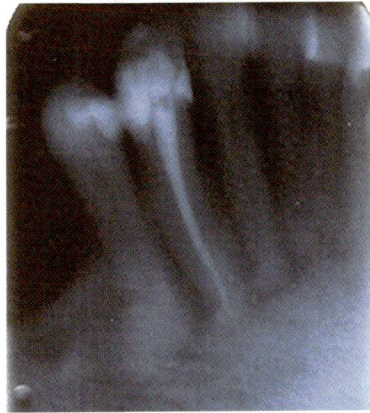
Fig. 4b: Post-op x-ray, #27.

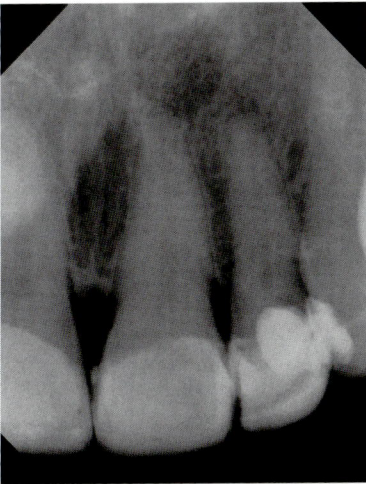
Fig. 5a: Pre-op x-ray, #10

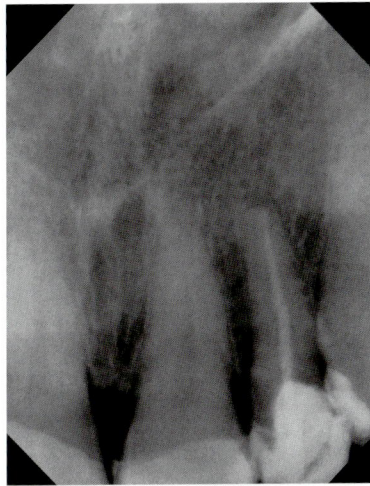
Fig. 5b: Post-op x-ray, #10

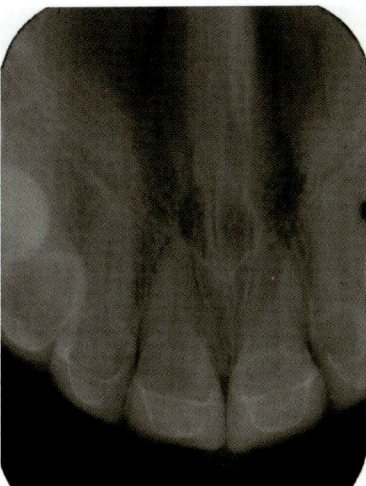
Fig. 6a: Pre-op x-ray, #8

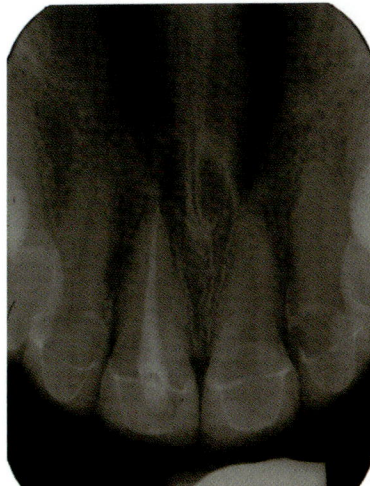
Fig. 6b: Post-op x-ray, #8

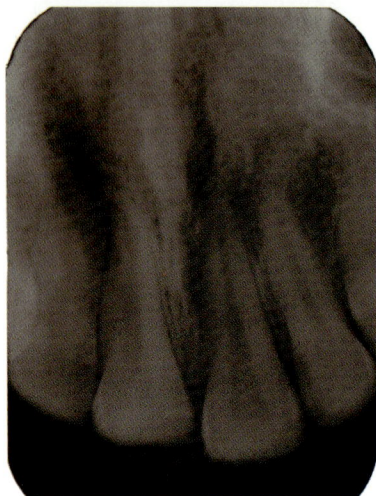

Fig. 7a: Pre-op x-ray, #8

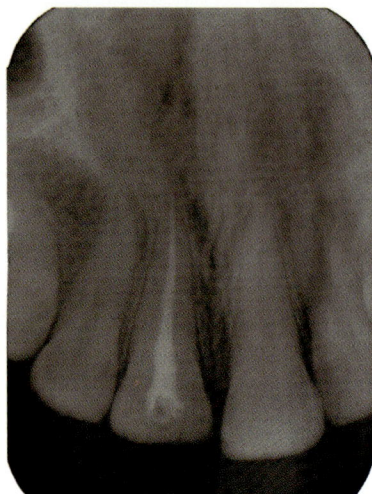

Fig. 7b: Post-op x-ray, #8

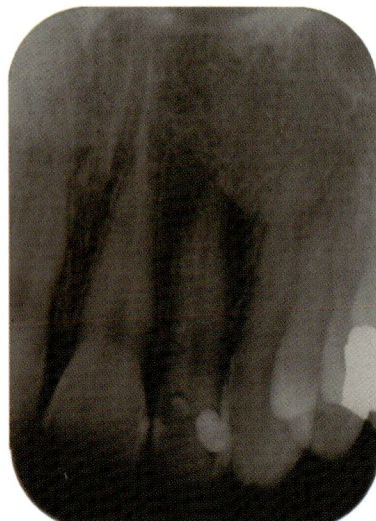

Fig. 8a: Pre-op x-ray, #10

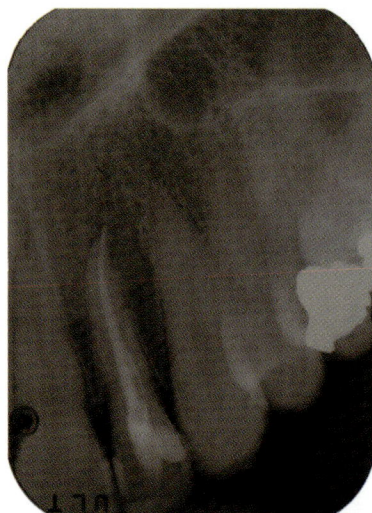

Fig. 8b: Post-op x-ray, #10

Bicuspid teeth:

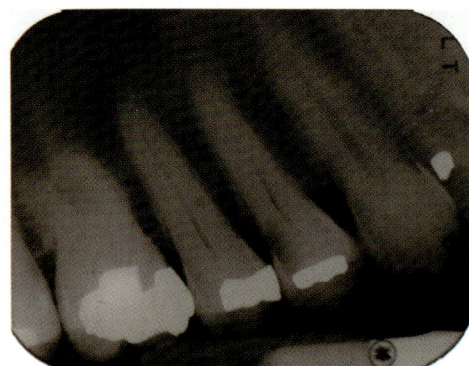

Fig. 9a: Pre-op x-ray, #5

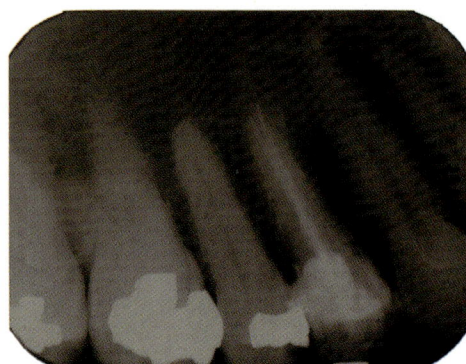

Fig. 9b: Post-op x-ray, #5

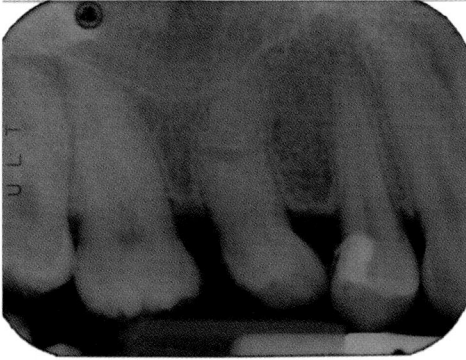

Fig. 10a: Pre-op x-ray, #5

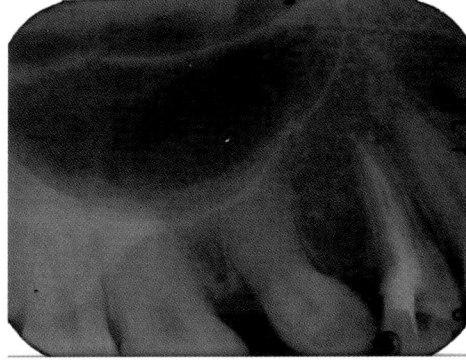

Fig. 10b: Post-op x-ray, #5

Posterior Teeth:

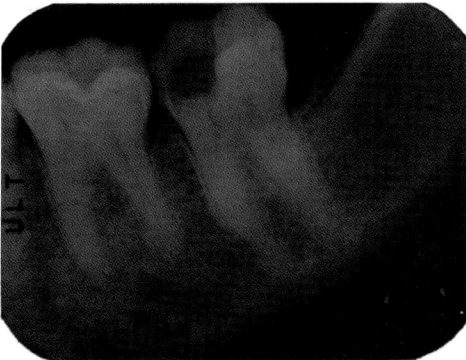

Fig. 11a: Pre-op x-ray, #18

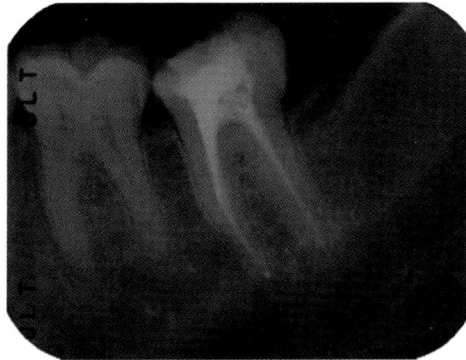

Fig. 11b: Post-op x-ray, #18

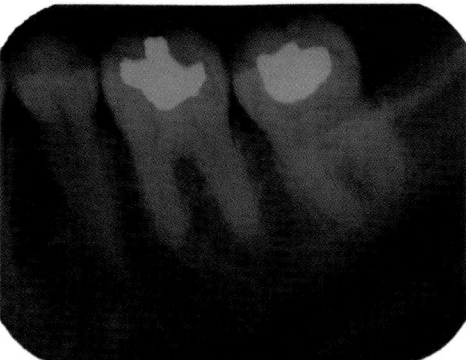

Fig. 12: Pre-op x-ray, #18

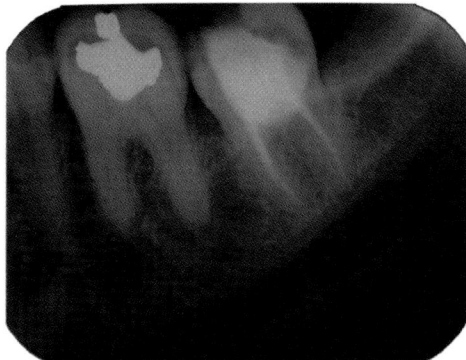

Fig. 12b: Post-op x-ray, #18

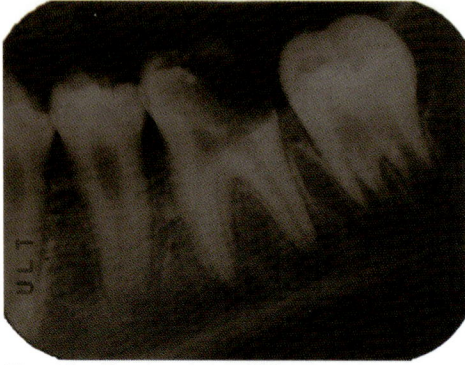

Fig. 13a: Pre-op x-ray, #19

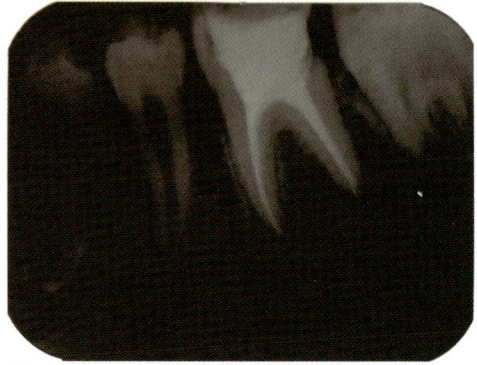

Fig. 13b: Post-op x-ray, #19

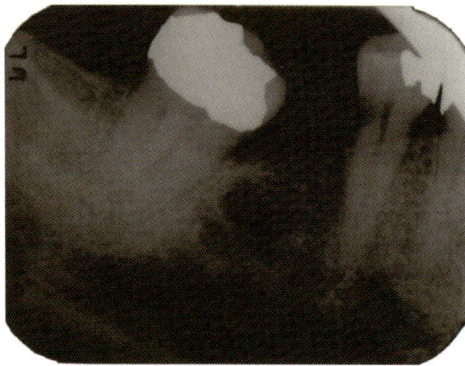

Fig. 14a: Pre-op x-ray, #31

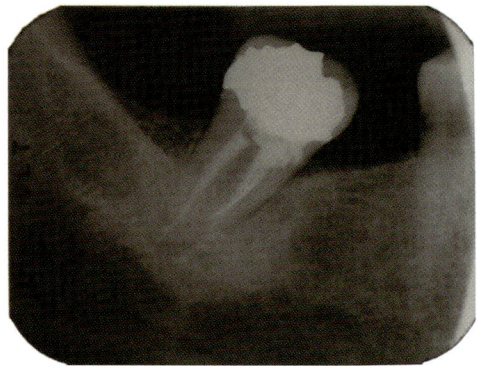

Fig. 14b: Post-op x-ray, #31

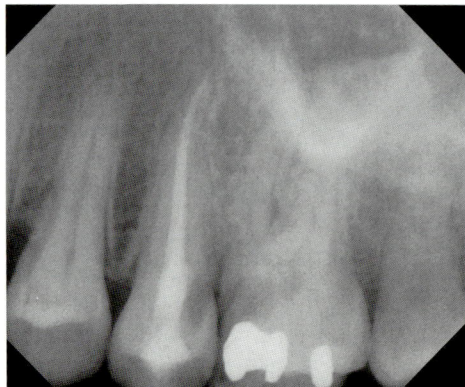

Fig. 15a: Pre-op x-ray, #14

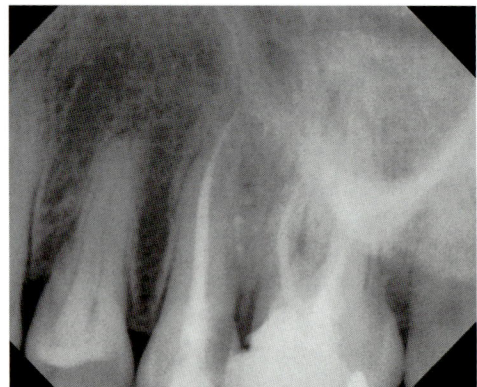

Fig. 15b: Post-op x-ray, #14

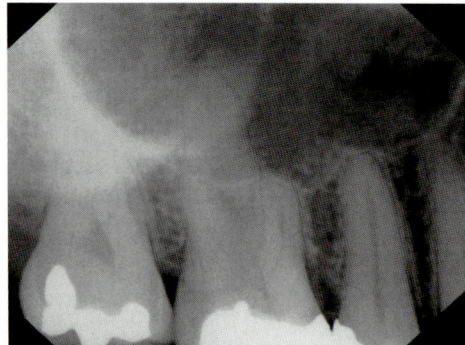

Fig. 16a: Pre-op x-ray, #3

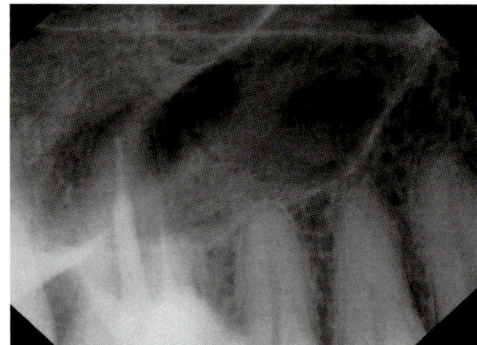

Fig. 16b: Post-op x-ray, #3

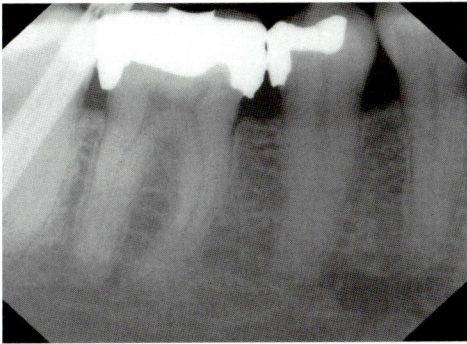

Fig. 17a:Pre-op x-ray, #30

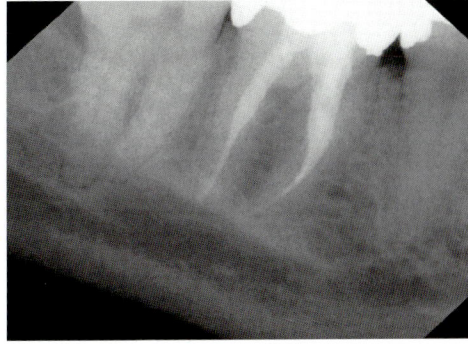

Fig. 17b: Post-op x-ray, #30

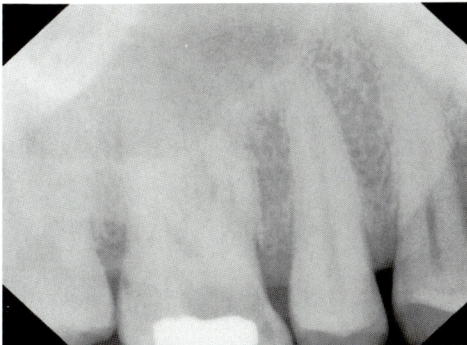

Fig. 18a: Pre-op x-ray, #3

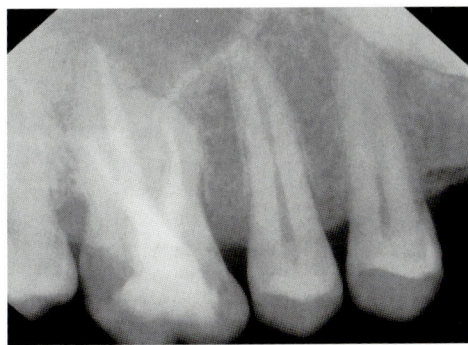

Fig. 18b: Post-op x-ray, #3

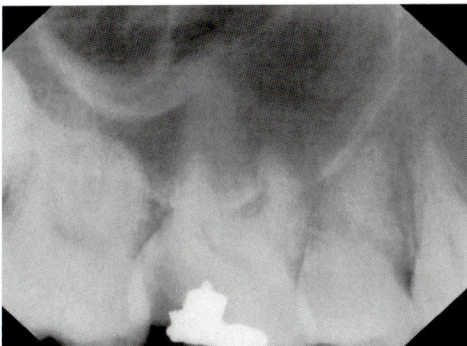

Fig. 19a: Pre-op x-ray, #3

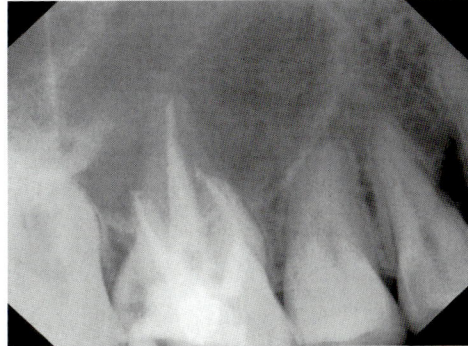

Fig. 19b: Post-op x-ray, #3

Periodontics

Introduction

Three common complaints from patients who undergo conventional periodontal root planing therapy are:

1.   Post-operative bleeding;
2.   Post-operative swelling; and
3.   Post-operative pain (which can sometimes last longer than seven days).

I have often heard patients say, "Had I known about these effects, I would not have gone ahead with the treatment." In conventional periodontal root planing therapy, patients are anesthetized using local anesthesia. The feeling of numbness lingers on for the rest of the day, causing dysfunction such as difficulty in speaking properly and difficulty in eating well.

During periodontal therapy, a sharp curette is used on the hard tissue side in order to remove calculus and plaque. Curettes have several disadvantages. Curettes remove healthy cementum, as well as diseased cementum. In addition, curettes open up dentinal tubules, resulting in patient complaints of sensitivity. The other side of sharp curettes remove granulation tissue from the pocket during the root planing procedure. The curettage and tearing of the soft tissue leads to histamine release, which results in bleeding, swelling, and pain. This is an experience that normally results from periodontal therapy.

Laser periodontal therapy, on the other hand presents a paradigm-shift from the conventional approach. Instead of using injection anesthesia, low-power laser analgesia is used. The patient experiences no needle and no immediate postoperative numbness or dysfunction. In laser periodontal therapy, light instrumentation by the Cavitron and curette therapy is used in order to remove calculus and plaque. However, the root planing and smoothing procedures are omitted from the procedure, thereby limiting the opening of dentinal tubules. The other side of the curette is dulled, so there is no concurrent curettage of the granulation tissue by a sharp instrument. In other words, there is no "tearing" of granulation tissue, and thus the patient experiences a reduced histamine release. As a result, there is less bleeding, less swelling and less pain. The granulation tissue will be surgically removed by the Er,Cr:YSGG laser system. Other advantages of using the Er,Cr:YSGG laser system for periodontal procedures include the "on-site" bactericidal effect at the treatment area, a reduced need for suturing, and the presence of low level laser therapy that reduces pain and promotes faster healing and faster regeneration.

There is also the option of performing some periodontal surgeries with a "closed flap" technique. In these closed-flap cases, "no shot, no pain" perio surgery can be performed. Depending on the severity of the disease, it may take multiple appointments to treat the moderate to advanced periodontitis. In this case, conventional open flap periodontal surgery may have an advantage: with open flap surgery, the case can be treated with one appointment for the surgery and another follow-up appointment for suture removal. As a result, patients do not need to schedule several appointments.

Patients should be well-educated on all of the pros and cons before choosing treatment that best suits each individual's need.

Closed-Flap Periodontal Therapy – Time Management

As a rule of thumb, you can expect to spend the following amounts of time on the different types of periodontal disease.

Type of Periodontal Disease	Duration of Procedure
Healthy (no inflammation)	1 hour
Type I Gingivitis	2-3 hours
Type II Beginning Periodontitis	2-4 hours
Type II-III Moderate Periodontitis	4-6 hours
Type III+ Advanced Periodontitis	6-8 hours
Type IV+ Severe Periodontitis	8-12 hours
Continual Care / Retreatment	1 hour

The impact of treatment on each patient will vary, depending on the patient's response to treatment as well as the patient's dietary habits. I find that the following flowchart explains the process of treatment quite well:

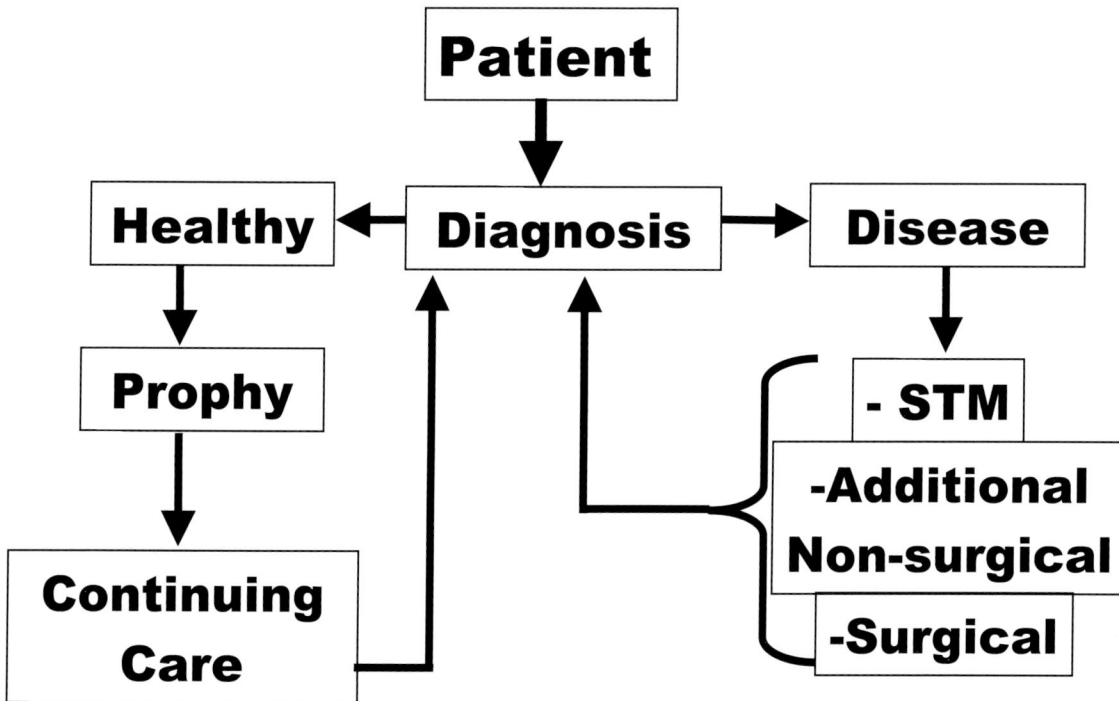

Throughout the clinical treatments described in this chapter, please refer to the following diagrams to assist you in the procedures.

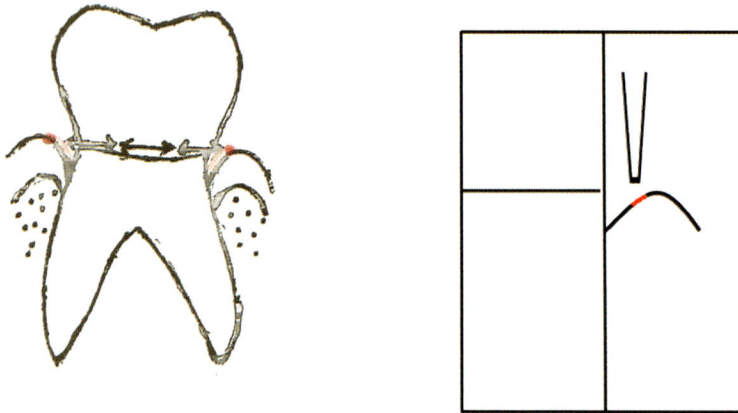

Fig. 1: The tip is aimed at the ablating diseased epithelium at the upper third (marginal gingiva) of the pocket.

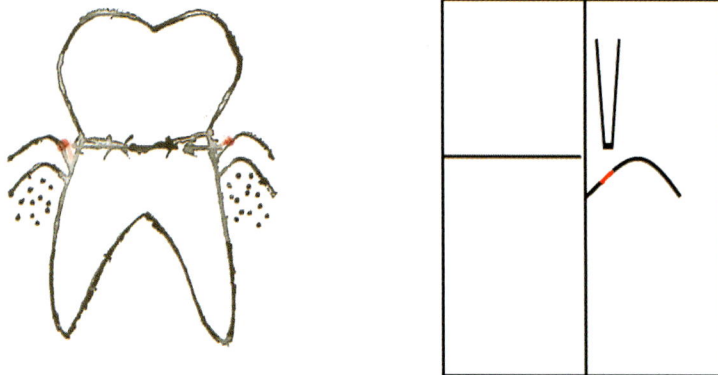

Fig. 2: The tip is aimed at the ablating diseased epithelium at the middle third of the pocket.

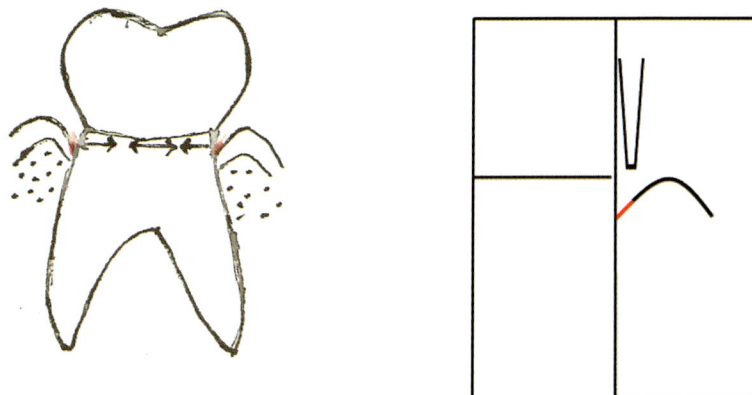

Fig. 3: The tip is aimed at ablating diseased epithelium at the basal third of the pocket. Special care must be taken to avoid violating the integrity of the basal area.

Closed Flap Er,Cr:YSGG Periodontal Therapy
(Minimally Invasive Periodontal Therapy)

In a typical laser periodontal appointment, the protocol for minimally-invasive closed flap therapy includes the following procedures:

- Laser analgesia
- Ultrasonic scaling
- Light hand instrumentation as needed
- Laser debridement and decontamination
- More ultrasonic scaling and light hand instrumentation (as needed)
- More laser debridement and decontamination
- Laser gingivectomy (removing granulation tissue inside the pocket)
- Laser de-epithelilization (similar to guided tissue regeneration in periodontal surgery) (see chapter on de-epithelilization)
- Antimicrobial irrigation
- Post-operative instructions / home-care instructions

Laser Parameters, Set 1: Pre-Conditioning (Laser Analgesia)

Waterlase MD laser system settings: MG-6 tip, 0.25W, 20% Water, 20% Air, 30 Hz
Other Er,Cr:YSGG laser system settings: G-6 tip, 0.25W, 15% Water, 15% Air

> Instead of using injection anesthesia, a low-power laser is used to prepare a quadrant of teeth for root planning.

> The procedure is similar to preparing the tooth for placement of rubber dams and clamp, placing amalgam restorations, performing pulpotomy without local anesthesia, or performing root canal therapy without local anesthesia. The low-power laser energy is applied to the cervical-sulcus area. The laser analgesia is applied to both the inner lining of gingiva and the cementum. The application should take approximately 15-30 seconds per site.

> (Note: Anterior teeth and bicuspids have two sites: buccal and lingual. An average molar has four sites: mesio-buccal, disto-buccal, mesio-lingual, and disto-lingual, and a large molar has six sites: three sites on the buccal and three on the lingual.)

> Calculus and plaque are removed by light instrumentation by using Cavitron and curettes (only the tooth side of the curette is sharpened). Do not smooth the root surface and do not remove granulation tissue.

Laser Parameters, Set 2: Debridement and Decontamination

Waterlase MD laser system settings: 0.75-1.25W, 9-11% Water, 11% Air, 30Hz, H mode
Other Er,Cr:YSGG laser system settings: 1.00W, 9% Water, 11% Air

Laser energy is then used to remove granulation tissue on the soft tissue side of the pocket. (Note: Adjust the parameters to provide the best result on the tissue and the maximum patient's comfort. As with other procedures in this book, always start at the lowest power setting and, if ablation is too slow, work your way up in 0.25W increments every 30 seconds of laser treatment.)

Place the tip, angled a little from being parallel to the long axis of the tooth, with the tip aimed at the gingiva. Since the laser cut is very shallow and ablates in a linear fashion, granulation tissue can be removed a small amount at a time. The laser gingival curettage (or gingivectomy) is performed a segment at a time. The tip is moved quickly in a back-and-forth motion, starting at the gingival crest position. After removing granulation tissue at the marginal gingival, it is easier to visually inspect the middle portion of the pocket. (See diagram.) After removing the granulation tissue from the middle region, the basal tissue can be evaluated. Then proceed to finish the gingivectomy at the basal region. Be careful when the fiber tip is near the base of the pocket. Do leave the tip in this area for too long, in order to avoid removing any attachment tissue. For pockets greater than 4mm where there is possible attachment loss and bone loss, the laser can be used to perform a de-epithelialization procedure in order to aim at regeneration of ligaments and bone from the connective tissue.

Laser Parameters, Set 3: Debridement, Decontamination and Low-Level Laser Therapy

Waterlase MD laser system settings: MG-6 tip, 0.25W, 9-11% Water, 11% Air, 30 Hz, H mode
Other Er,Cr:YSGG laser system settings: G-6 tip, 0.25W, 9% Water, 11% Air

Move the fiber tip in a horizontal, back-and-forth direction in the periodontal pocket. This procedure is aimed at debridement, cleaning and decontamination of periodontal pocket. This is followed by flushing out debris using an irrigation syringe filled with Chlorhexidine or Tetracycline.

In subsequent treatments, unresolved pockets will be treated again with a similar approach described above, until all pockets are eliminated.

Case 1: An Example of Treatment for Type II Periodontal Disease

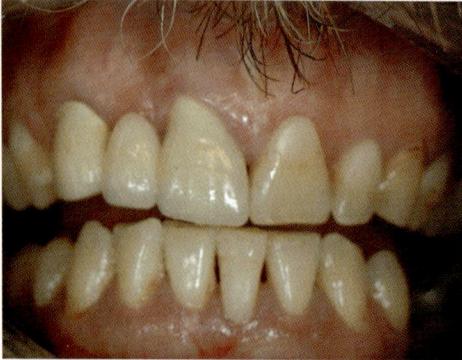
Fig. 1: Pre-op. Frontal view.

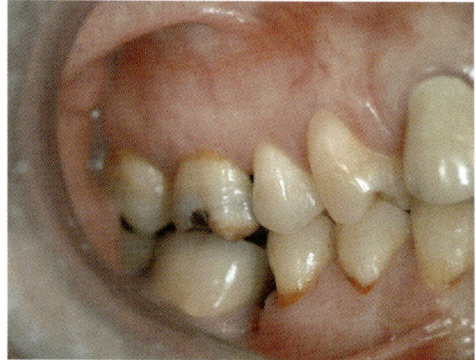
Fig. 2: Pre-op. View of right side.

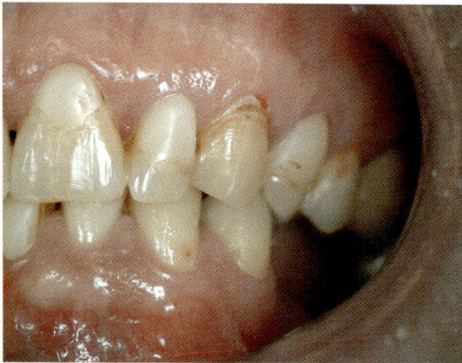
Fig. 3: Pre-op. View of left side.

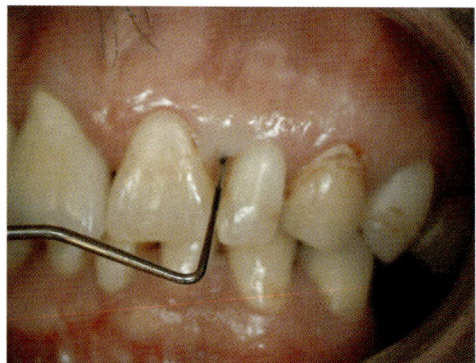
Fig. 4: #10, mesio-facial pocket showing a 5mm pocket.

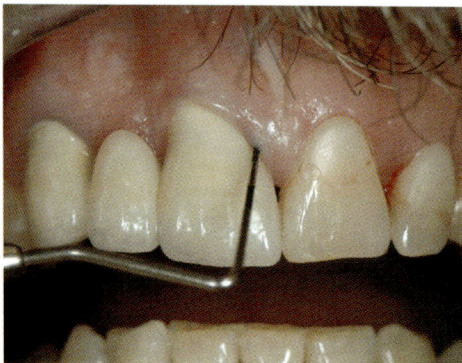
Fig. 5: # 8, mesio-facial pocket showing a 4mm pocket.

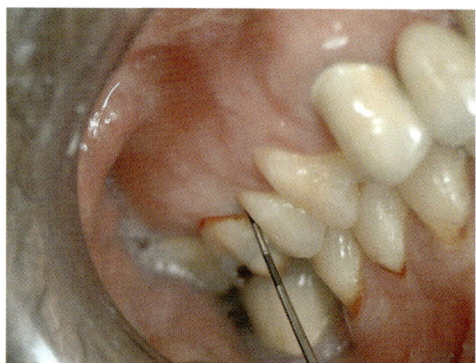
Fig. 6: #3, mesio-buccal pocket showing a 4mm pocket.

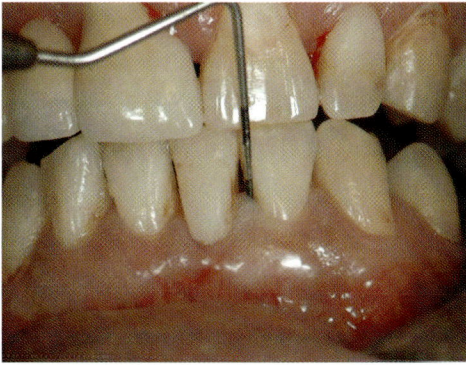

Fig. 7: #23, mesio-facial pocket.

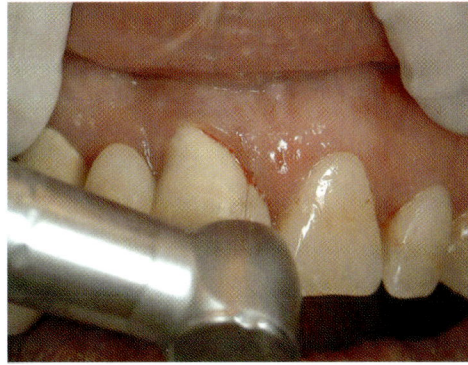

Fig. 8: After light instrumentation using Cavitron® and curettes, laser energy is used to perform a closed-flap periodontal surgery. A G-6 tip (or Z-6 or C-6) is used with the M-2 Waterlase for periodontal gingivectomy. The setting is 1.00W, 9% Water, 11% Air. A similar technique is used to remove granulation tissue, debride and decontaminate the pockets.

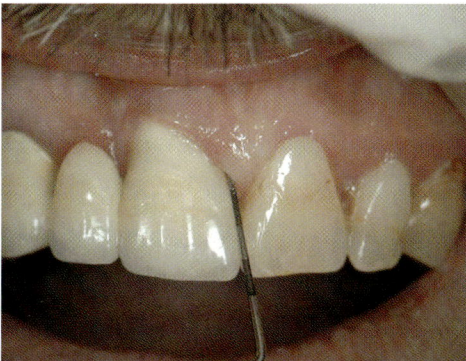

Fig. 9: Post-op, approximately 6 weeks. # 8, mesio-facial showing a 2mm sulcus and healthy gingiva.

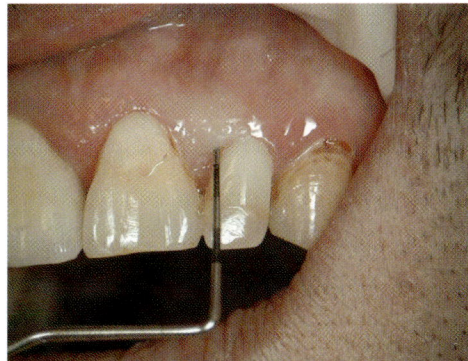

Fig. 10: Post-op, approximately 6 weeks. #10, mesio-facial showing a 2mm sulcus and healthy gingiva.

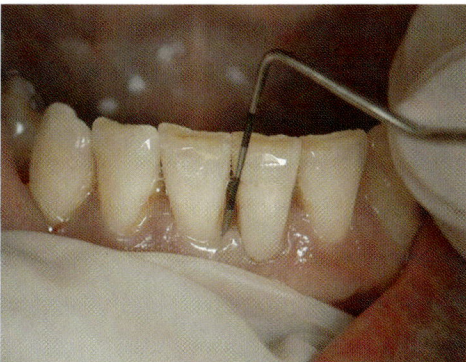

Fig. 11: Post-op, approximately 6 weeks. #24, mesio-facial showing a 2mm sulcus and healthy gingival.

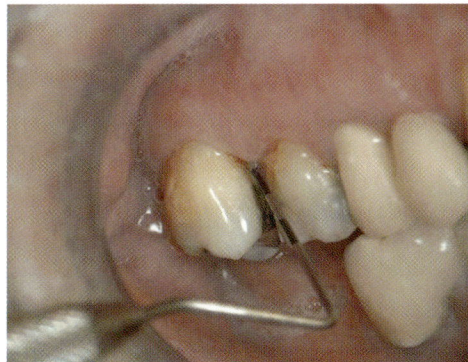

Fig. 12: Post-op, approximately 6 weeks. #2, mesio-facial showing a 2mm sulcus and healthy gingiva.

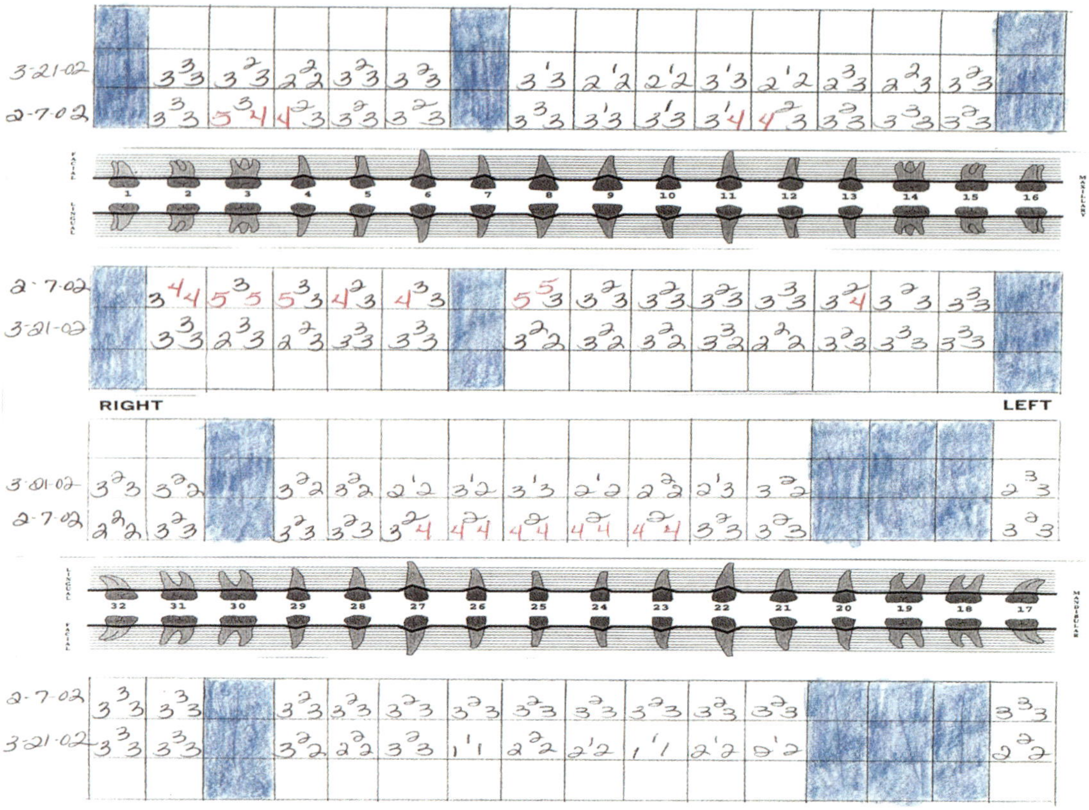

Fig. 13: Chart

Case 2: Type III Periodontal Disease, Treatment of Mandibular Right Quadrant

Below is a typical appointment of a Type III periodontal disease treatment (an example of treatment to one quadrant of teeth with generalized Type III periodontal disease).

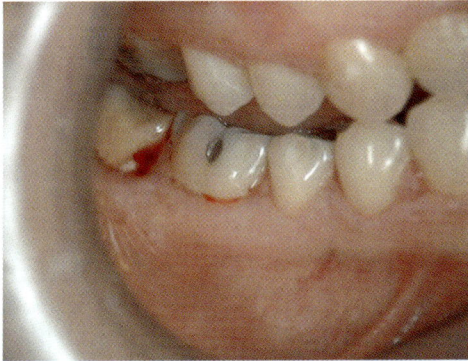

Fig. 1: Pre-op. Type III periodontal disease is diagnosed on the mandibular right quadrant, showing attachment loss and bone loss.

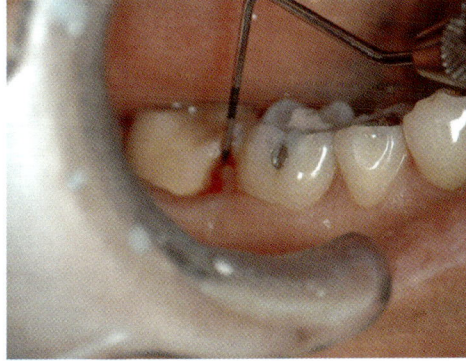

Fig. 2: A 5mm periodontal pocket is noted at the mesio-buccal corner of tooth #31.

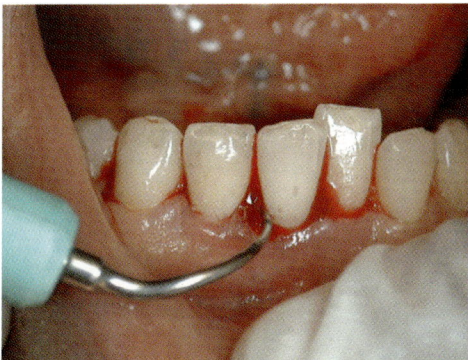

Fig. 3: After laser analgesia is applied to all periodontal pockets in the mandibular right quadrant, using a G-6 tip with a setting of 0.25W, 15% Water, 15% Air, 15-30 seconds per site, light instrumentation is used to remove calculus and plaque by Cavitron® and curettes.

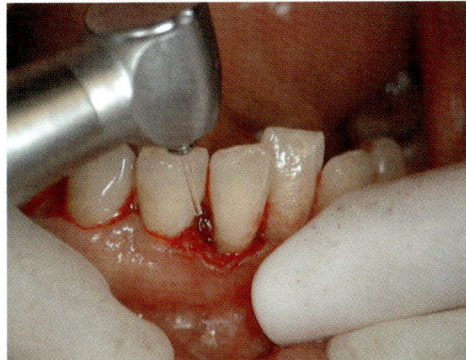

Fig. 4: Laser gingivectomy is used to remove diseased epithelium in the periodontal pockets. The setting is 1.00W, 9% Water, 11% Air. This is followed by laser de-epithelialization (outside periodontal pockets). The setting is same as laser gingivectomy.

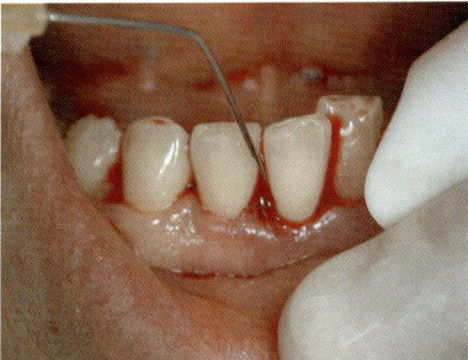

Fig. 5: Irrigation is performed by using

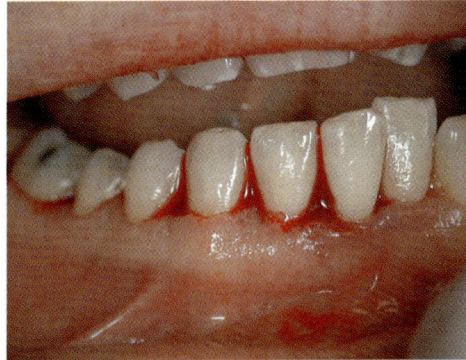

Fig. 6: Immediate post-op of the anterior teeth.

chlorhexidine in a syringe.

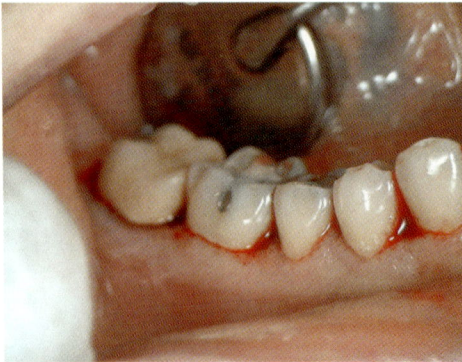

Fig. 7: Immediate post-op of the posterior teeth.

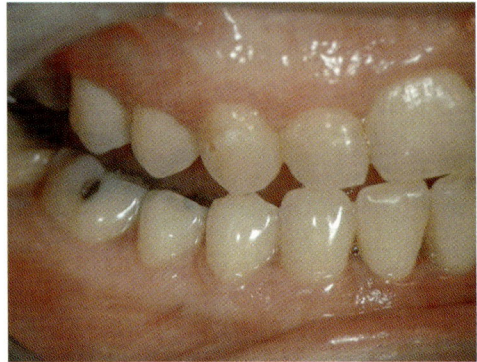

Fig. 8: Post-op, approximately 1.5 months, showing a healthy periodontal condition.

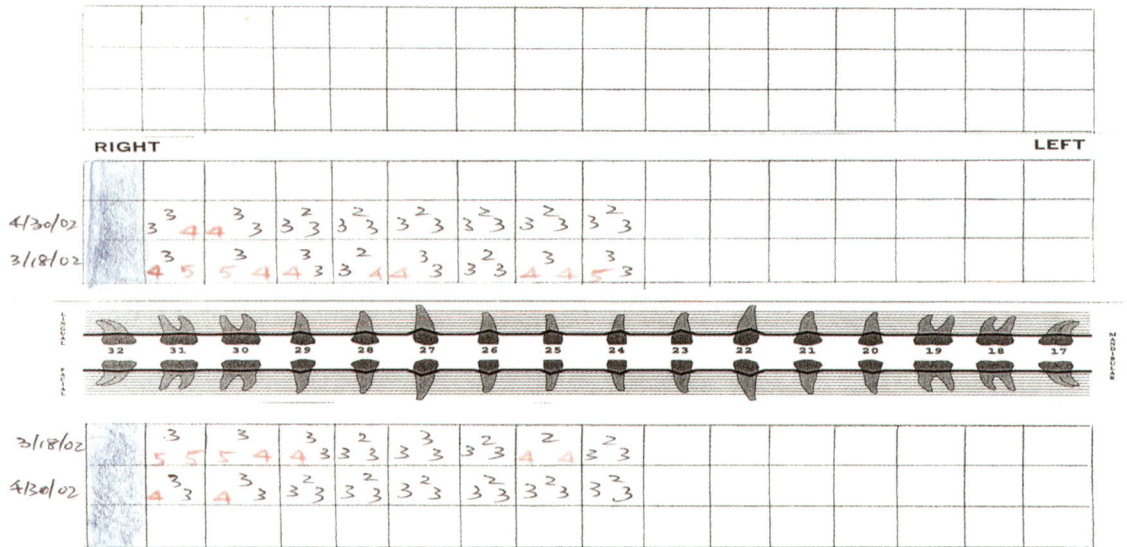

Fig. 9: Chart.

Case 3: Type III Periodontal Disease Therapy of All Four Quadrants

Below is an example of laser-assisted periodontal surgery (closed-flap) on four quadrants of late Type III periodontal disease. Laser procedures, as well as the timing of techniques, are discussed below.

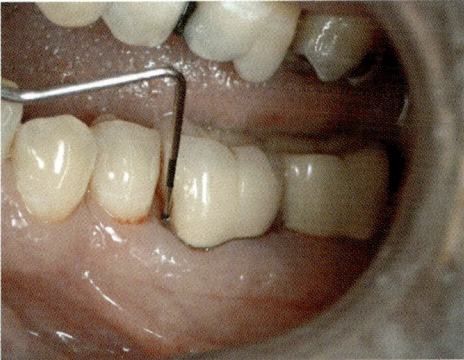

Fig. 1: Pre-op. 6mm pocket is noted at the mesio-buccal area of #19.

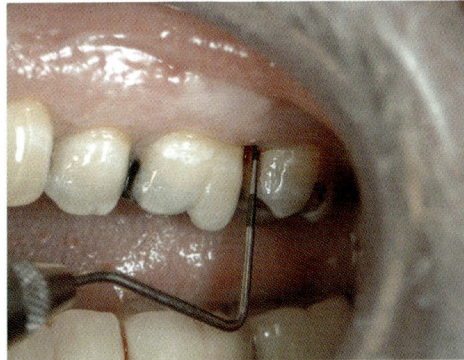

Fig. 2: Pre-op. 5mm pocket is noted at the disto-buccal area of #14.

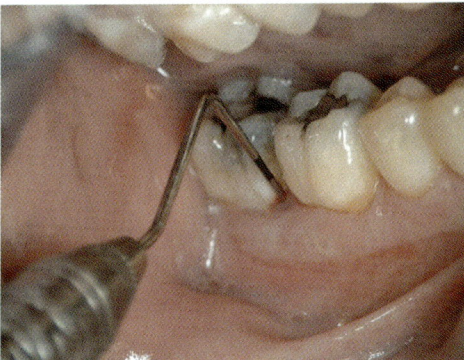

Fig. 3: Pre-op. 5mm pocket is noted at the mesio-buccal area of #31.

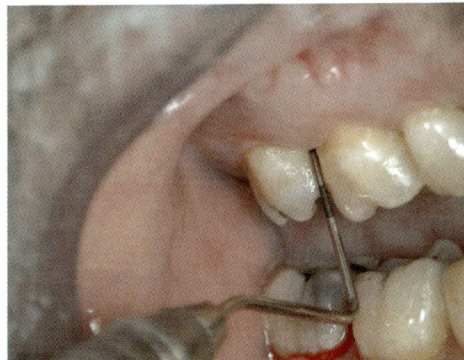

Fig. 4: Pre-op. 6mm pocket is noted at the disto-buccal area of #3.

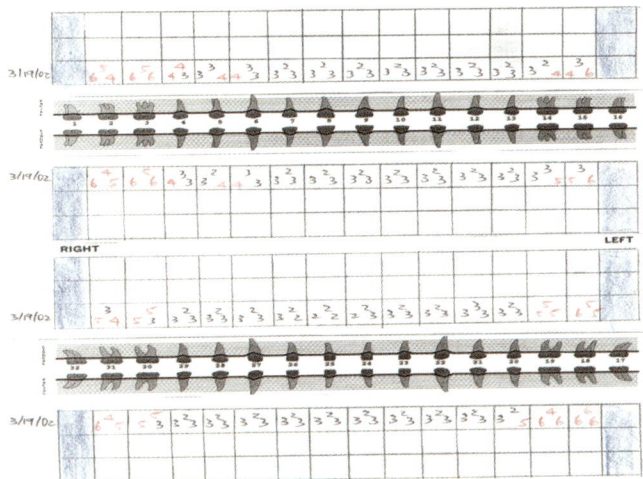

Fig. 5: Pre-op periodontal charting of this late Type III periodontal disease case.

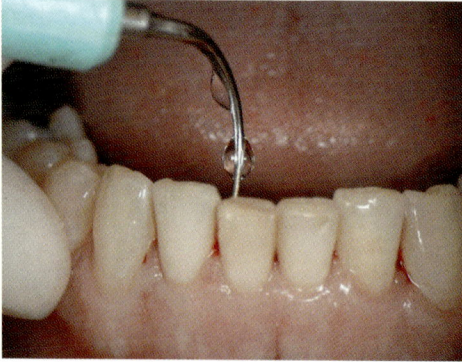

Fig. 6: In the first appointment after laser analgesia has completed for the mandibular right quadrant (using a G-6 tip, 0.25W, 15% Water, 15% Air, 15-30 seconds per site), light instrumentation is used to remove calculus and plaque. Cavitron and curettes are used.

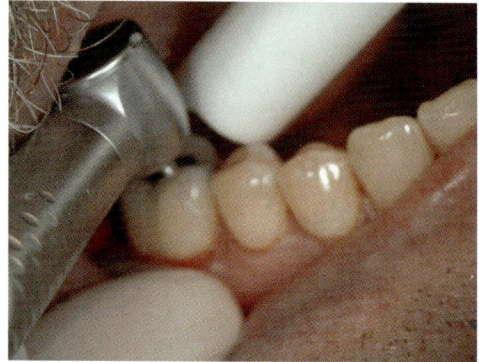

Fig. 7: Laser gingivectomy and de-epithelialization are being performed to remove diseased epithelium, using a G-6 tip. The setting is 1.00W, 9% Water, 11% Air.

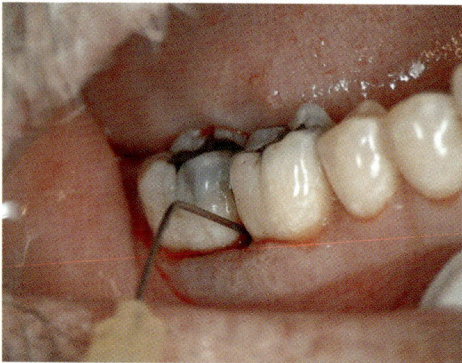

Fig. 8: Irrigation of the treated pockets is done with a chlorhexidine rinse in a syringe. The first appointment has been completed.

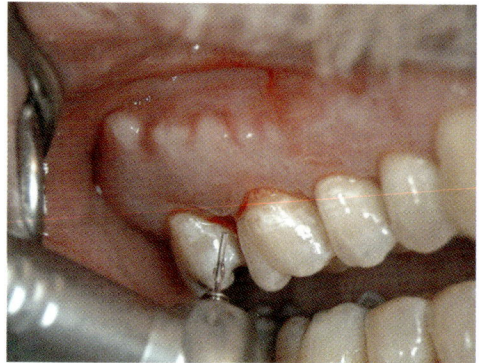

Fig. 9: In the second appointment, similar protocol as used in the first appointment is followed in the maxillary right quadrant. "Touch up" treatment is performed on the mandibular right quadrant.

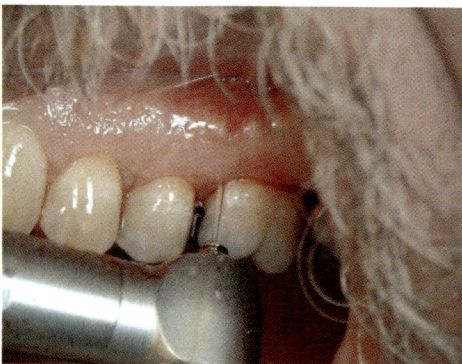

Fig. 10: In the third appointment, similar protocol as used in the first appointment is followed in the maxillary left quadrant. "Touch up" is performed on mandibular right and maxillary right quadrants.

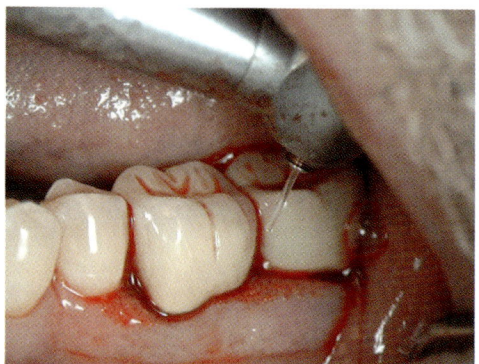

Fig. 11: In the fourth appointment, similar protocol as used in the first appointment is followed in the mandibular left quadrant. "Touch up" is performed on the other previously treated quadrants.

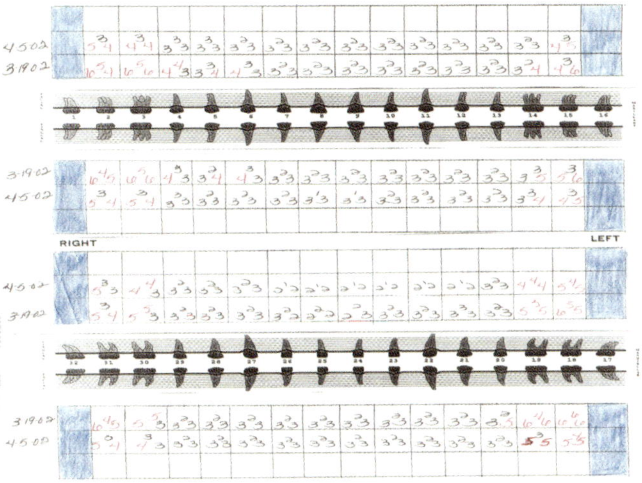

Fig. 12: Perio chart showing progress.

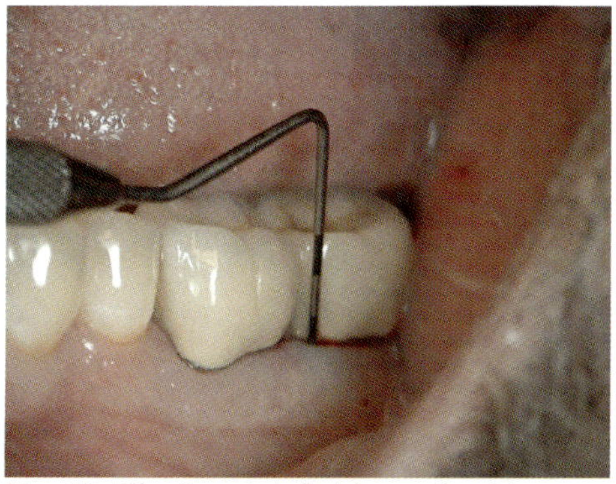

Fig. 13: The 6mm pocket is resolved to a 3mm healthy sulcus.

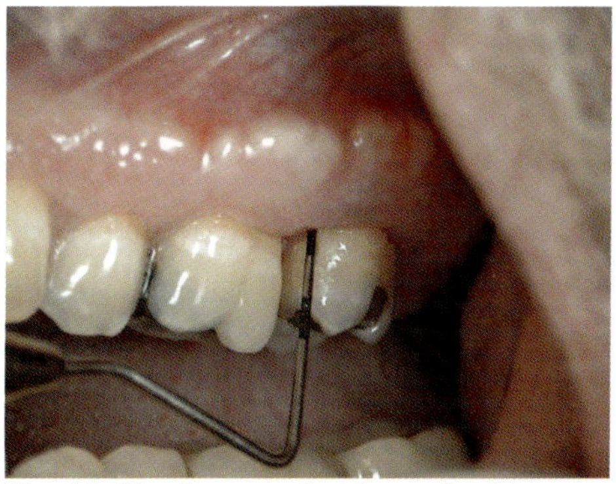

Fig. 14: The 5mm pocket is resolved to a 2.5mm healthy sulcus.

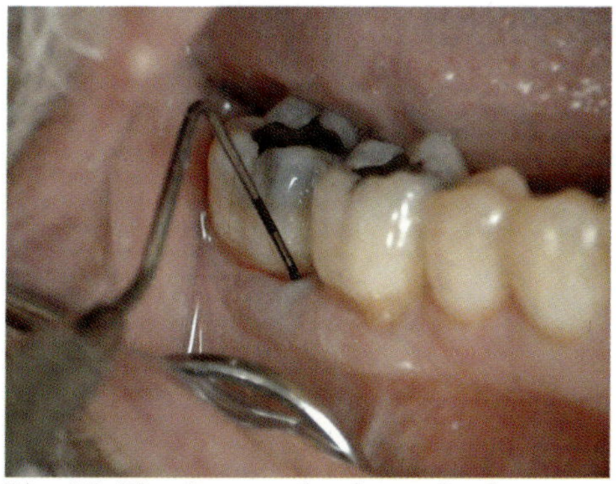

Fig. 15: The 5mm pocket is resolved to a 3mm healthy sulcus.

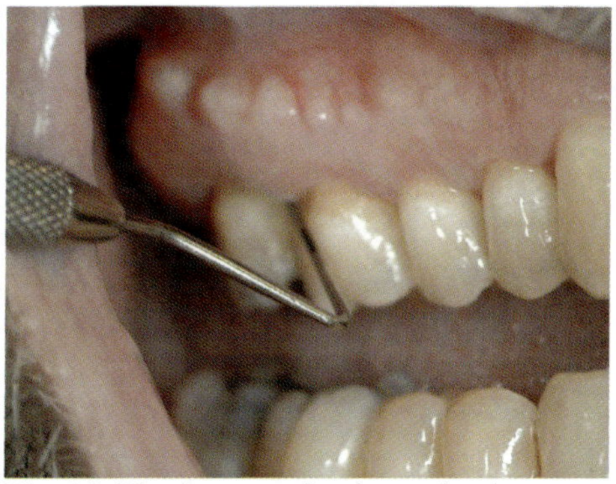

Fig. 16: The 6mm pocket is resolved to a 3mm healthy sulcus.

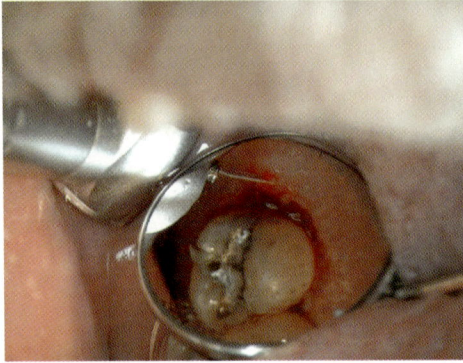

Fig. 17: In the fifth appointment, distal wedge periodontal surgery is performed at #15 using a MC-6 (9mm). The setting is 1.50W, 7% Water, 11% Air.

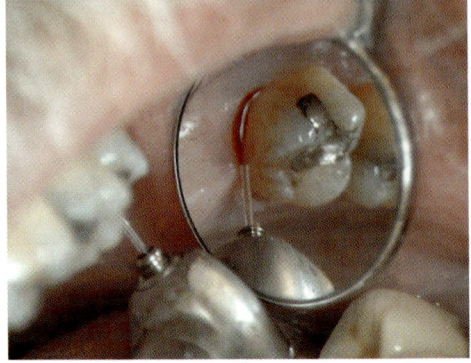

Fig. 18: The laser gingivectomy extends to disto-lingual area of #15.

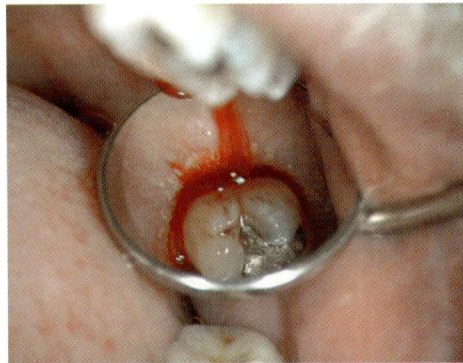

Fig. 19: Immediate post-op after distal wedge periodontal surgery at the distal of #15.

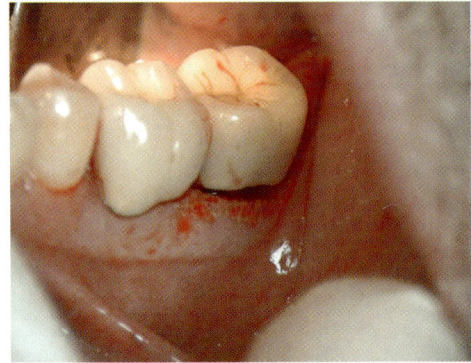

Fig. 20: In the fifth appointment, distal wedge periodontal surgery is also performed at #18.

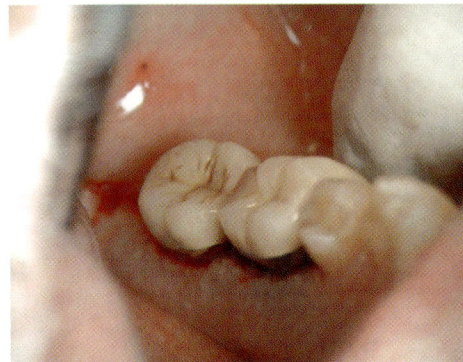

Fig. 21: In the sixth appointment, distal wedge periodontal surgery is performed at #31 using similar protocol as in Fig. 18.

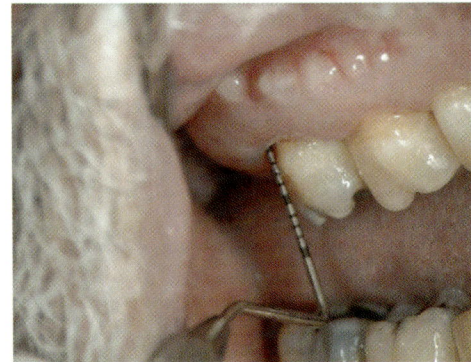

Fig. 22: Four weeks post-op showing healthy gingiva in the maxillary right quadrant.

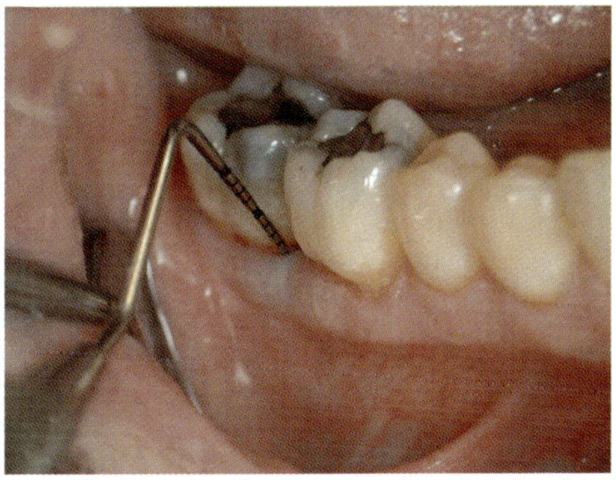

Fig. 23: Four weeks post-op showing healthy gingiva in the mandibular right quadrant.

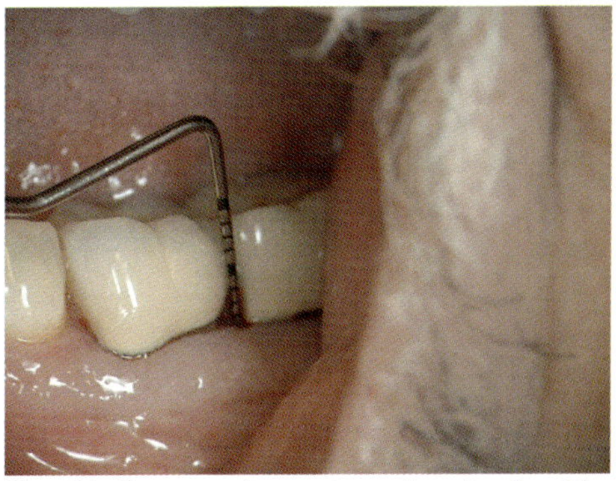

Fig. 24: Four weeks post-op showing healthy gingiva in the mandibular left quadrant.

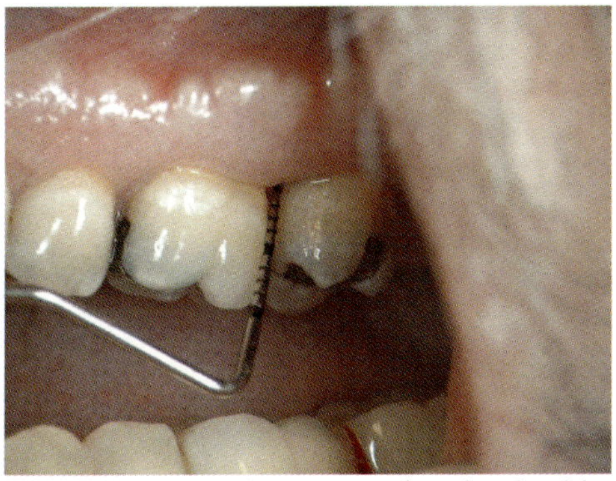

Fig. 25: Four weeks post-op showing healthy gingiva in the maxillary left quadrant.

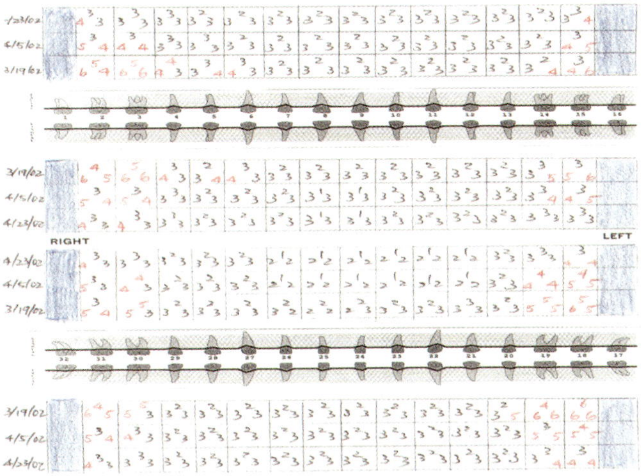

Fig. 26: Perio chart showing progress.

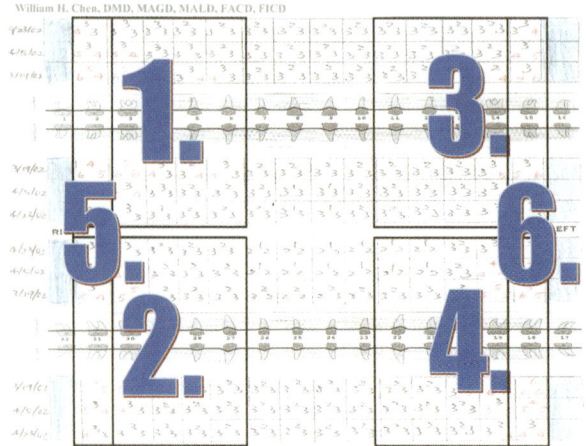

Fig. 27: The numbered blocks represent appointments. For the first appointment, use the protocol described in Fig. 6-8. For the second appointment, follow similar protocol as used in the maxillary right quadrant. "Touch up" treatment is performed on appointment site one. For the third appointment, use protocol in the maxillary left quadrant. "Touch up" is performed appointment sites one and two. In the fourth appointment, follow similar protocol as used in the mandibular left quadrant. "Touch up" is performed on the other previously treated quadrants. In the fifth appointment, distal wedge periodontal surgery is performed at #15 and #18. In the sixth appointment, distal wedge periodontal surgery is performed at #31 and #2.

De-Epithelialization

This concept is developed based on the success of guided tissue regeneration (GTR), in which a membrane is placed in the surgically-treated pocket to keep the epithelial cells from growing down into the pocket and forming a long junction epithelium. When this happens, there is no connective tissue regrowth. The membrane serves as a barrier to the epithelial tissue, allowing time for the connective tissues to regenerate periodontal ligament, cementum and bone to the previously diseased root surfaces.

Laser de-epithelialization is used to prevent epithelium from growing. This allows time for the connective tissue to regenerate periodontal ligaments, cementum, and bone to the root surface.

Laser energy can be used to de-epithelialize periodontal pockets over 4mm in depth.

Laser Parameters, Set 1: De-Epithelialization

Waterlase MD laser system settings: MG-6 tip, 1.00-1.50W, 7% Water, 11% Air, 30 Hz
Other Er,Cr:YSGG laser system settings: G-6 tip, 0.75-1.25W, 7% Water, 11% Air

> The surface ablation of the gingiva is extended 4-5mm outside the pocket. An added benefit of this setting is that it also offers a biostimulation effect. Since de-epithelialization is conducted with a low-power laser setting, it also serves as a LLLT on the gingiva that will result post-operative pain attenuation and more rapid wound healing.

> To finish the root planing therapy, chlorhexidine is used to irrigate the treated pockets. No suturing is required. Post-operative instructions should include the following, if you do not already include these in your recommendations:
> 1. Do not brush your teeth for 24 hours.
> 2. Do not eat anything spicy, messy or sharp for 24 hours.
> 3. Do not rinse your mouth with alcohol-based mouthwash for 24 hours.
> 4. Resume normal activities, including good oral hygiene, after 24 hours.

The patient should return for a follow-up visit in 2-3 weeks. Another quadrant of pockets will be treated, and touch-up treatment should be given to pockets that have not been resolved from the previous treatment. Deeper pockets may require additional gingivectomy and de-epithelialization. It can take several appointments to treat advanced pockets. The time management of the closed-flap approach needs to be planned well in order to maximize the efficiency of each appointment.

Case 1: Type IV Periodontal Disease Therapy, Site specific

The following case used the Er,Cr:YSGG to debride, decontaminate and de-epithelialize the epithelium. The therapy was successful in reducing 8mm pockets to a size of 3mm and restoring healthy periodontal tissue with formation of new attachment.

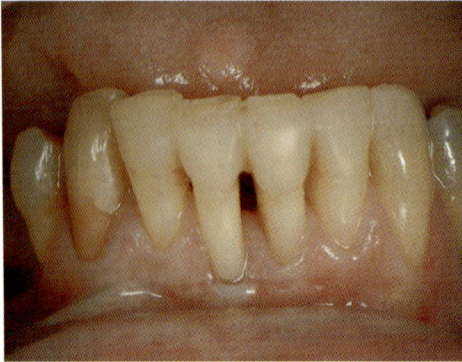

Fig. 1: Pre-op #24 and #25 show severe periodontitis with severe recession and mobility.

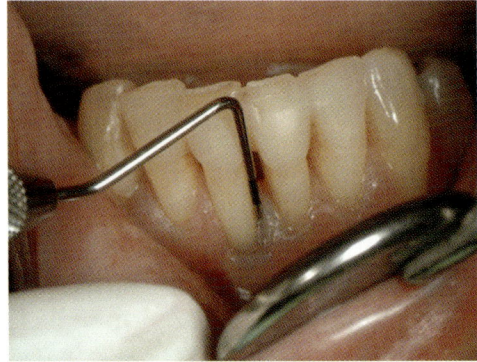

Fig. 2: 8.5mm pocket is present at the mesio-facial area of #25. Two and a half wall defect noted in #25.

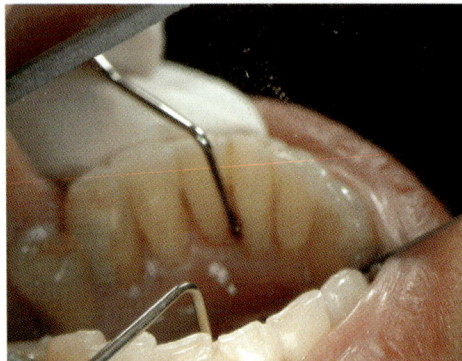

Fig. 3: 6.5mm pocket is present at the disto-lingual area of #24. Two and a half wall defect is noted in #24.

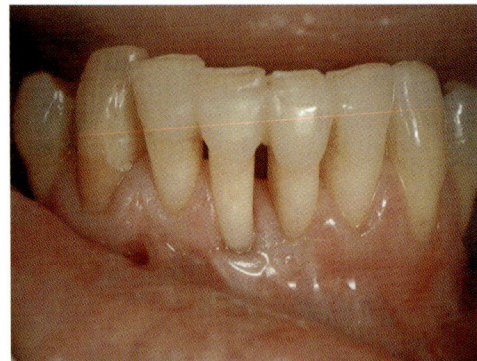

Fig. 4: After calculus and plaque are removed, laser gingivectomy is used to remove diseased epithelium in the pockets and de-epithelialize outside the pocket. A G-6 tip is used with a setting of 1.00W, 9% Water, 11% Air.

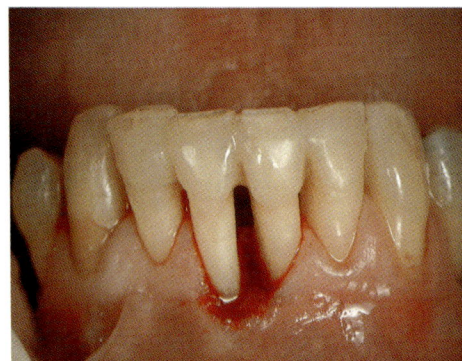

Fig. 5: Immediate post-op after laser gingivectomy and de-epithelialization.

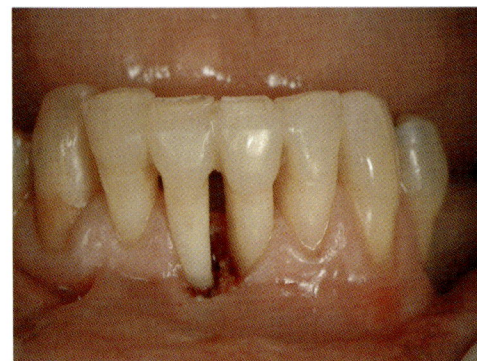

Fig. 6: One week post-op. The surgical site is healing.

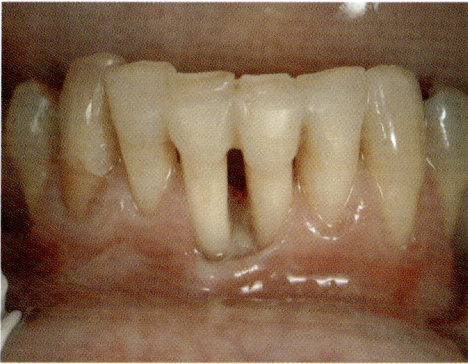

Fig. 7: Three weeks post-op. Some down growth of epithelial tissue is noted.

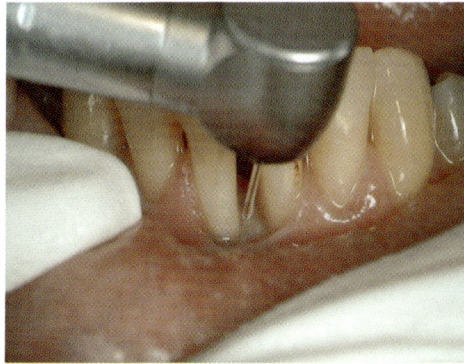

Fig. 8: Laser gingivectomy and de-epithelialization is repeated using same setting as in Fig. 4.

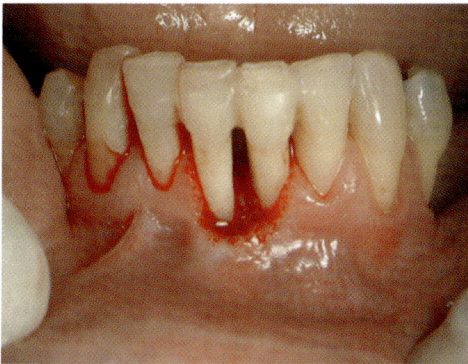

Fig. 9: Immediate post-op after the second laser periodontal surgery (closed-flap). Similar surgery is repeated two more times at two-week intervals.

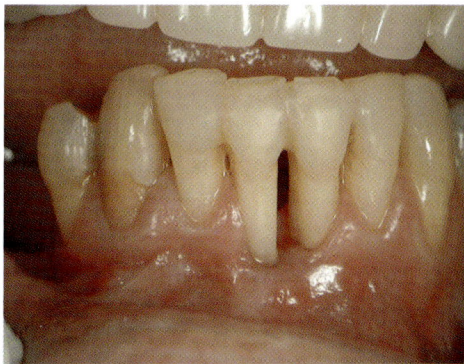

Fig. 10: Four weeks after the fourth periodontal surgery, the periodontal tissue of # 24 and #25 appears healthy.

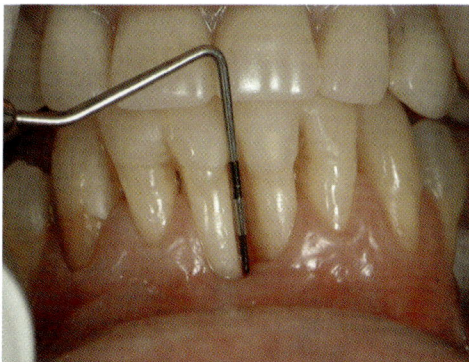

Fig. 11: 18 months post-op. 2.5mm sulcus is present at the mesio-facial area.

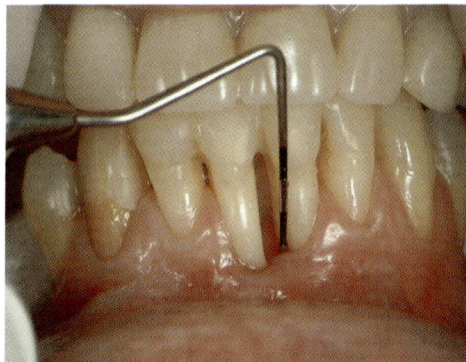

Fig. 12: 18 months post-op. 2.5mm sulcus is present at the mesio-facial area.

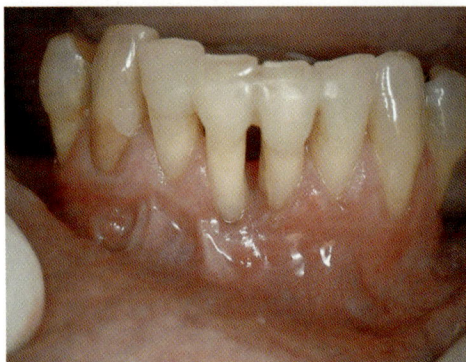

Fig. 13: 18 months post-op. Healthy
periodontal condition is present.

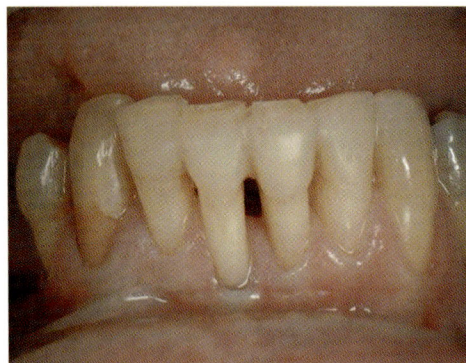

Fig. 14a: Pre-op condition

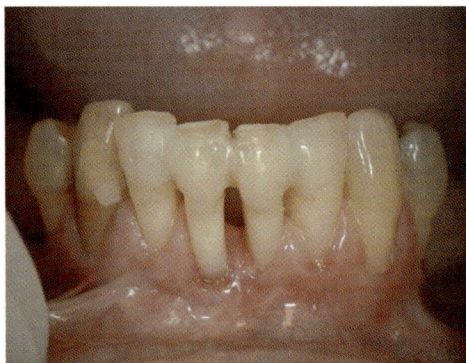

Fig. 14b: Post-op condition at 18 months.

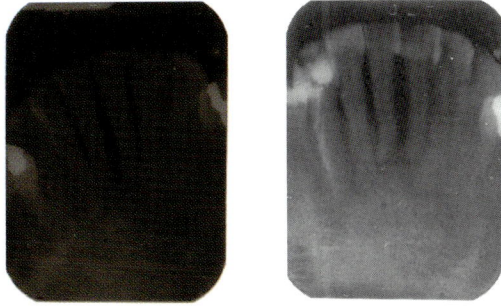

Fig. 15: Pre-op and 18 months post-op X-rays. New bone and new attachment are found to be present #24 and #25. The laser- assisted periodontal surgery (closed-flap) is successful in a seemingly hopeless case.

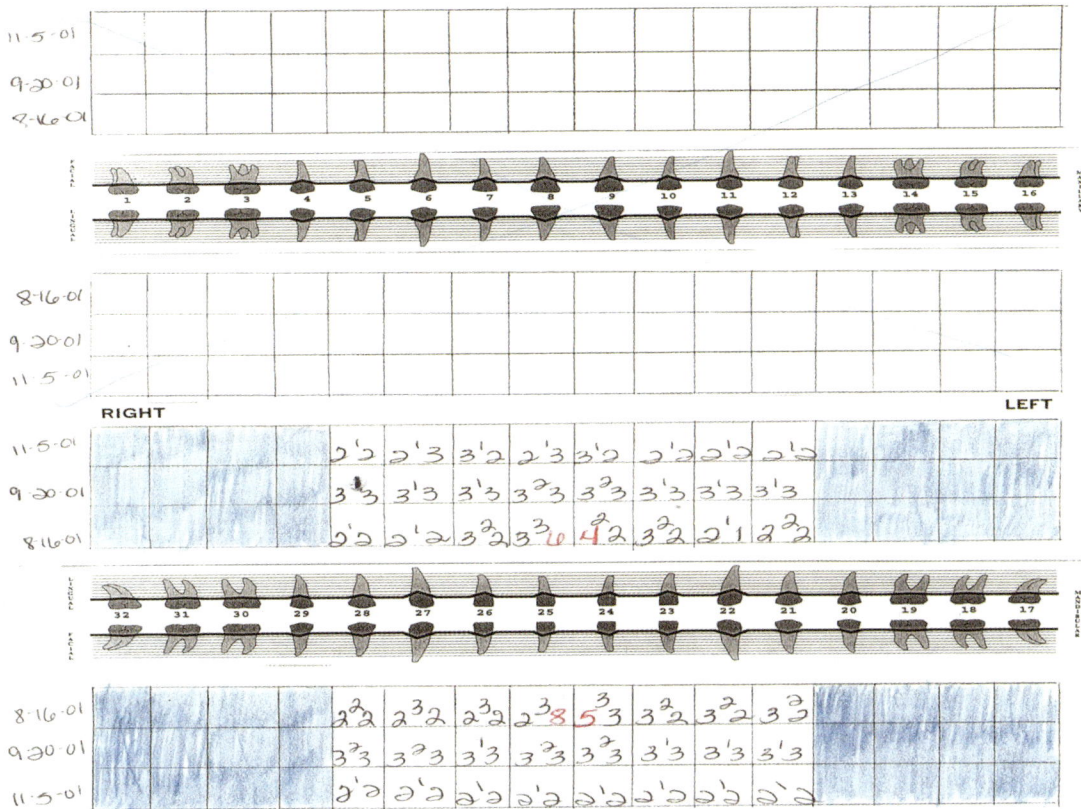

Fig. 16: Periodontal charting pre and post treatment.

Mandibular Molar Furcation Therapy
Using Er,Cr:YSGG and Enamel Matrix Derivative

Laser energy is used here for partial incision of flap, removing granulation tissues, debridement and decontamination of the furcation area and LLLT. An enamel matrix derivative (EMD) will serve as a biologic regenerative material and is used in this procedure instead of bone graft and membrane barrier. EMD promotes regeneration of cementum, connective tissue attachment and bone regeneration.

Laser Parameters, Set 1: Incision of Flap

Waterlase MD laser system settings: MT-4 tip, 2.00W, 7% Water, 11% Air, 30 Hz
Other Er,Cr:YSGG laser system settings: T-4 tip, 1.25-1.50W, 7% Water, 11% Air

Use the laser to perform an incision of flap. While the laser should be your first choice of tool, there may be occasions where access is limited and esthetic is critical. In these situations, it may be preferable to use a #12 scalpel.

After reflecting the mucogingival tissue, Cavitron® and periodontal surgical curettes are used to remove calculus and plaque on the root and in the furcation area.

Laser Parameters, Set 2: Remove Granulation Tissue

Waterlase MD laser system settings: MG-6 tip, 2.00W, 7% Water, 11% Air, 30 Hz
Other Er,Cr:YSGG laser system settings: G-6 tip, 1.50W, 7% Water, 11% Air

Use the surgical periodontal curette to grossly remove granulation tissue in the furcation area. Next, use the Er,Cr:YSGG laser to remove the remainder of the granulation tissue adhered to the furcation and the alveolus bone in the area.

Laser Parameters, Set 3: Odontoplasy/Osteoplasty

Waterlase MD laser system settings: 2.00W, 60% Water, 80% Air, 30 Hz
Other Er,Cr:YSGG laser system settings: 1.50-1.75W, 30% Water, 30% Air

Use the Er,Cr:YSGG to perform debridement, decontamination and smoothing of the bone and furcation of the roots.

This is followed by treatment with EDTA. Use saline solution for two minutes to rinse the site clear of EDTA. After the furcation area is suction-dried, enamel matrix derivative is applied to the furcation from the apical area up to the coronal region. Make sure the entire furcation surface is covered with enamel matrix derivative. The soft tissue is then re-adapted to the alveolus and the tooth. The flap is placed more coronally to cover the furcation. Resorbable sutures are used to hold the gingival tissue over the furcation.

Laser Parameters, Set 4: Soft Tissue Treatment

Waterlase MD laser system settings: MC-12 tip, 1.50W, 0% Water, 11% Air, 30 Hz, defocused at 3-5mm
Other Er,Cr:YSGG laser system settings: C-12 tip, 1.25W, 0% Water, 11% Air

Direct Er,Cr:YSGG laser energy in a defocused mode of 3-5mm from the surgical site and apply LLLT to the areas on both sides of the suture. A periodontal dressing (Barricade) is placed over the furcation area. This dressing will be removed in one week.

Post-Operative Care

After completing the procedures described above, instruct your patient as follows:

1. Do not brush the treated area for three weeks.
2. Rinse the treated area daily with 0.2% Chlorhexidine solution for three weeks.
3. Avoid muscle traction or other trauma to the treated area for three weeks.
4. The sutures and periodontal dressing will be removed by the doctor in one week.
5. Recall maintenance care and check in two to three months.
6. After three weeks, the patient may brush the treated area lightly; two to three months post-surgery, the patient may resume regular hygiene of the treated area.

Case 1: Furcation Surgery, Mandibular Molar, Open Flap, MD Regular HP with MG-6 Tip

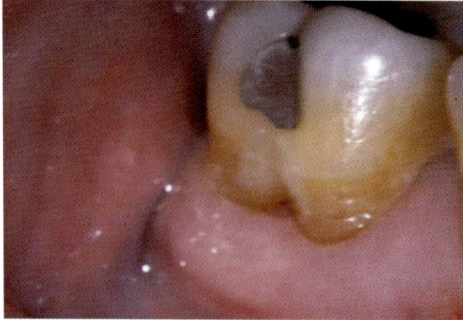

Fig. 1: Pre-op. Tooth #30 has a buccal furcation.

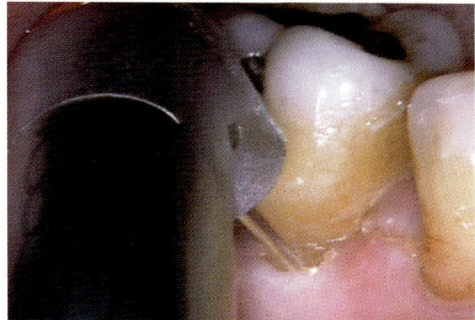

Fig. 2: Er,Cr:YSGG laser is used to make the initial incision for an apically-positioned flap.

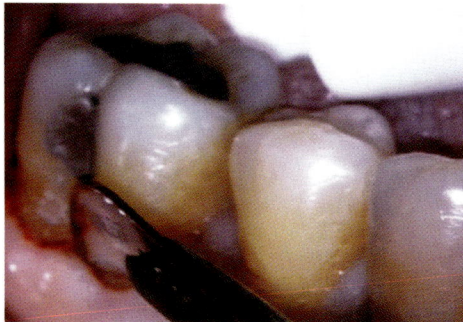

Fig. 3: Due to limited access, a #12 scalpel is used to complete the incision for flap from the distal of #30 to the mesial of #29.

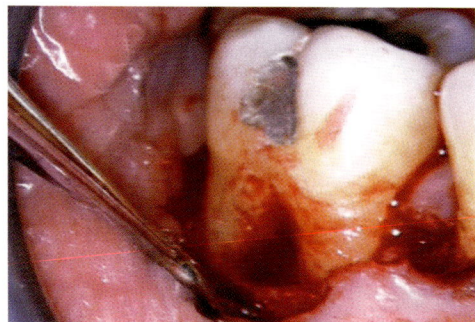

Fig. 4: Furcation is uncovered.

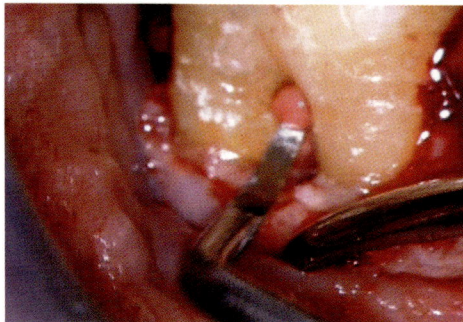

Fig. 5: A periodontal surgical curette is used to remove gross granulation tissue.

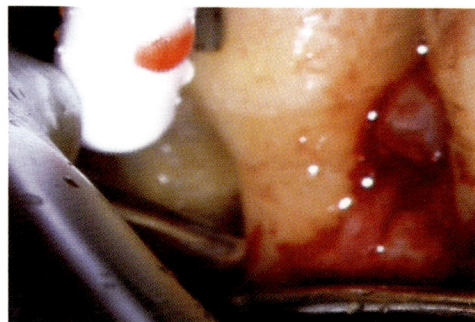

Fig. 6: The Er,Cr:YSGG is used to remove granulation tissue, some calculus and plaque.

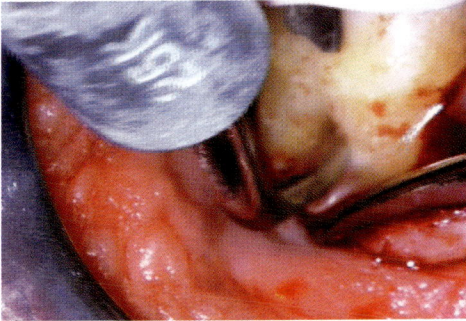

Fig. 7: A Cavitron is used to remove calculus and plaque.

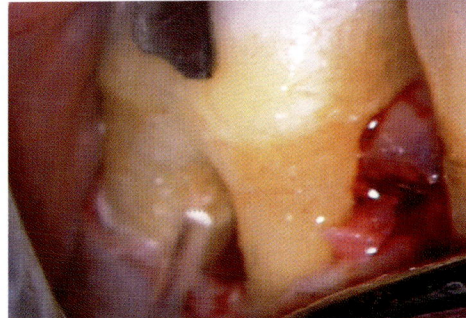

Fig. 8: The Er,Cr:YSGG is used to remove all tenacious tissue at furcation and to perform odontoplasty.

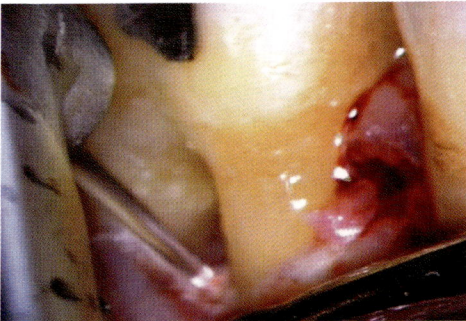

Fig. 9: The Er,Cr:YSGG is used to perform osteoplasty.

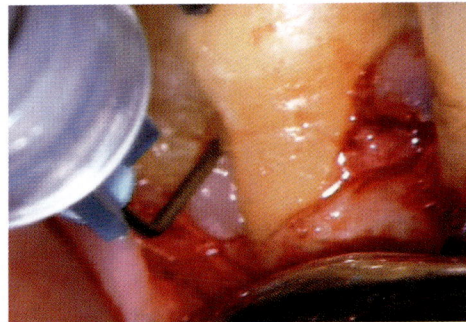

Fig. 10: EDTA is applied to furcation through syringe.

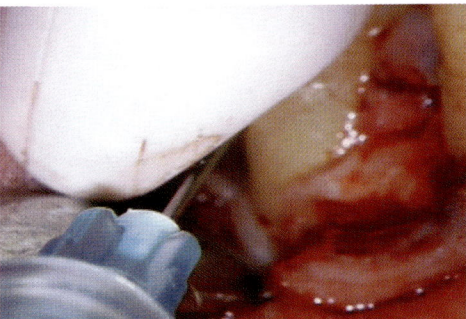

Fig. 11: EDTA is washed out by saline through a syringe.

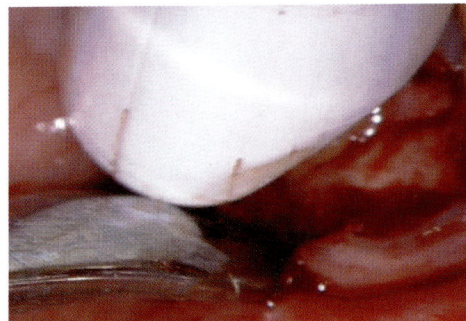

Fig. 12: Furcation is suction-dried.

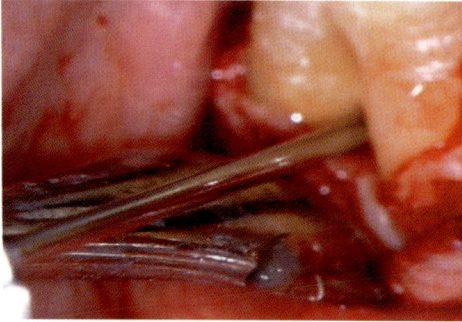

Fig. 13: EMD is placed at the surface of the furcation starting at the apical area.

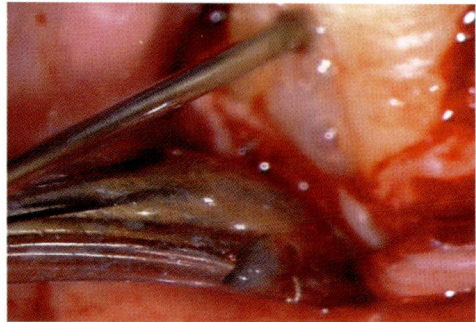

Fig. 14: EMD is placed at the surface of the furcation all the way to the coronal area.

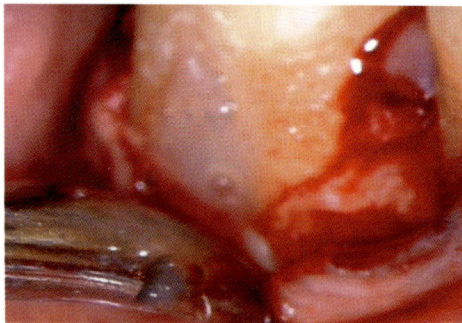

Fig. 15: EMD placement is complete.

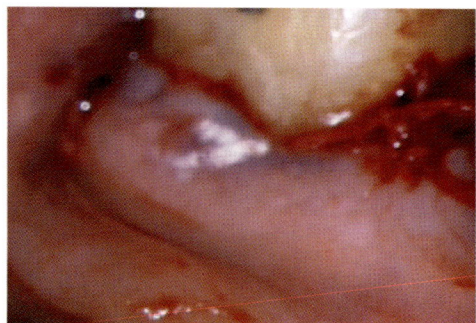

Fig. 16: Resorbable vicryl suture is placed with the gingiva covering the furcation area.

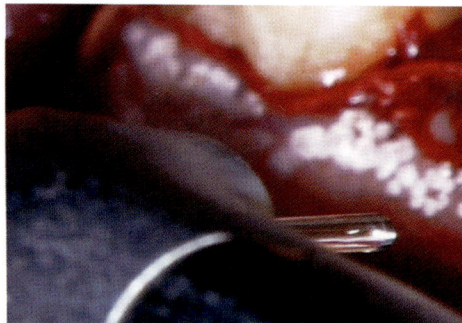

Fig. 17: Laser energy is directed over the sutured area.

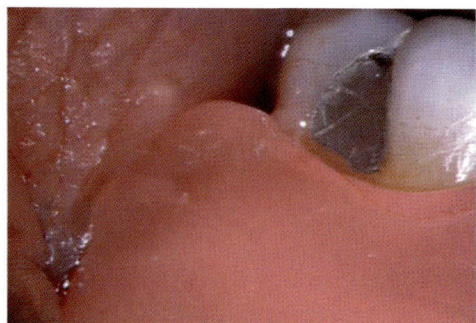

Fig. 18: Periodontal dressing is cured and the furcation surgery completed.

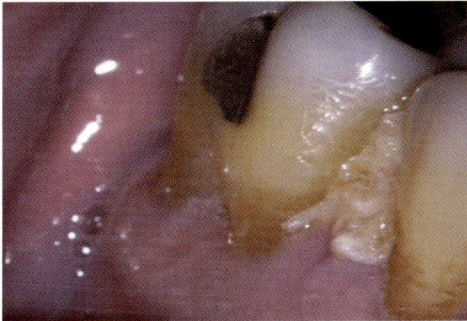
Fig. 19: Post-op. 20 days.

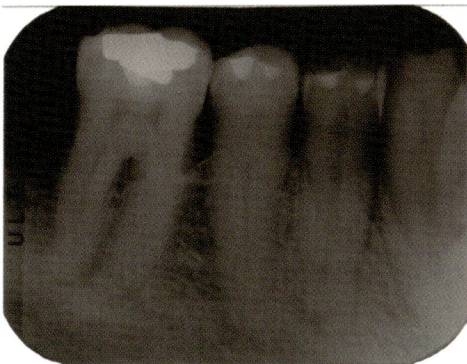
Fig. 20: Pre-operative x-Ray

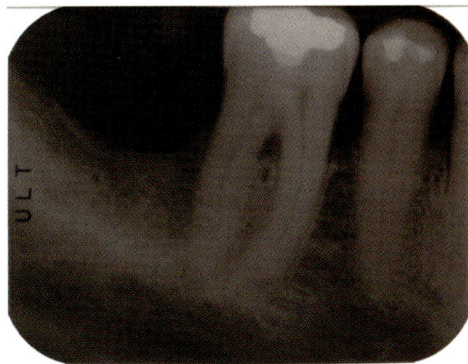
Fig. 21: Post-operative x-Ray

Case 2: Furcation Surgery, Mandibular Molar, Open Flap, MD Gold HP with MZ-5 Tip

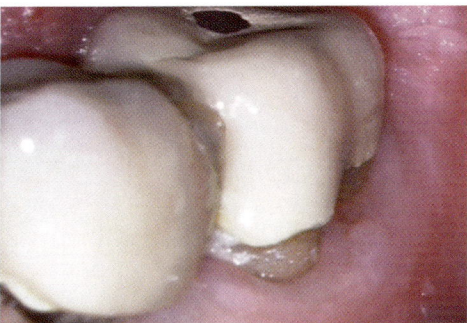
Fig. 1: Pre-op. Class II furcation is noted at buccal of #19.

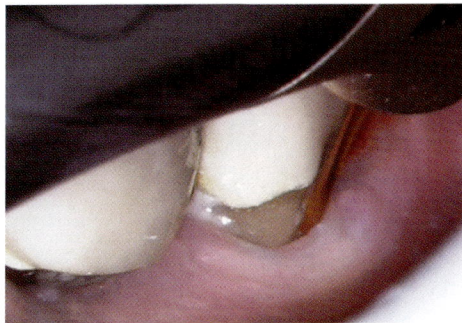
Fig. 2: A MZ-5 tip in a MD Gold Handpiece is used to make an incision for a flap. The setting is 2.25W, 20% Water, 11% Air, 50 Hz, S mode.

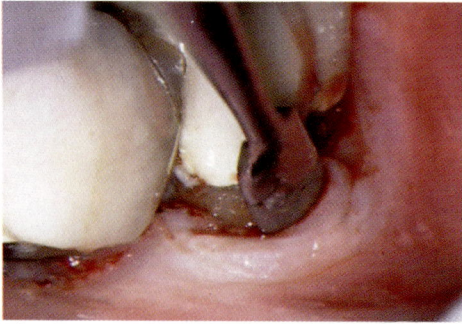
Fig. 3: An open flap is being elevated.

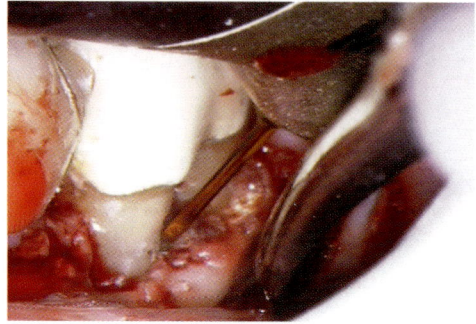
Fig. 4: The laser is used to remove granulation tissue in the furcation area. The setting is 1.25W, 15-20% Water, 11% Air, 30 Hz.

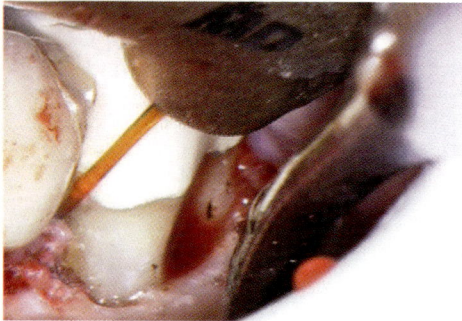
Fig. 5: The laser is used to remove granulation tissue in the mesial pocket of #19.

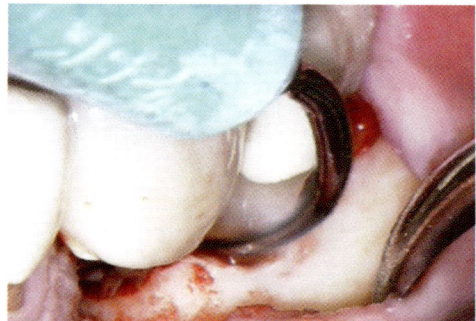
Fig. 6: The Cavitron is used to remove calculus in the furcation area as well as in the mesial pocket.

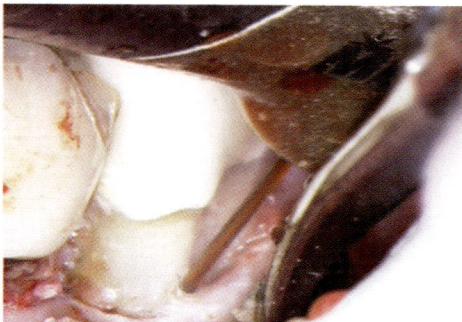
Fig. 7: The Laser is used to debride and clean the root and bone surface. The setting is 1.00W, 60% Water, 15% Air.

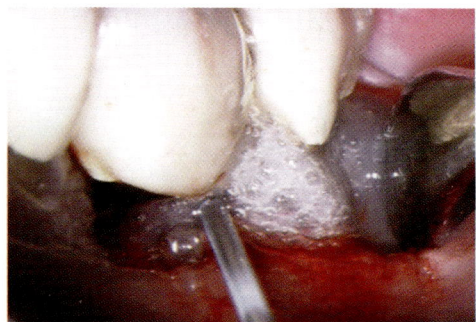
Fig. 8: Pregel (EDTA) is applied to the furcation and mesial pocket.

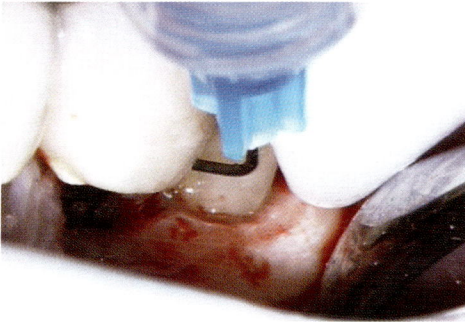

Fig. 9: Saline rinse applied for 2 minutes.

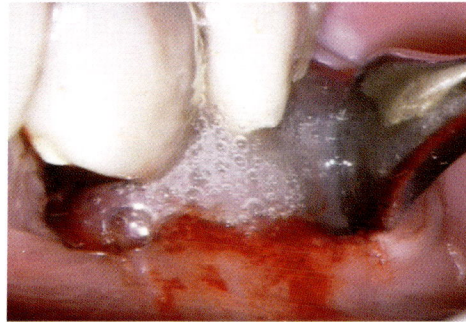

Fig. 10: EMD is placed in the furcation and the mesial pocket.

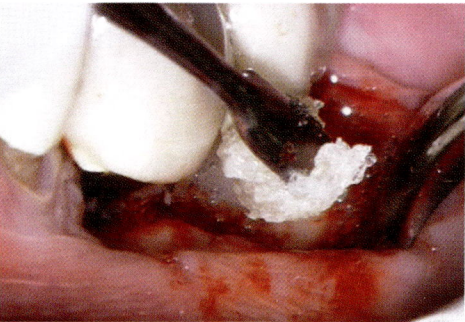

Fig. 11: Bone graft (dried freeze irradiated bone) is placed in the furcation.

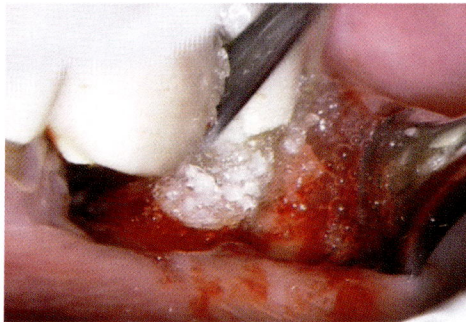

Fig. 12: Bone graft is placed in the mesial pocket.

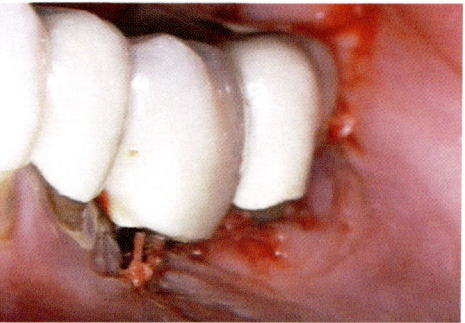

Fig. 13: Interrupted sutures have been placed.

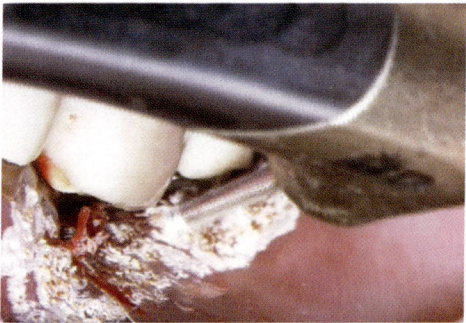

Fig. 14: Laser biologic band-aid is applied, using a MC-12 tip and a setting of 1.50W, 0% Water, 11% Air, 30 Hz, defocused 5 mm.

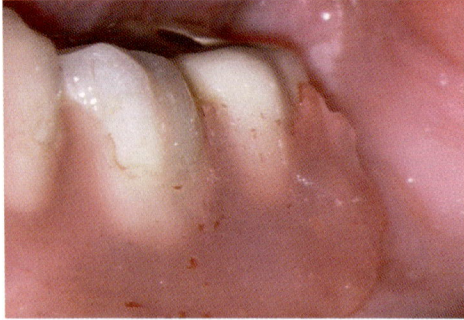

Fig. 15: Periodontal dressing is in place.

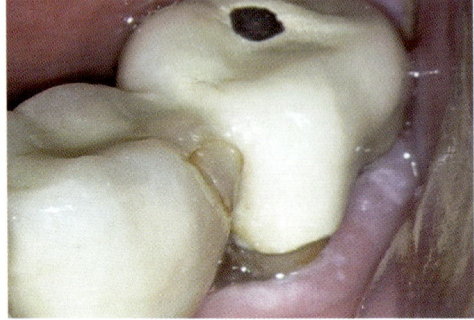

Fig. 16: One week post-op.

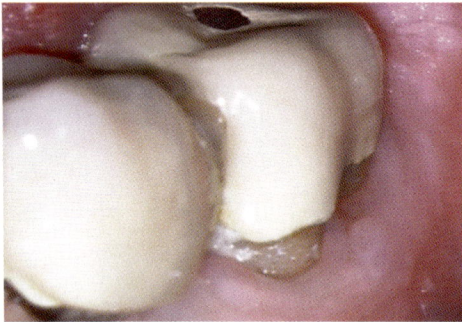

Fig. 17: Three weeks post-op.

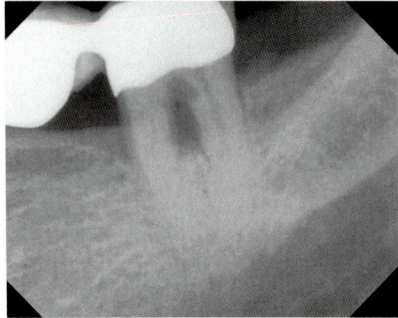

Fig. 18: Pre-operative X-ray

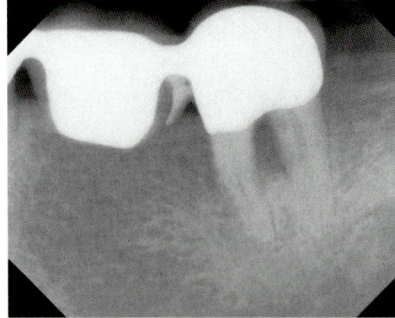

Fig. 19: After X-ray

Open-Flap Periodontal Surgery Using Biology-Based Regenerative Material – Enamel Matrix Derivative (EMD)

Enamel Matrix Derivative (EMD) promotes periodontal regeneration by mimicking the biological processes involved in nascent tooth development, including the development of the root and the supporting tissues.

In this clinical case, there is gingival recession that results in exposing several millimeters of cementum. Instead of using a free gingival graft, EMD is used.

Coronally Advanced Flap with EMD Application

After profound local anesthesia is administered, the root surface is treated with Cavitron®, then curetted and debrided with the laser. Next, make sulcular incisions bilaterally at the site of the recession. The incision is extended into the interdental areas lateral to the recession site.

Laser Parameters, Set 1: Laser Incision for Flap

Waterlase MD setting: MT-4 tip, 1.00-2.00W, 7-11% Water, 11% Air, 30 Hz

Horizontal incisions are made a couple of millimeters coronal to the level of the soft tissue margin of the recession. Next, make two vertical divergent incisions at the end of the lateral extensions of the horizontal incisions. The vertical release incisions direct apically into the lining mucosa.

A full-thickness flap is raised until the mucogingival junction is reflected several millimeters apical to the bone dehiscence.

Laser Parameters, Set 2: Laser Preparation of a Coronally Advanced Flap

Waterlase MD setting: MG-6, MZ-6 or MC-6 tip, 1.00-1.75W, 7-11% Water, 11% Air, 30 Hz

Use the laser to make a horizontal cut through the periosteum to raise a split-thickness flap. This allows the flap to be coronally positioned to cover the recession area. De-epithelialization of the interdental papillae is done by laser to create a connective tissue bed for suturing the coronally advanced flap.

Laser Parameters, Set 3: Debridement and Cleaning of Root Surface

Waterlase MD setting: MG-6 or MZ-6 tip, 0.75-1.00W, 60% Water, 80% Air, 30 Hz

Use the laser to debride and clean the exposed root surface.

Apply EMD such that it fully covers the exposed root surface. Next, raise the flap coronally to cover the root surface and secure the flap at the CEJ level by suturing the flap into the de-epithelialized recipient bed. The vertical incisions are closed with 4-0 black silk sutures.

Laser Parameters, Set 4: Biologic Band-Aid

Waterlase MD setting: MC-12 tip, 1.5W, 0% Water, 11% Air, 30 Hz

Use the laser to apply a "biologic band-aid" to the surgical site. Next, apply a light-cured periodontal dressing (Barricade). Both sutures and dressings are removed at a one-week post-operative follow up appointment.

Post-Operative Care

After completing the procedures described above, instruct your patient as follows:

1. Do not brush the surgical site for 3-4 weeks.
2. Rinse the surgical site two times daily with 0.1%-0.2% Chlorhexidine solution for antiseptic purposes.
3. Do not brush the teeth for 24 hours immediately following the operation.
4. Do not eat or drink anything hot for 24 hours.
5. Do not eat or drink anything messy or spicy for 24 hours.
6. After the initial healing period, use a rolling-stroke method to clean the teeth in order to minimize apically-directed trauma on the gingival margin.
7. Make a post-operative follow-up appointment once a month.
8. Make a maintenance appointment once every 3 months.
9. Do not allow sub-gingival probing of the treated area until 4-6 months post-surgery.

Case 1: Root Coverage Using Enamel Matrix Derivative with No Tissue Graft

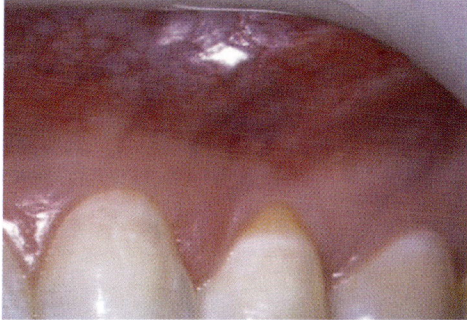

Fig. 1: Tooth # 12 shows several mm of gingival recession exposing cementum. Periodontal condition is otherwise healthy.

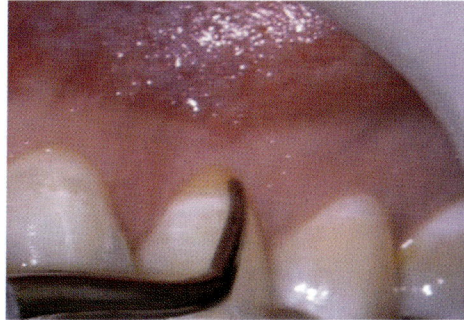

Fig. 2: After profound local anesthesia is administered, perform light instrumentation with the Cavitron to remove plaque and calculus.

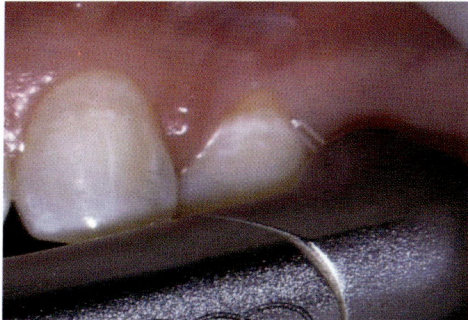

Fig. 3: The laser is used to debride and clean the root surface.

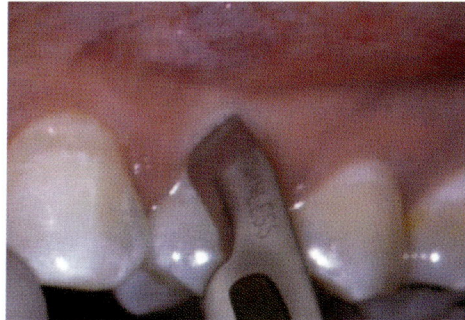

Fig. 4: A scalpel blade is used to make an incision for a flap at the mesial half of #12.

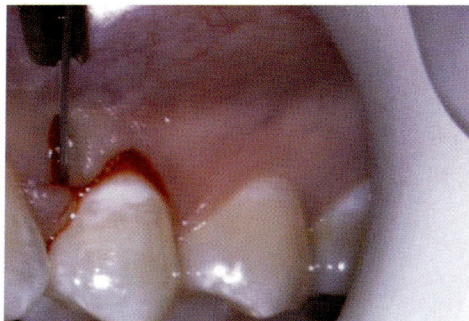

Fig. 5: A vertical relief incision is made mesial to #12.

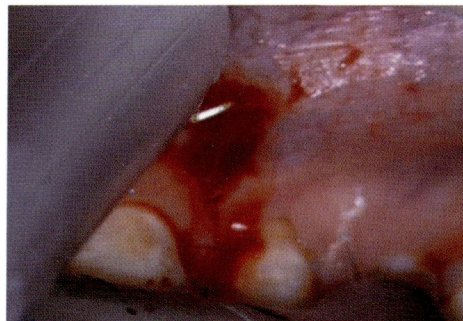

Fig. 6: A vertical relief distal to #12 is made by the laser. A MG-6 (MZ-6, MT-4 or MC-6) tip is used. The setting is 1.75W, 11% Water, 11% Air, 30 Hz.

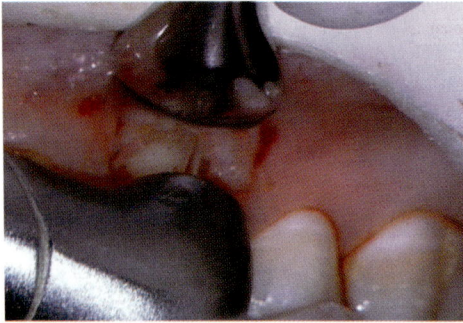

Fig. 7: A partial thickness relief is made to prepare the flap. The MG-6 tip is used with a setting of 2.00W, 11% Water, 11% Air, 30 Hz.

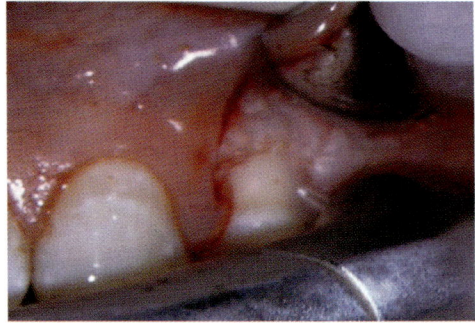

Fig. 8: The cementum is treated with the laser for debridement and cleaning. The setting is 1.00W, 60% Water, 80% Air, 30 Hz.

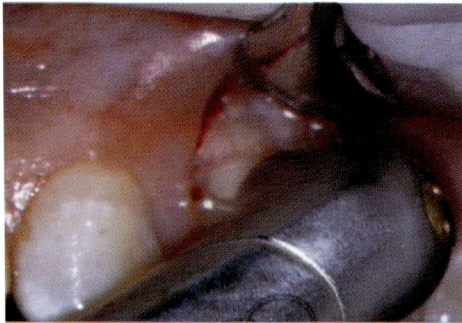

Fig. 9: De-epithelialization is performed at the mesial and the distal area to prepare for the covering of the cementum. The setting is 1.75W, 7% Water, 11% Air, 30 Hz.

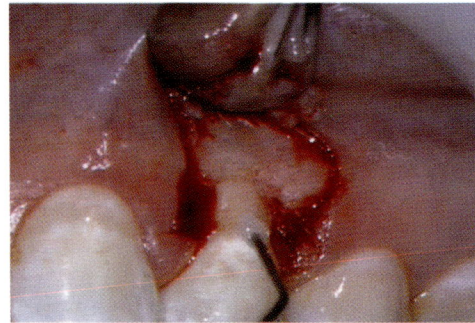

Fig. 10: Pregel (EDTA solution) is applied to the cementum.

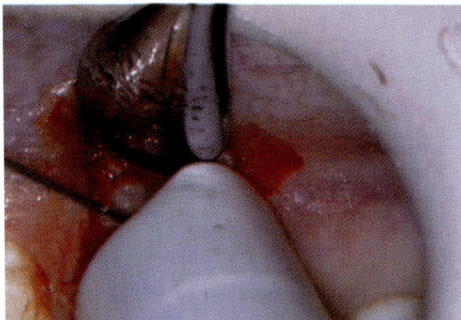

Fig. 11: A saline rinse is used to remove and cleanse the site of Pregel.

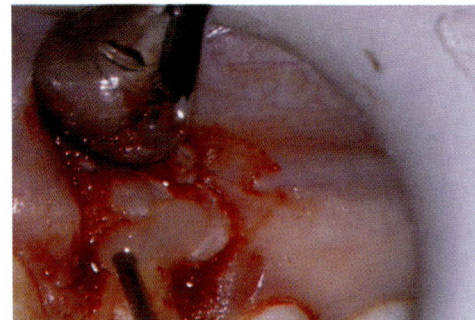

Fig. 12: An enamel matrix derivative is applied to the cementum.

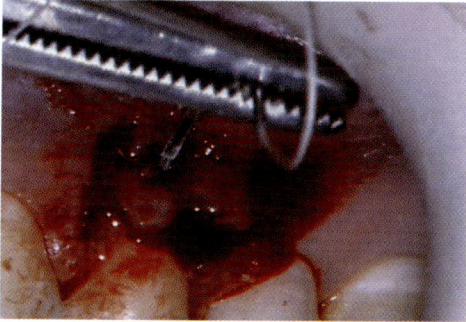

Fig. 13: The flap is lifted to cover the exposed cementum. Interrupted 4-0 black silk is placed.

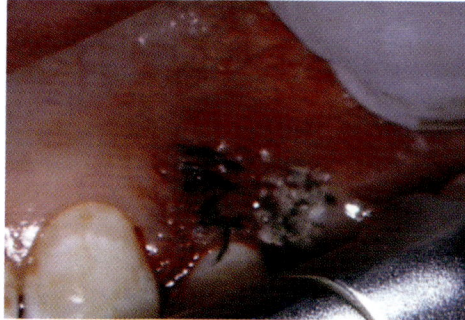

Fig. 14: A biologic band-aid is applied by a setting of 1.25W, 0% Water, 11% Air, 30 Hz, in a defocused mode.

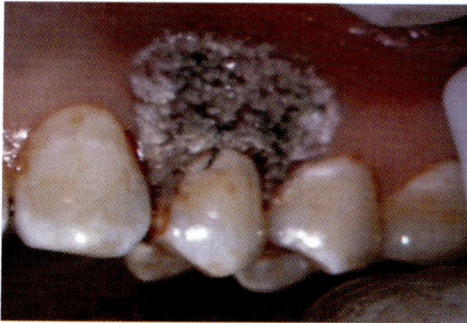

Fig. 15: The biologic band-aid is complete.

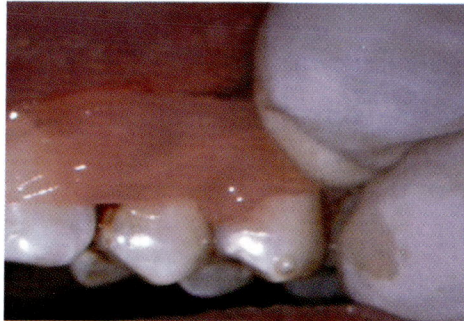

Fig. 16: A barricade (a light cured periodontal dressing) is placed.

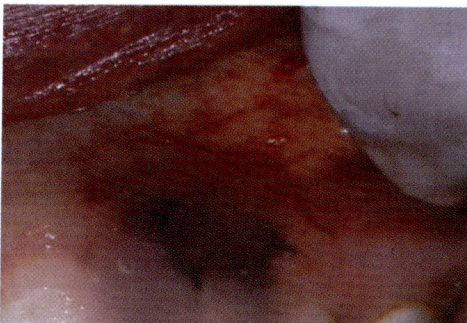

Fig. 17: Immediate post-op.

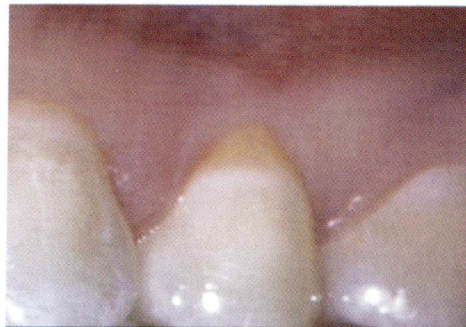

Fig. 18.1: Pre-op.

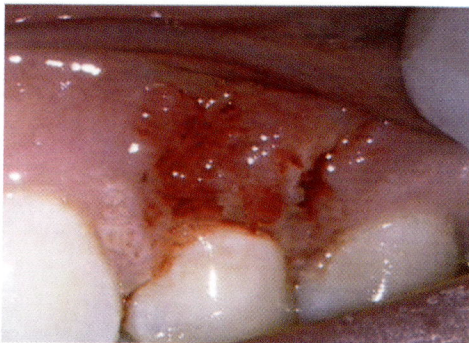

Fig 18.2: Post-op, 1 week.

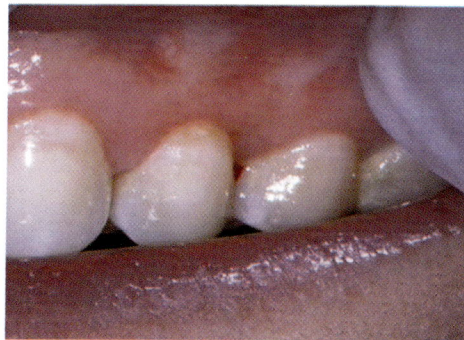

Fig. 18.3: Post-op, 6 weeks.

Oral Surgery

Introduction

In oral surgery, the laser offers significant patient benefits at one significant cost. For any oral surgical procedures, especially those that involve ablation of bone (whether the procedures involve impacted third molars, removal of a torus or placement of an implant), the tradeoff for generally reduced post-operative pain, edema and swelling is the duration of time it takes to complete a procedure. The laser is not as fast as a drill or saw (and if this is one of the rare instances where general anesthetic is being administered, or there are other pressing time concerns, the laser may not be an appropriate selection for the clinician), but it has been my experience that patients find that the benefits of the laser outweigh the negatives. The post-operative patient condition is always superior to that when surgery is performed with scalpels, drills or a saw.

Crown Lengthening

Before we discuss the details of the techniques used in crown lengthening, we need to understand the importance of the biologic width. Violating the biologic width may result in gingival inflammation and periodontal involvement. It can even lead to the loss of the supporting tissue and loss of the tooth. Sometimes doctors can get carried away with creating an esthetic smile design and can overlook the management of the integrity of the biologic width. As a result, some procedures that look esthetically pleasing may not last due to poor biological condition. Crown lengthening is performed to provide tooth length for the proper restoration of a tooth without compromising the periodontium.

A tooth being considered for surgical crown lengthening must be evaluated carefully. Ideally there should be a total of 5mm of gingiva (3mm free and 2mm attached). Bone sounding is a procedure that is performed clinically to determine the existing periodontal condition of the tooth under evaluation. By probing through the sulcus, the CEJ of the tooth may be located. Apical to the CEJ, the probe may locate the alveolar crest. Ideally, it should be approximately 2mm apical to the CEJ. When it is closer to or covering the CEJ, bone reduction is indicated. Another aspect of evaluation of the alveolar crest is the thickness. This sometimes becomes difficult – an open or partially open flap evaluation may be necessary.

The decision whether or not to use local anesthesia should depend on whether successful bone sounding can be tolerated without local anesthesia. Apply concentrated topical (EMLA or Tac-gel) to the gingiva and the sulcus. Leave the gel on for at least 3½ minutes before the bone sounding procedure is performed. If the patient cannot tolerate the procedure with only the help of an application of concentrated topical anesthetic gel, give the patient injection anesthesia as well. On the other hand, if the patient can tolerate the evaluation procedure, there is a good chance the crown lengthening procedure can be done without injection of anesthesia.

In addition to esthetic improvement, crown lengthening is also indicated for the following reasons:

1. Restoring teeth with caries in the subgingival area.
2. Restoring teeth with fractures in the subgingival area.
3. Restoring teeth that are shortened by extensive fracture or caries.
4. Restoring teeth with anatomical short clinical crowns.
5. Restoring teeth shortened by incomplete exposure of the natural crown.

Contraindications:

1. Teeth that are not restorable because of caries that have reached the pulp.
2. Teeth that are not restorable because of the extension of fractures deep below the gingival crest.
3. Teeth that are not restorable because of a severe loss of tooth structure from bruxism or accident. This may cause displacement of adjacent teeth and may cause loss of mesial-distal dimensions.
4. Situations in which adjacent teeth would be compromised either esthetically or functionally.

Soft Tissue Crown Lengthening

Laser Parameters, Set 1: Outline the Surgical Site

Waterlase MD laser system settings: MG-6 tip, 0.50W, 0% Water, 11% Air, 30 Hz
Other Er,Cr:YSGG laser system settings: G-6 tip, 0.5W, 0% Water, 11% Air

A concentrated topical gel (Tac-gel) is used for 3½ minutes before bone sounding. If the patient can tolerate it, no injection is needed. After the bone sounding procedure, determine the height of soft tissue to be removed. Use a MG-6 tip with a setting of 0.5W, 0% Water, 11% Air to mark the outline of the soft tissue to be removed. This serves as a blue print for the laser surgery.

Laser Parameters, Set 2: Soft Tissue Reduction

Waterlase MD laser system settings: MG-6 tip, 0.50-1.25W, 7% Water, 11% Air, 30 Hz
Other Er,Cr:YSGG laser system settings: G-6 tip, 0.50-1.25W, 7% Water, 11% Air

Continue to ablate the outlined tissue with the laser. If necessary, increase the power by 0.25W to improve cutting efficiency; however, ensure that the patient is comfortable with the final laser setting.

If a veneer or crown prep is needed for the tooth, use the laser to remove soft tissue, one segment at a time, by following the outline, with the tip placed perpendicular to the gingival and with a slow back-and-forth sweeping motion. If there is no plan for restoring the tooth, the tip is placed parallel to the long axis of the tooth to avoid ablation on hard tissue underneath the gingiva. The technique involves removing 1mm of soft tissue at a time. Due to the pulsed mode, the cutting may produce a relatively uneven margin. The back-and-forth sweeping motion helps to improve the quality and straightness of the margin. A higher pulse rate (50 Hz) may also be used to finish smoothing the gingival margin. A lower power gives better control of the accuracy of the surgical procedure.

Laser Parameters, Set 3: Finishing the Marginal Gingiva

Waterlase MD laser system settings: 1.00W, 7% Water, 11% Air, 50 Hz
Other Er,Cr:YSGG laser system settings: 0.50W, 7% Water, 11% Air

After the lengthening procedure has been completed, reduce the power and place the tip at an angle to fashion the marginal gingiva to a knife-edge configuration.

Laser Parameters, Set 4: Hemostasis

Waterlase MD laser system settings: MG-6 tip, 2.25W, 1% Water, 11% Air, 50 Hz, S mode
Other Er,Cr:YSGG laser system settings: C-6 tip, 0.50W, 2-3% Water, 11% Air

If coagulation is necessary, aim the tip at the margin. Move the tip quickly in a sweeping motion to coagulate and smooth the margin. This is followed by a gentle rinsing and air spray to reveal a refined finish of the surgery. The CEJ should line up with the marginal gingiva.

Soft Tissue and Hard Tissue Crown Lengthening

Repeat soft tissue crown lengthening, Laser Parameters Set 1 to Set 4. Continue on as follows:

Laser Parameters, Set 5: Bone Reduction

Waterlase MD laser system settings: MZ-6 tip, 1.50-2.50W, 60% Water, 80% Air, 30 Hz
Other Er,Cr:YSGG laser system settings: Z-6 tip, 1.50-2.50W, 60% Water, 65% Air

Apply concentrated topical (Tac-gel) to sulcus. Use bone sound to determine where the alveolus bone margin is. If the measurement from the marginal gingiva to the alveolus bone is less than 3mm, bone reduction procedure is necessary to attain the proper biological zone.

The MZ-6 tip is marked with an indelible pen 3mm from the end of the tip. Let the marking dry up before using the tip. Use a "tap-cut, tap-cut, tap-cut, smooth, smooth" technique. With the power setting described in this parameter, tap the bone lightly to feel where the bone level is. Withdraw the tip from the sulcus approximately to cut. Move the tip directly along the outline of the gingiva. After three times of "tap-cut", the tip should be 1mm defocused from the bone level. Move the tip back and forth along the area tapped and cut earlier. The same routine continues on to the next segment of the bone until the tip reaches the other proximal side. Notice the marking on the tip being immersed into the sulcus as laser energy reduces the bone. When the marking of the MZ-6 tip lines up with the marginal gingiva, the bone level is 3mm from the marginal gingiva. Use an explorer to feel the bone to make sure the reduction is done with a smooth finish. Use the laser on any rough area that has been detected, in order to smooth and improve the bone margin.

Flush and clean up the sulcus with irrigation with chlorhexidine in a syringe. This completes the crown lengthening procedure.

Case 1: Soft Tissue Crown Lengthening

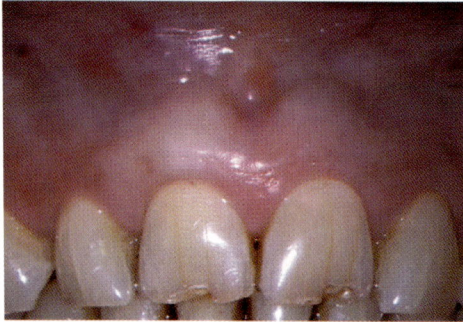

Fig. 1: Pre-op. The patient has short clinical crown with a "gummy smile."

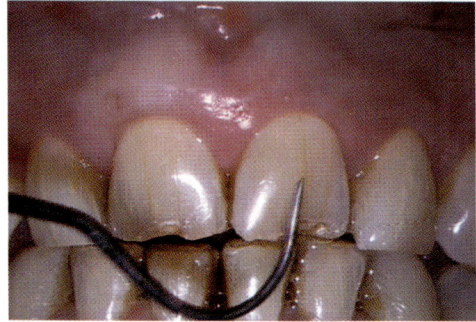

Fig. 2: Bone sounding is performed to determine how far subgingival the CEJ is.

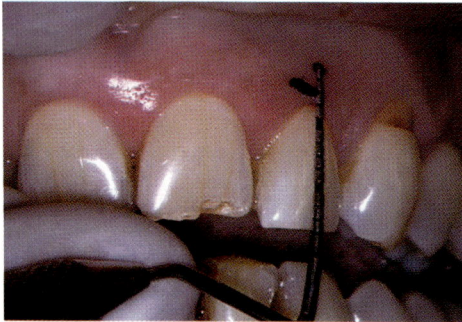

Fig. 3: An ink mark is placed at the CEJ. Bone sounding continues to locate the alveolus bone level. Another ink mark is made to indicate the alveolus bone level.

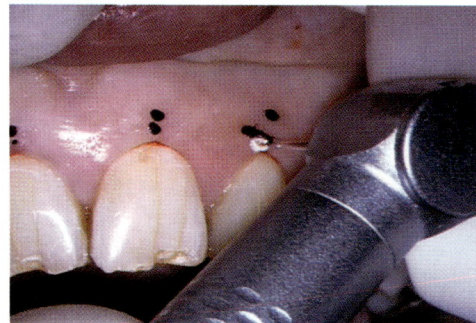

Fig. 4: A G-6 tip is used with a parameter of 0.50W, 0% Water, 11% Air to mark the soft tissue to be ablated. This lines up the CEJ with the new marginal gingiva.

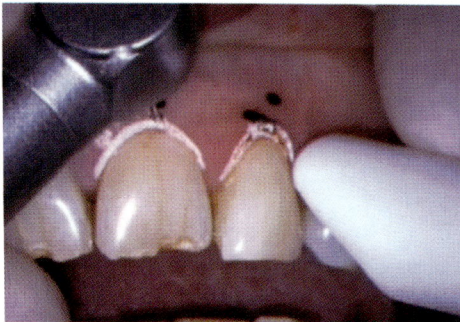

Fig. 5: The outline of the new marginal gingiva is made on all six anterior teeth.

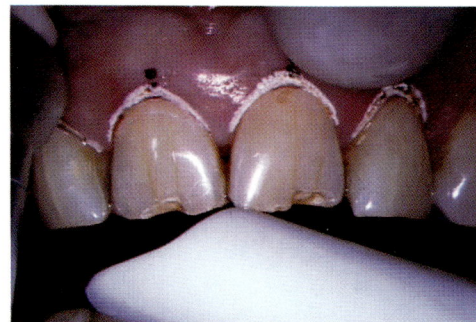

Fig. 6: Detailed design of the "zenith point" is included.

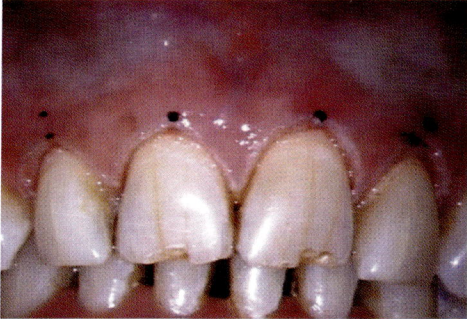

Fig. 7: A G-6 tip is used with 1.00W, 7% Water, 11% Air to ablate the soft tissue of #8 and #9 to be at the same level lined up with the CEJ.

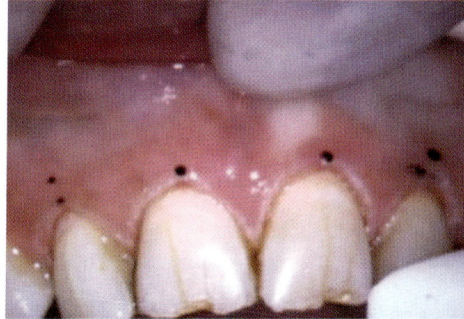

Fig. 8: The soft tissue crown lengthening is complete.

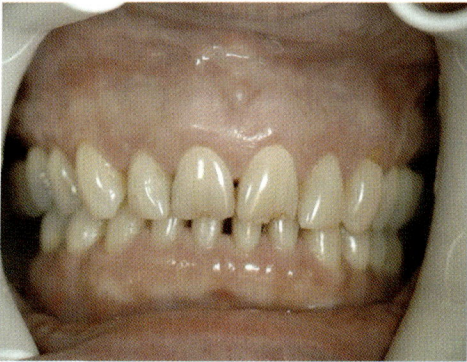

Fig. 9: One month post-op.

Case 2:
Soft and Hard Tissue Crown Lengthening (Closed Flap Technique)

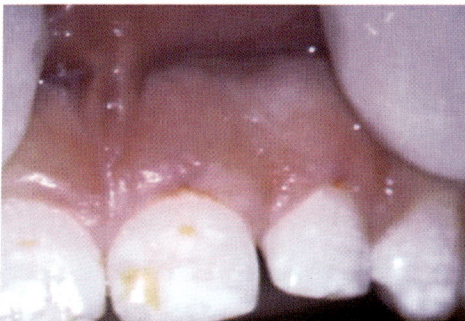

Fig. 1: Pre-op. Concentrated topical (Tac-gel) is used on 7-10 before bone sounding. Tac-gel is used on gingiva and gingival sulcus for three minutes.

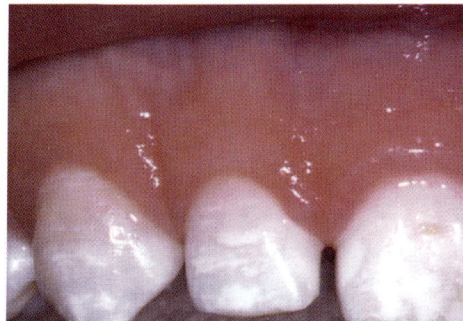

Fig. 2: Pre-op of #7 and 8.

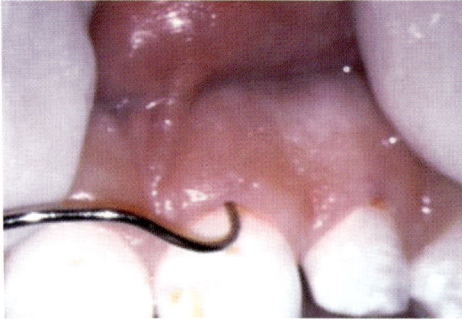

Fig. 3: An explorer is used to bone sound. CEJ is about 1.5mm from the marginal gingiva.

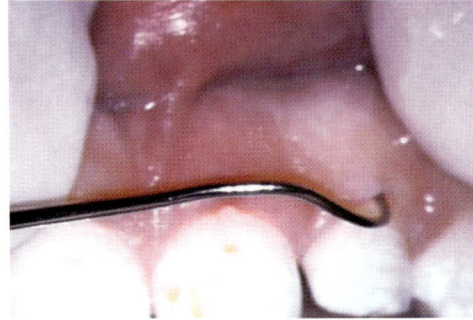

Fig. 4: Bone sounding is performed on #10, as well as #7 and #8.

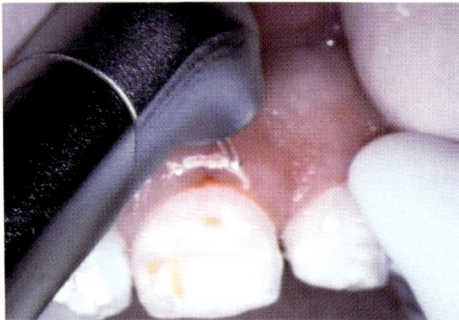

Fig. 5: Using an MG-6 tip with 0.50W, 0% Water, 11% Air, 30 Hz, soft tissue outline is made. It marks the amount of soft tissue to be removed.

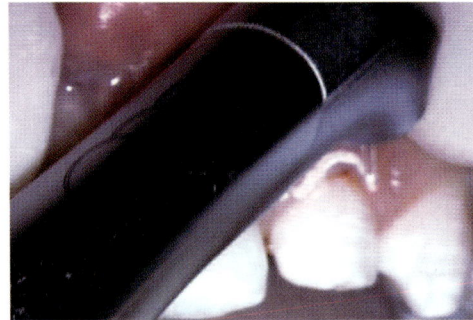

Fig. 6: The outline of soft tissue to be removed continues with teeth #10, #7 and #8.

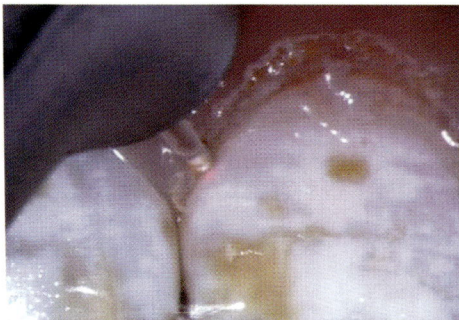

Fig. 7: Soft tissue crown lengthening is done with a MG-6 tip at a setting of 1.25W, 11% Water, 11% Air, 30 Hz. This continues on until the marginal gingiva lines up with the CEJ.

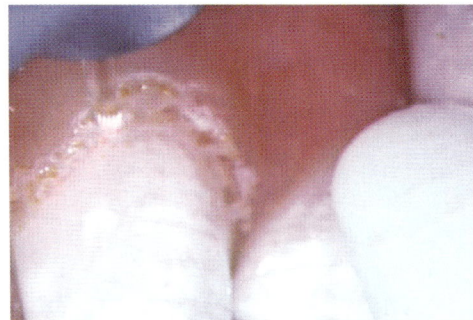

Fig. 8: The soft tissue crown lengthening continues on with #10.

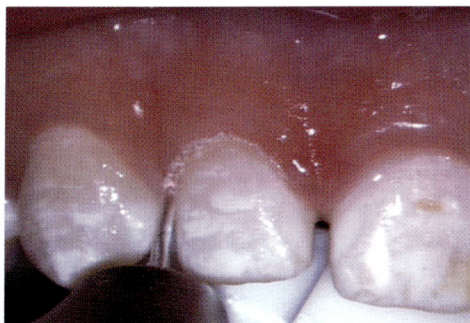

Fig. 9: The soft tissue crown lengthening continues on with #7 and #8.

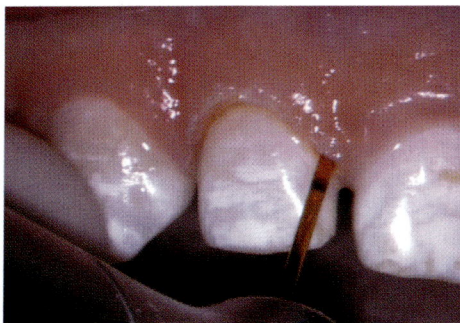

Fig. 10: After bone sounding to locate the crest of the bone, about 2mm of bone is to be reduced to reach the proper biologic zone.

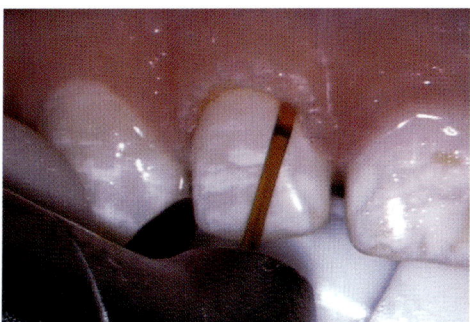

Fig. 11: A MZ-6 tip marked at 3mm with an indelible ink is used. The "bone tapping" technique is used to reduce bone to 3mm subgingival level. The setting is 2.00W, 60% Water, 80% Air, 30 Hz.

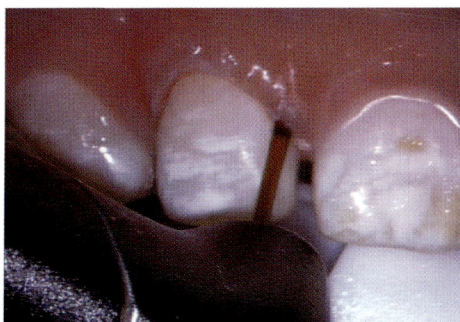

Fig. 12: Bone reduction continues until the mark levels with the marginal gingiva. The bone crest is now 3mm from the marginal gingiva. A similar technique and setting are used to perform bone reduction for #8, #9 and #10.

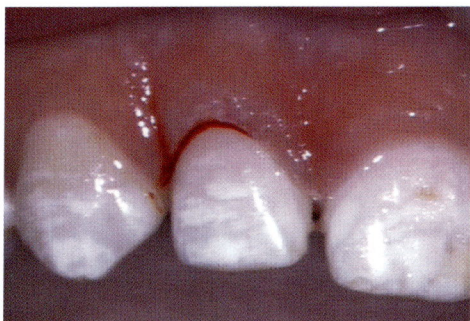

Fig. 13: Immediate post-op of #7 and #8.

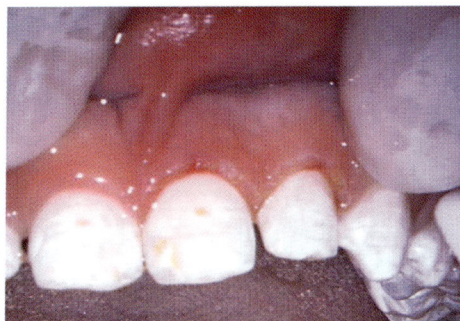

Fig. 14: Immediate post-op of #8, #9 and #10.

Case 3:
Soft Tissue Crown Lengthening (16 Units)
Laser Veneer Preparation, Laser Hemostasis (Before Cementation) and
Laser Debridement (Before Cementation)

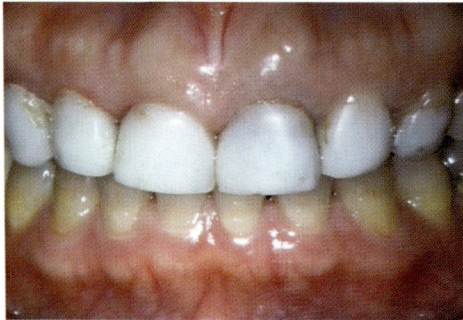

Fig. 1: Old and worn composite veneers are treatment planned to be replaced by eight unit porcelain veneers in the maxilla (#5-#12) and eight more units of new porcelain veneers will be placed in the mandible.

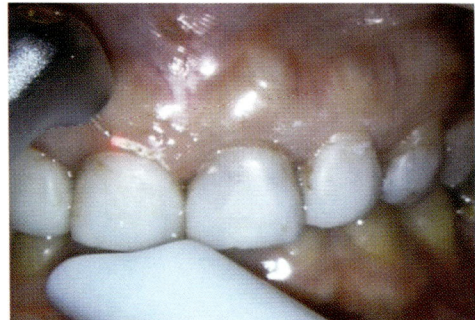

Fig. 2: After bone sounding, soft tissue crown lengthening is indicated in selective areas. The tip is MG-6, at a setting of 0.25W, 0% Water, 11% Air, 30 Hz to mark the soft tissue to be reduced.

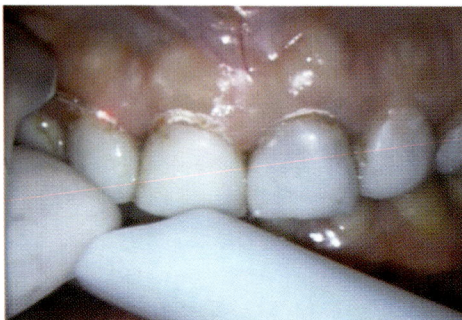

Fig. 3: The pre-treatment is performed on #7-#10.

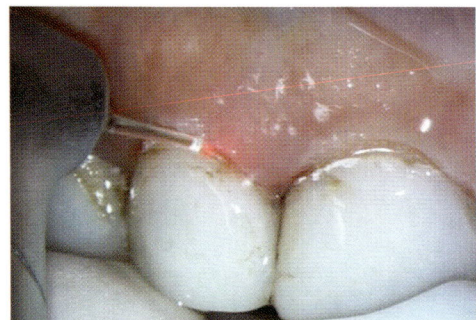

Fig. 4: The soft tissue crown lengthening is performed with a MG-6 tip, at 0.50W, 11% Water, 11% Air, 30 Hz. The gumline above #7 is receiving soft tissue reduction.

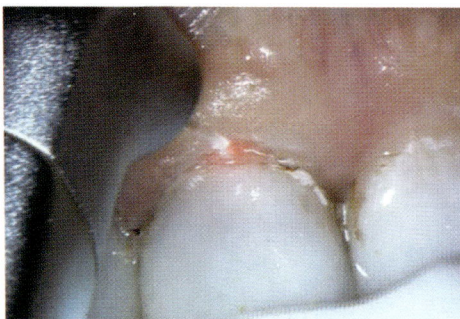

Fig. 5: Soft tissue crown lengthening is performed on #8.

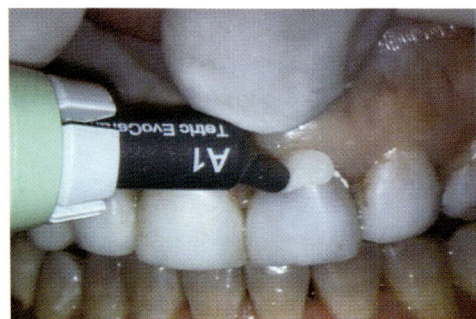

Fig. 6: After crown lengthening, composite is added to #7-#10 at the gingival area to simulate the final restoration.

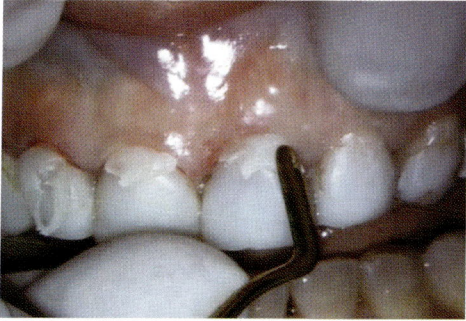

Fig. 7: The margins are scalped precisely before a template mold is taken for the fabrication of temporary veneers.

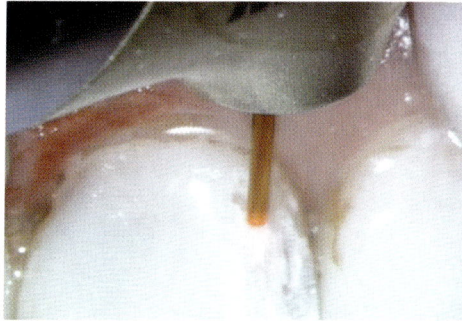

Fig. 8: This is followed by veneer preparation of the eight units from #5-#12. A MZ-5 in a MD Gold Handpiece is used at 4.50W, 60% Water, 11% Air, 15 Hz, to perform the veneer prep.

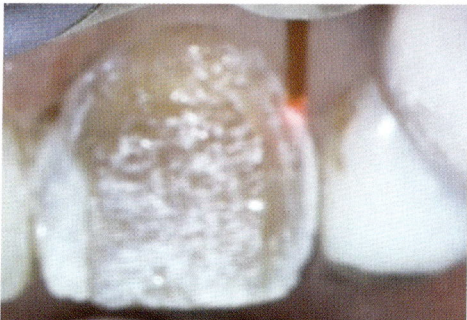

Fig. 9: The outline of the veneer preparation is performed by the laser.

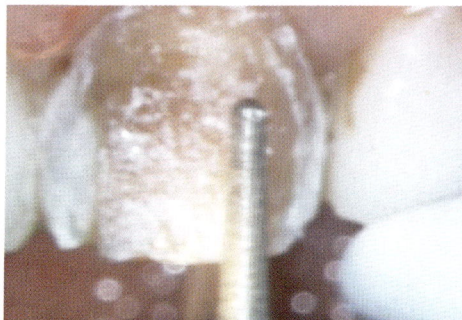

Fig. 10: A high-speed diamond bur in an electric handpiece is used to finish and complete the veneer prep.

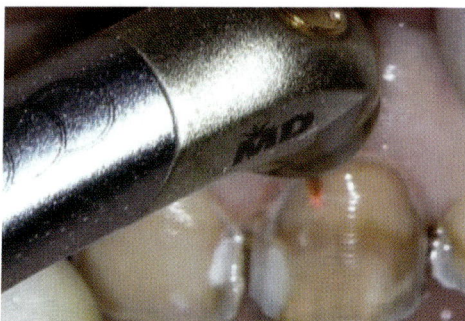

Fig. 11: The laser is used to remove smear and debris and to finish the preparation. The setting is 1.00W, 60% Water, 80% Air, 40 Hz.

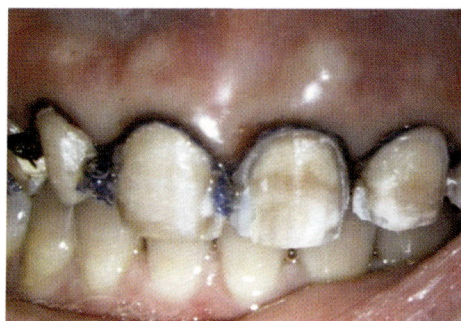

Fig. 12: A retraction cord is used before impression. (The exact marginal gingiva contour is not to be violated).

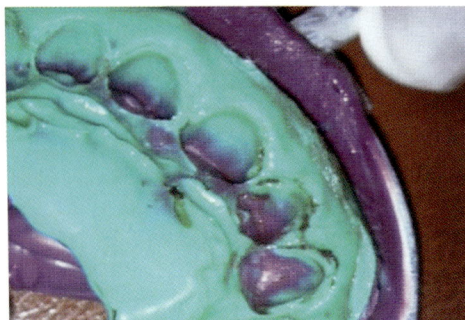

Fig. 13: Addition silicone impression is taken.

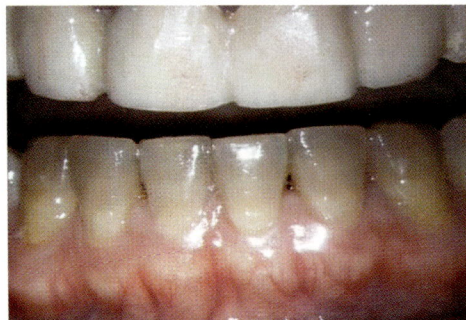

Fig. 14: Pre-op for lower eight units.

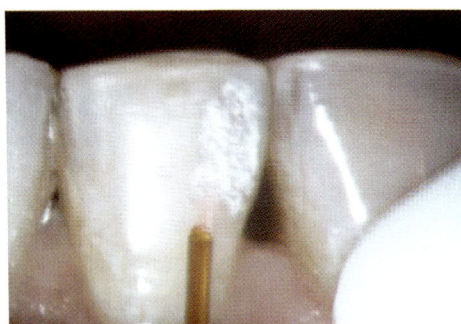

Fig. 15: Initial veneer preparation is performed with the laser using a MZ-5 tip in a MD Gold Handpiece. The setting is 3.50W, 60% Water, 80% Air, 15 Hz.

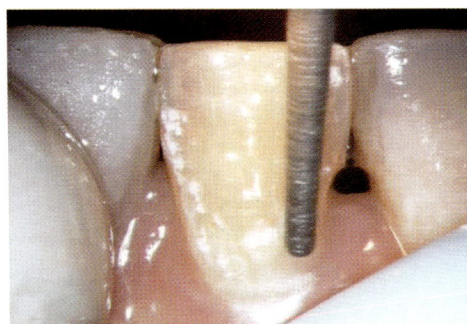

Fig. 16: The veneer prep is finished with a high-speed diamond.

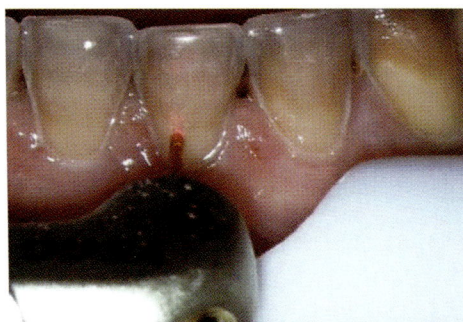

Fig. 17: Smear and debris are removed by laser at 1.00W, 60% Water, 80% Air, 40 Hz.

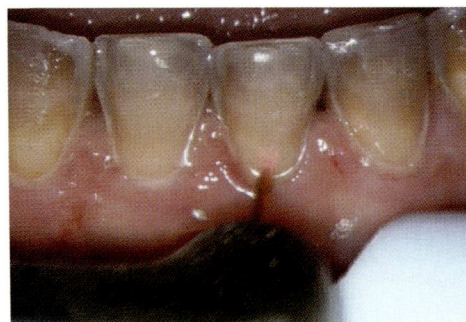

Fig. 18: Soft tissue crown lengthening is performed in selective area.

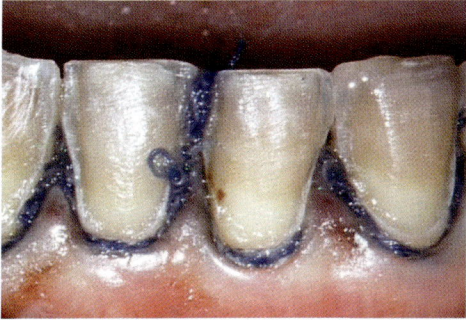

Fig. 19: Cord is packed before final impression.

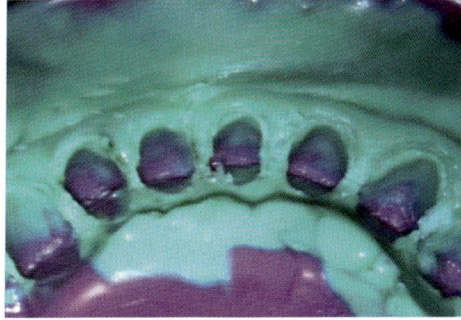

Fig. 20: Addition silicone impression of the eight unit veneers to be made.

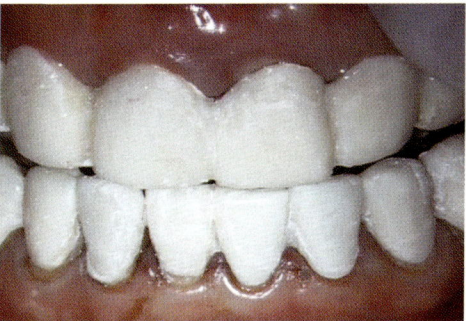

Fig. 21: Immediate post-op with 16 units of temporary veneers.

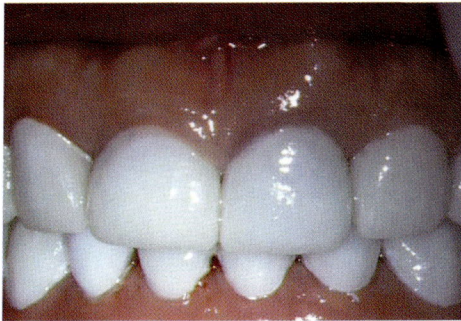

Fig. 22: Post-op with the final restorations cemented.

Case 4: Soft Tissue Crown Lengthening, M2 with G-6 Tip

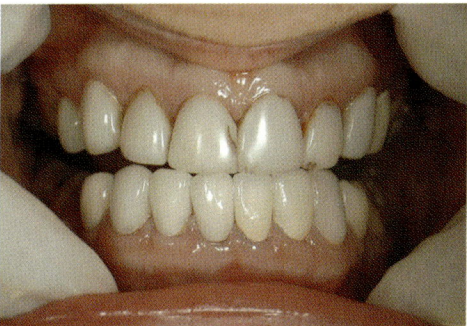

Fig. 1: Pre-op. New porcelain veneers are planned in the treatment due to fractures in the veneer. Improvement of the gingival line is planned for better esthetic result.

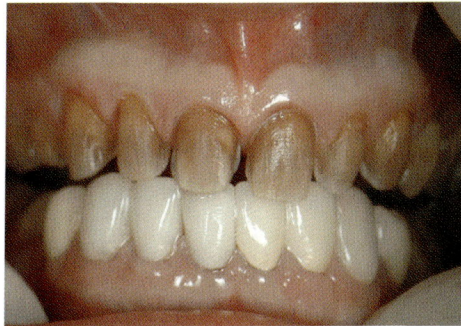

Fig. 2: Old porcelain veneers have been removed. #8 and #9 could use better zenith points to improve character and #10 could use more recontouring.

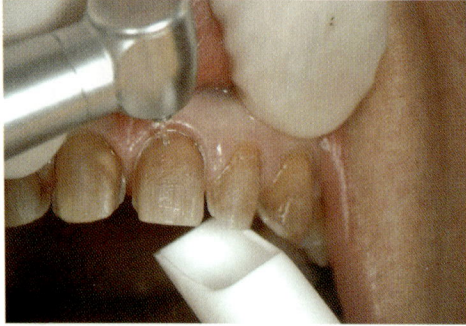

Fig. 3: A G-6 (or Z-6 or C-6) tip is used to recontour gingiva on #9. The setting is 1.00W, 7% Water, 11% Air.

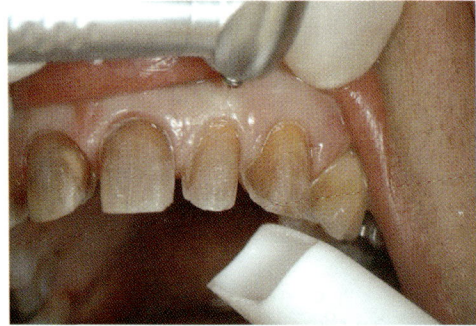

Fig. 4: #10 gingival recontouring is done to improve the esthetic line.

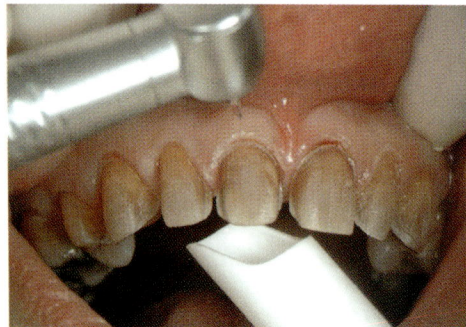

Fig. 5: #8 gingival recontouring is done with the same setting as in Fig. 3.

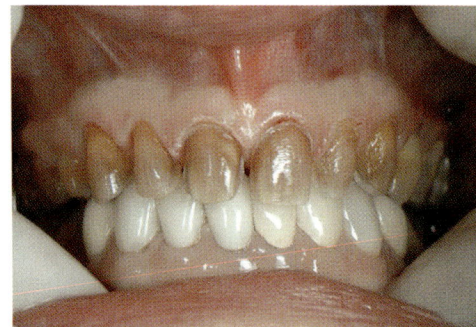

Fig. 6: Immediate post- op.

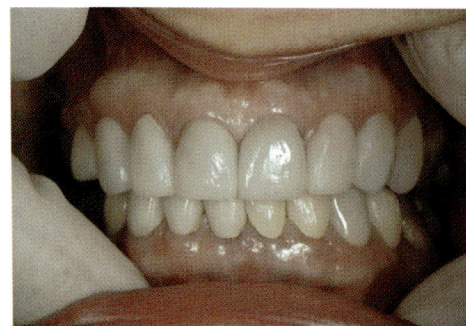

Fig. 7: Post-op. New porcelain veneers have been placed.

Case 5:
Soft and Hard Tissue Crown Lengthening (Troughing Technique)
(Newest Technique Invented by Dr. Bret Dyer from Houston, Texas)

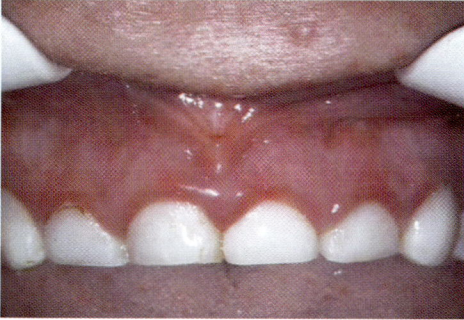

Fig. 1: Pre-op. Gingivitis is present due to poor biological zone. Patient also complains about having a "gummy smile."

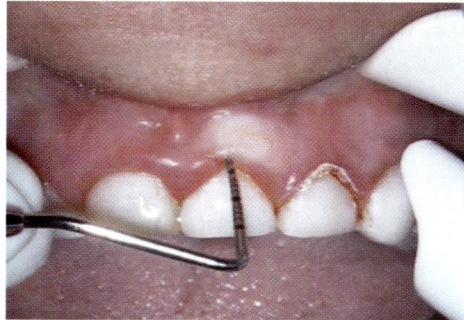

Fig. 2: Profound anesthesia is obtained by local anesthesia with injection. Bone sounding is done to locate the CEJ.

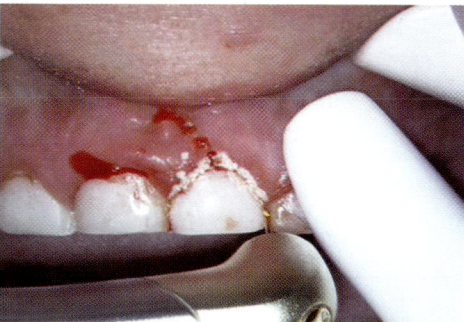

Fig. 3: A dry setting is used to mark the soft tissue that is to be reduced. A MZ-5 in a MD Gold Handpiece is used with a setting of 0.25W, 0% Water, 11% Air, 30 Hz.

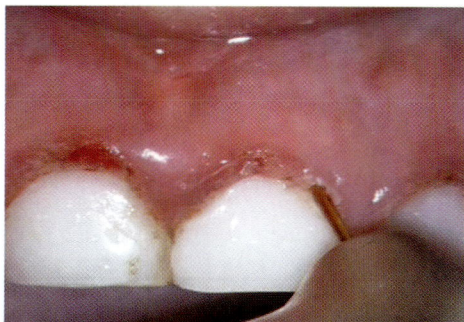

Fig. 4: Since new composite veneers are treatment planned, the tip is placed perpendicular to the long axis of teeth for the soft tissue crown lengthening. The setting is 1.00W, 11% Water, 11% Air, 30 Hz.

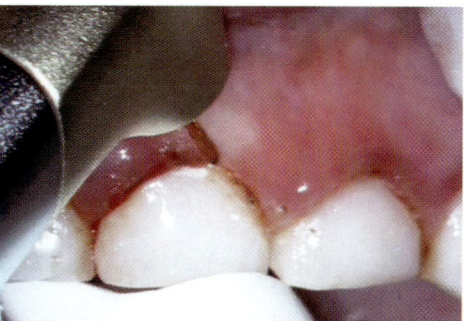

Fig. 5: The soft tissue crown lengthening is in progress.

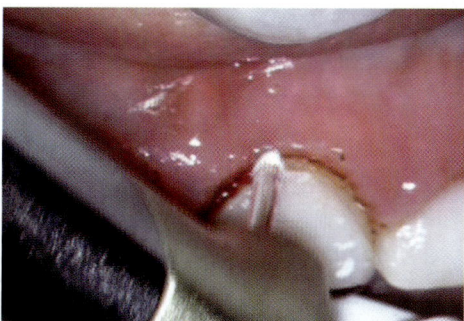

Fig. 6: Beveling of the marginal gingiva is performed with a MC-12 tip placed at approximately 45° to give a knife-edge finish to the marginal gingiva. The setting is 0.75-1.75W, 11% Water, 11% Air, 50 Hz.

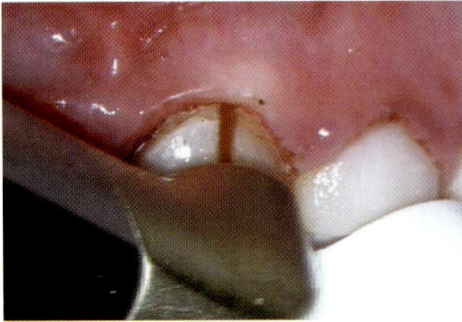

Fig. 7: This is followed by troughing to create a space between the gingiva and the root. The tip is MZ-5 and the setting is 1.00-1.50W, 15% Water, 11% Air, 30 Hz.

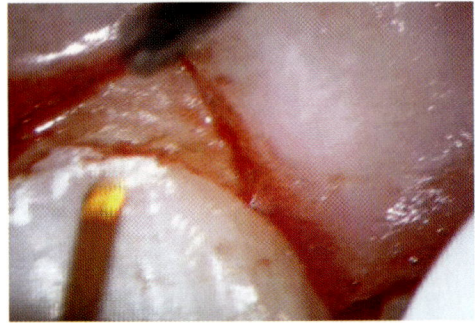

Fig. 8: Bone sounding is done with direct vision under high magnification. Bone reduction is performed with a MZ-5 tip with direct vision. The setting is 2.50-4.00W, 60% Water, 15% Air, 20-50 Hz.

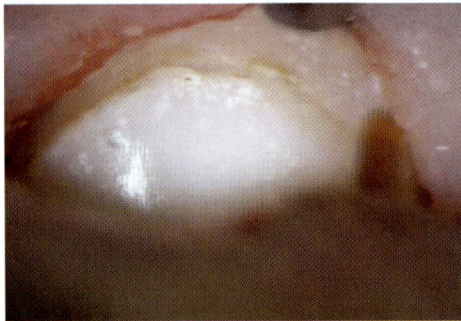

Fig. 9: The bone reduction continues until new bone level is ≈ 4mm from the marginal gingiva.

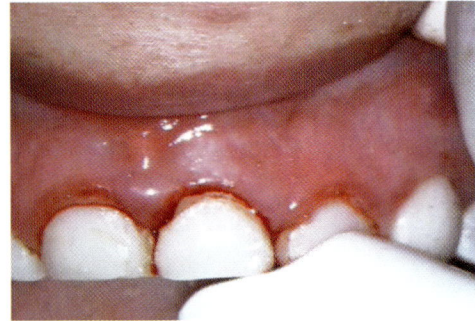

Fig. 10: Immediate post-op after soft and bony crown lengthening.

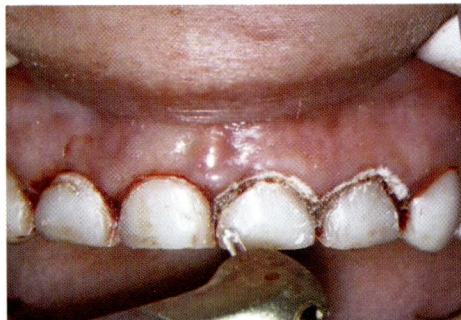

Fig. 11: Biologic band-aid is applied using the MC-12 tip at 1.25W, 0% Water, 11% Air, 30 Hz.

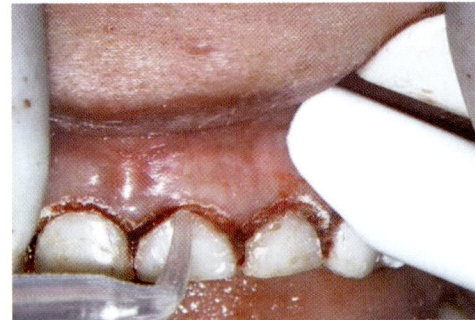

Fig. 12: Tissue adhesive (cyanoacrylate such as Iso-dent) is used to adhere the soft tissue onto hard tissue.

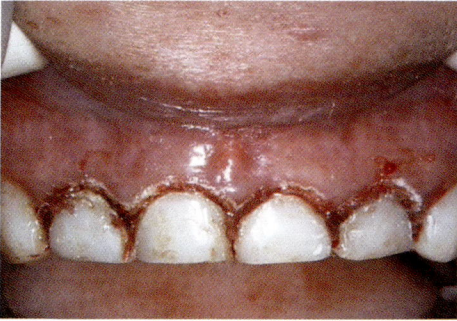

Fig. 13: Immediate post-op, #7-10.

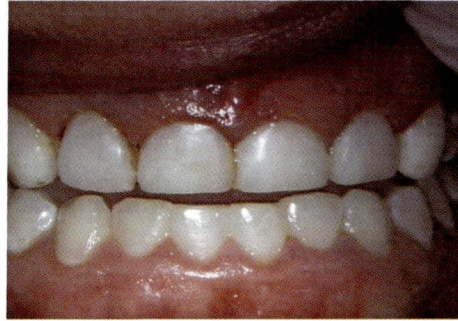

Fig. 14: Three week post-op after new composite veneers are placed.

Laser-Assisted Tooth Extraction

The Er,Cr:YSGG laser system may be used for any extraction that requires more than elevators to subluxate the tooth before exodontia. Laser-assisted extractions help to preserve bone and reduce post-operative complications such as bleeding, swelling, and pain. In proposed implant sites that require extraction, exodontia should be performed with the least amount of bone removal. Laser involvement is most beneficial in the preservation of bone integrity for future implant procedures.

Laser-Assisted Tooth Extraction
Technique #1: Troughing Technique

Laser Parameters, Set 1: Troughing and Cutting of Ligaments

Waterlase MD laser system settings: MZ-4 tip, 2.50W, 60% Water, 15% Air, 20 Hz
Other Er,Cr:YSGG laser system settings: Z-4 tip, 2.50W, 40% Water, 15% Air

The tip is lined up along the long axis of the tooth, with the tip slightly angled aiming towards the tooth. Using a slow motion and a back-and-forth sweeping fashion, aim the tip at cutting ligament attachments. This is similar to troughing the alveolus around the tooth.

The surgical procedure will extend into approximately 1/2 to 2/3 of the root until the tooth is loose. With some pressure by an elevator, sublexation is performed. The tooth can be removed by a pair of forceps. This procedure is minimally invasive to the alveolus and preserves bone for future implant placement. The use of the laser in this surgery also reduces the release of histamine. That results in less bleeding, less swelling and less pain.

Laser Parameters, Set 2: Smoothing Bone

Waterlase MD laser system settings: MZ-4 tip, 1.50W, 60% Water, 15% Air, 40 Hz
Other Er,Cr:YSGG laser system settings: Z-4 tip, 1.00W, 30% Water, 30% Air

The 20 Hz pulsing of the laser may have produced some rough bone. We now use a higher frequency and lower power laser energy to smooth the bone gently.

Laser Parameters, Set 3: Hemostasis

Waterlase MD laser system settings: MC-12 tip, 1.50W, 0% Water, 11% Air, 30 Hz
Other Er,Cr:YSGG laser system settings: C-12 tip, 1.50 W, 0% Water, 11% Air

After suture is placed at the extraction site, the tip is defocused 3-5mm and aimed at the bleeding soft tissue to coagulate. Biostimulation is also applied to the tissue by a low-level laser.

Laser-Assisted Tooth Extraction
Technique #2: Slot Technique

Laser Parameters, Set 1: Bone Troughing

Waterlase MD laser system settings: MZ-6 tip, 2.50-4.00W, 60% Water, 80% Air, 20 Hz
Other Er,Cr:YSGG laser system settings: Z-6 tip, 2.50-4.00W, 60% Water, 65% Air

The tip is lined up along the long axis of the tooth at the mesial area, with the tip slightly angled towards the tooth. A bone slot is produced at the mesial area of the tooth. This is about 2mm in depth. This is used as a "purchase slot" for the elevator to subluxate the tooth. When the tooth is loose, a pair of forceps is used to remove the tooth. The procedure is also minimally invasive considering there is no need to prepare a flap.

Laser Parameters, Set 2: Biologic Band-Aid

Waterlase MD laser settings: MZ-6 tip, 1.25 W, 0% Water, 11% Air, 30 Hz
Other Er,Cr:YSGG laser system settings: Z-6 tip, 1.00W, 0% Water, 11% Air

After a suture is placed at the extraction site, the tip is defocused 3-5mm and aimed at the bleeding soft tissue to coagulate the tissue. Biostimulation is also applied to the tissue by a low-level laser.

Case 1: Troughing Technique

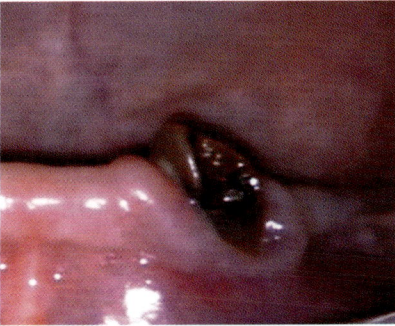

Fig. 1: Pre-op. Mandibular left cuspid is treatment planned to be removed. A mandibular block and a long buccal are given.

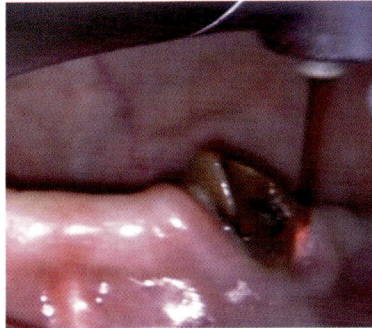

Fig. 2: A MZ-6 (9mm) long tip is used to ablate ligaments around the tooth. The laser setting is 6.00W, 75% Water, 90% Air, 20 Hz.

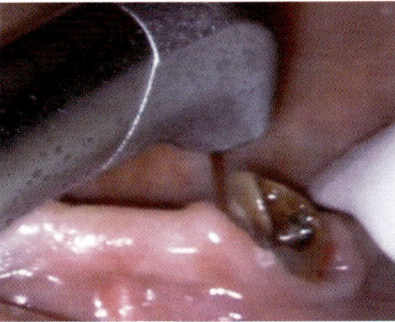

Fig. 3: The tip ablates its way into ½ to 2/3 of the root length.

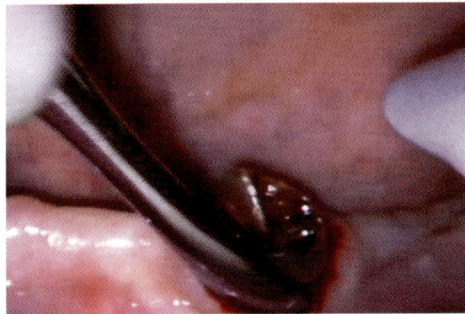

Fig. 4: A periosteal elevator is used to subluxate the tooth.

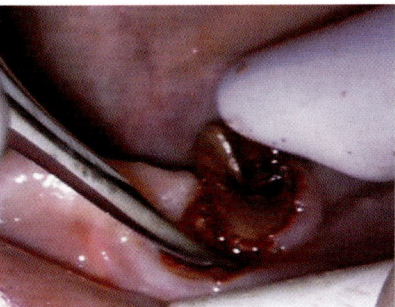

Fig. 5: The tooth is easily elevated out of the socket.

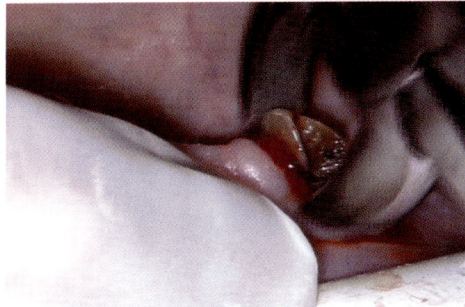

Fig. 6: A forcep is used to remove the tooth.

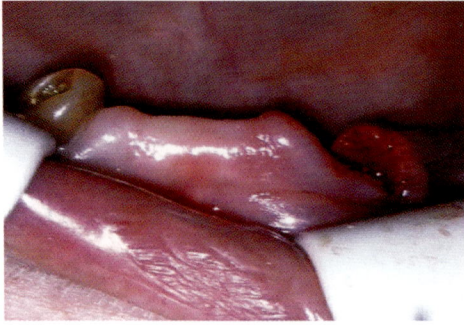

Fig. 7: Not much bleeding is noted after the laser-assisted exodontia.

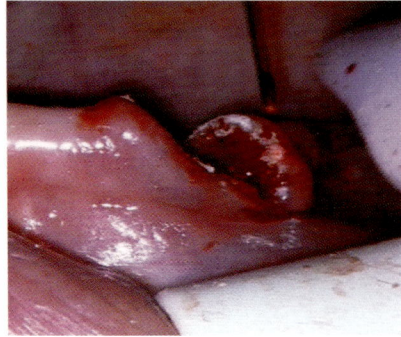

Fig. 8: A biologic band-aid procedure is performed. The laser setting is 1.25W, 0% Water, 11% Air, 30 Hz.

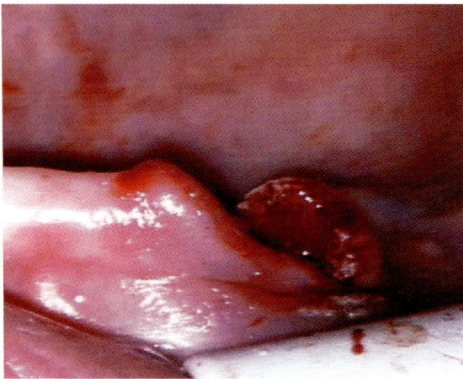

Fig. 9: Post-op after biologic band-aid.

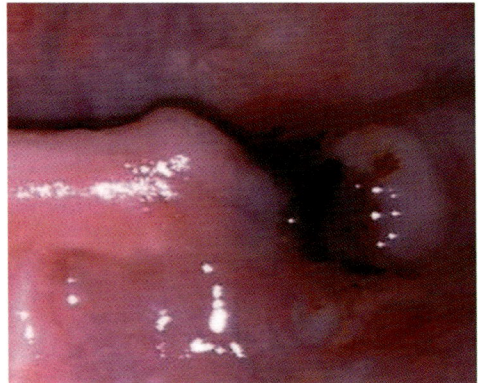

Fig. 10: Post-op at 24 hours.

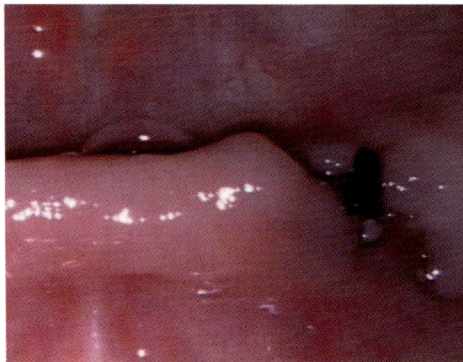

Fig. 11: Post-op at 4 days. Note the pink tissue is healthy.

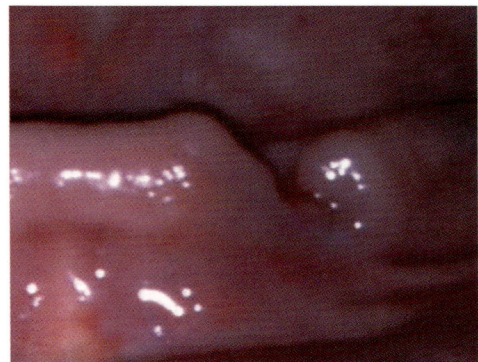

Fig. 12: Post-op at 1 week.

Case 2: Slot Technique

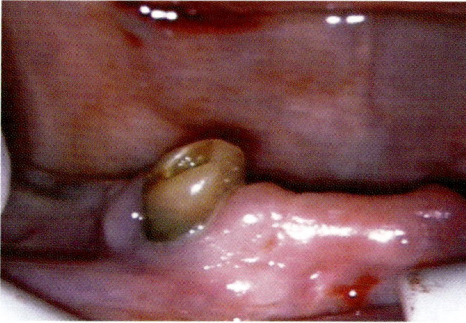

Fig. 1: Pre-op. #27 treatment planned to be extracted.

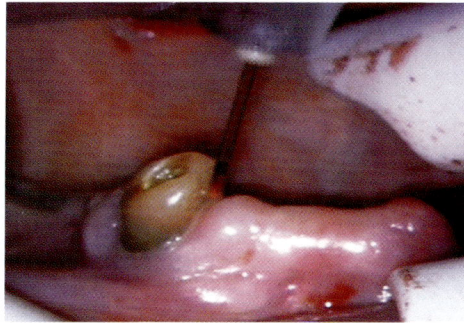

Fig. 2: After profound local anesthesia has been administered, a MD Handpiece with a MZ-6 (9mm) is used to trough the gingiva and prepare a slot preparation at the mesial area of #27. The setting is 4.50W, 60% Water, 80% Air, 20 Hz.

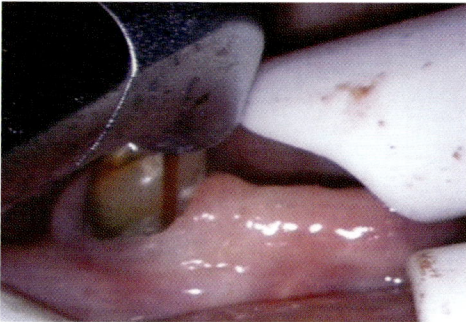

Fig. 3: The slot preparation is about 2-3mm into the bone.

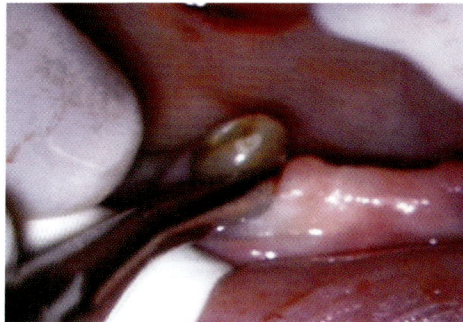

Fig. 4: A 301 elevator is placed into the bone slot, which serves as a "purchase point" to allow the elevator to subluxate #27.

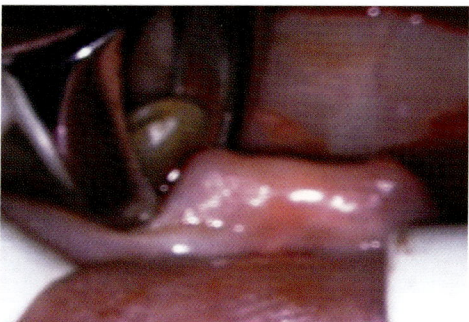

Fig. 5: The tooth is easily removed by a forcep.

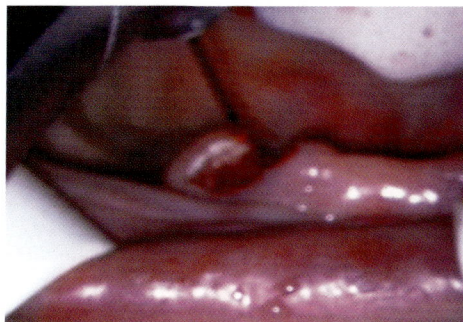

Fig. 6: A biologic band-aid is performed by the laser using 1.25W, 0% Water, 11% Air, 30 Hz, defocused to about 5mm.

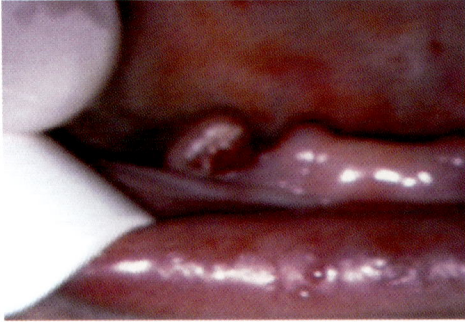

Fig. 7: Immediate post-op.

Impacted Third Molar Extraction

Laser Parameters, Set 1: Incision for Flap

Waterlase MD laser system settings: MT-4 tip, 2.00W, 7% Water, 11% Air, 30 Hz
Other Er,Cr:YSGG laser system settings: T-4 tip, 1.50W, 7% Water, 11% Air

Prepare an incision for a flap using the laser. Starting distal to second molar, make an incision mesial of the second molar on the buccal side. The technique for making the incision involves a back-and-forth sweeping motion over a 2-3mm segment of tissue at a time. A vertical relief is optional. In reflecting the flap, notice the soft tissue should come away from the alveolus with ease.

Laser Parameters, Set 2: Osteotomy

Waterlase MD laser system settings: MG-6 tip, 6.00W, 60% Water, 80% Air, 20 Hz
Other Er,Cr:YSGG laser system settings: G-6 tip, 6.00W, 75% Water, 90% Air

The reduction of bone starts from distal of the third molar and then the buccal surface. It also involves removing bone mesial to the third molar. This will create a "purchase slot" for the elevator to subluxate the third molar.

If sectioning of the tooth is needed, use a high-speed rotary instrument to section the tooth. Any additional bone reduction is performed by using laser energy.

Laser Parameters, Set 3: Alveoplasty

Waterlase MD laser system settings: 2.50-4.00W, 60% Water, 80% Air, 30 Hz
Other Er,Cr:YSGG laser system settings: 2.00-4.00W, 60% Water, 65% Air

After removal of the impacted third molar (by forceps or elevator), use the laser to smooth the bone edges. This is followed by suture placement.

Laser Parameters, Set 4: Hemostasis

Waterlase MD laser system settings: 1.25W, 0% Water, 11% Air, 30 Hz, H mode
Other Er,Cr:YSGG laser system settings: 1.00W, 0% Water, 11% Air

The tip is aimed at bleeding soft tissue at a defocused distance, 3-5mm. Coagulation and biostimulation are applied to the soft tissue extraction site.

Case 1: Laser-assisted Extraction of Partial Impacted Mandibular Molar, MD Regular HP with MG-6 Tip

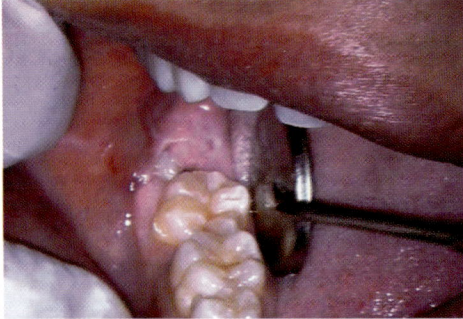

Fig. 1: Pre-op. Assessment of the right mandibular third molar shows a partial bony-impacted tooth.

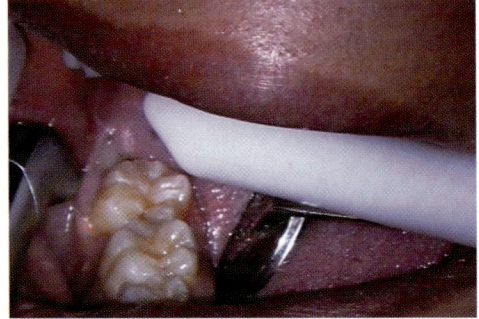

Fig. 2: A MT-4 tip is used to make the incision for flap. The setting is 2.50W, 7% Water, 11% Air, 50 Hz. The incision is from distal of the tooth to mesial of right mandibular second molar where a vertical relief is made.

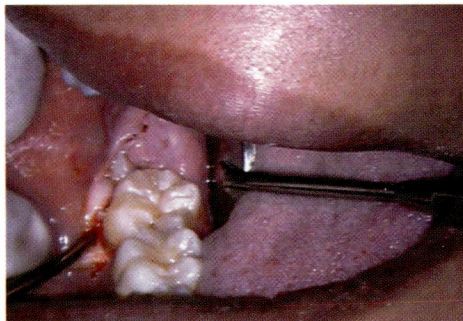

Fig. 3: A periosteal elevator is used to retract the mucogingival tissue.

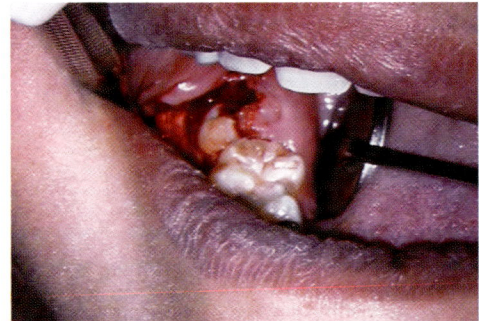

Fig. 4: The impacted third molar is revealed.

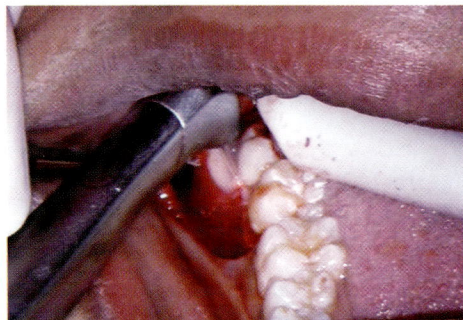

Fig. 5: A MG-6 tip is used for osteotomy to better expose the crown. The setting is 6.00W, 60% Water, 65% Air, 20 Hz.

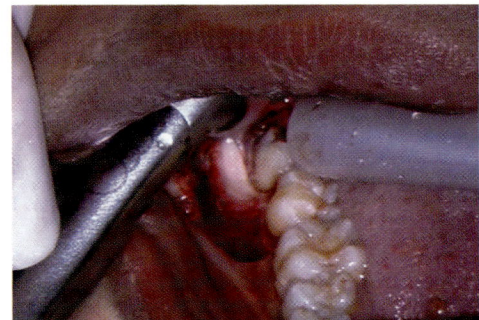

Fig. 6: The bone reduction includes the mesial and buccal areas of the crown.

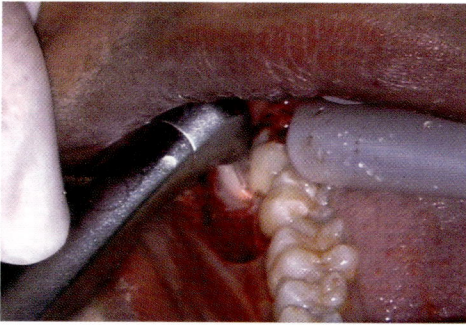

Fig. 7: The bone reduction extends from the buccal to distal areas of the crown.

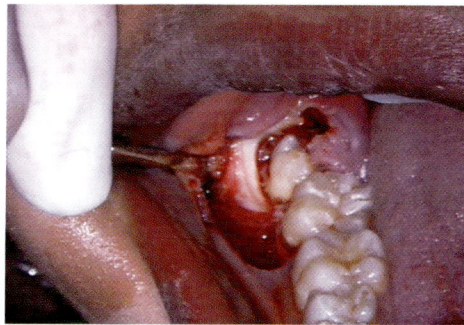

Fig. 8: Bone reduction of the impacted third molar is complete.

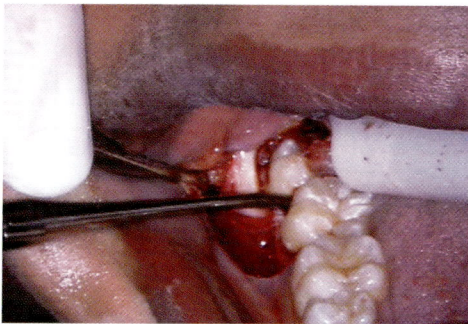

Fig. 9: Subluxation of the tooth starts with a periosteal elevator.

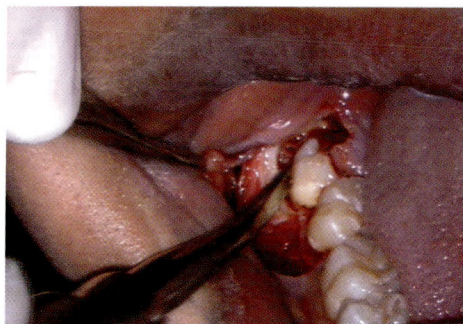

Fig. 10: The subluxation of the tooth is continued using 301 and 302 straight elevators from mesial and buccal areas.

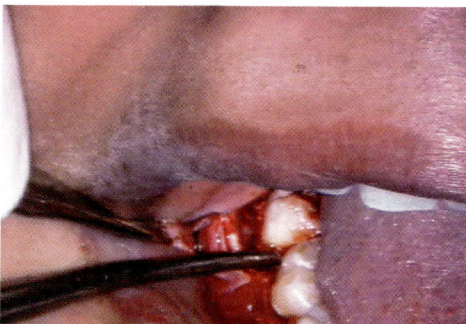

Fig. 11: The tooth is elevated on its way out of the socket.

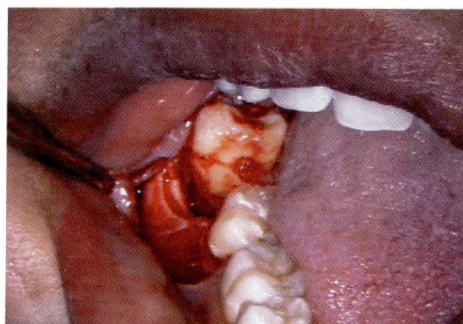

Fig. 12: The tooth is ready to be removed by forceps.

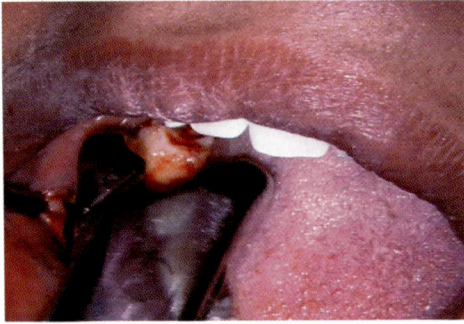

Fig. 13: Forceps are used to remove the tooth.

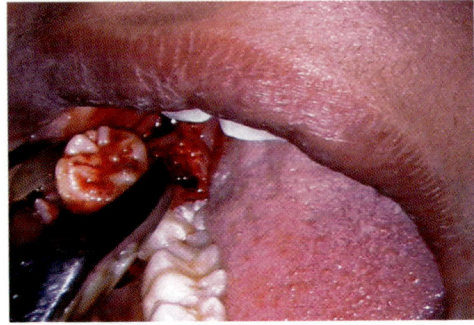

Fig. 14: The tooth is removed from the socket.

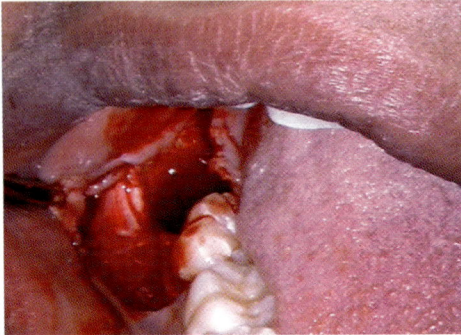

Fig. 15: Minimal bleeding is noted at the surgical site.

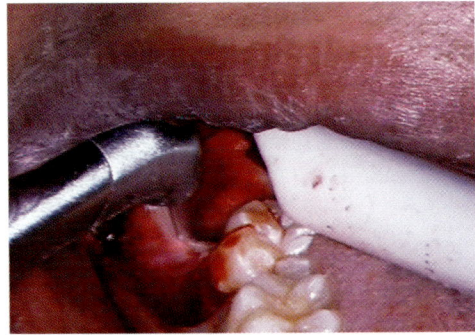

Fig. 16: The setting of 2.50W, 60% Water, 65% Air, 40 Hz is used to smooth bone.

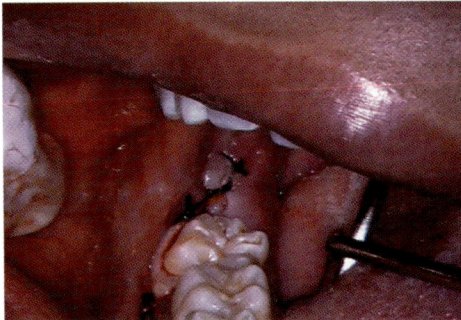

Fig. 17: 3-0 black silk is used to close the surgical site.

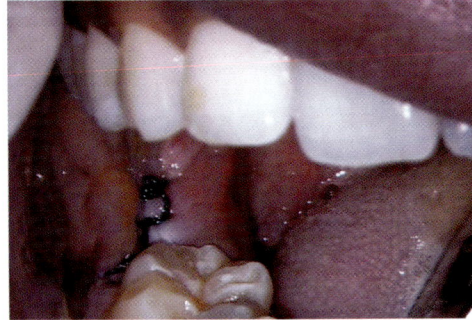

Fig.18: 24-hour post-op. No secondary bleeding is noted. No post-op complications can be seen.

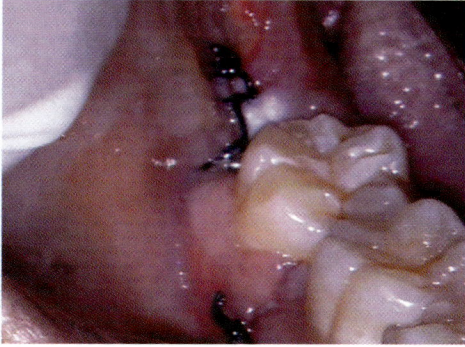

Fig. 19: Three-day post-op. The surgical site is healing well.

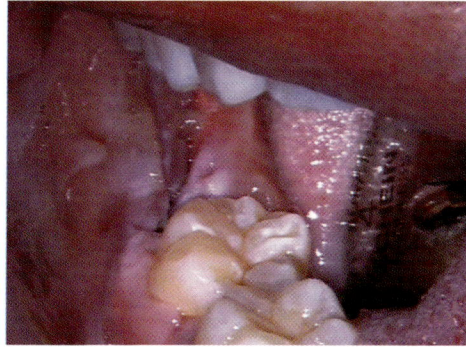

Fig. 20: One-week post-op. Sutures have been removed, with good healing noted.

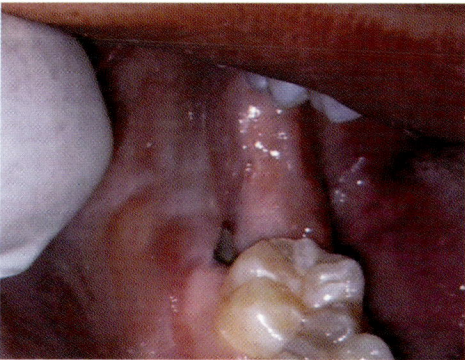

Fig. 21: Two-week post-op follow up.

Lingual Torus Removal

Laser Parameters, Set 1: Incision for Flap

Waterlase MD laser system settings: MT-4 tip, 2.00W, 7% Water, 11% Air, 30 Hz
Other Er,Cr:YSGG laser system settings: T-4 tip, 1.50W, 7% Water, 11% Air

A full thickness flap is prepared by laser energy with a vertical relief made 4-5mm from the torus.

Laser Parameters, Set 2: Osteotomy

Waterlase MD laser system settings: MG-6 tip, 6.00W, 60% Water, 80% Air, 20 Hz
Other Er,Cr:YSGG laser system settings: G-6 tip, 6.00W, 75% Water, 90% Air

After reflecting the tissue, laser is used to perform a bone osteotomy. From the occlusal surface, place the tip parallel to the alveolus surface, and mark an outline of the torus in the bone. For small tori, this outline will be deepened until the torus is hanging by the apical portion of the bone. A chisel can be used to separate the torus from alveolus. The last tissue attached can be ablated by the laser. For large tori, extend the outline on the occlusal area vertically at the mesial and distal area. This is followed by sectional cuts dividing the large torus into several smaller tori. These tori are removed individually similar to removing small tori.

Laser Parameters, Set 3: Smooth Edge and Base of Alveolus; Segment Torus

Waterlase MD laser system settings: MC-3 tip, 2.50-4.00W, 60% Water, 80% Air, 30-40Hz
Other Er,Cr:YSGG laser system settings: C-3 tip, 2.50-4.00W, 60% Water, 65% Air

Use the laser to smooth the alveolus surface and edge.

Bone files can be used, but use laser energy to finish with debridement and decontamination.

Laser Parameters, Set 4: Hemostasis

Waterlase MD laser system settings: MG-6 tip, 1.25W, 0% Water, 11% Air, 30 Hz
Other Er,Cr:YSGG laser system settings: G-6 tip, 1.00W, 0% Water, 11% Air

After suturing the surgical site, use the laser to treat a band of 4-5 mm of the mucogingival tissue on both sides of the cut. This low-level laser therapy serves as a bandage and will have the effect of pain attenuation, in addition to better and faster wound healing.

Case 1: Mandibular Lingual Torus Removal , MD Regular HP with MG-6 and MC-3 Tips

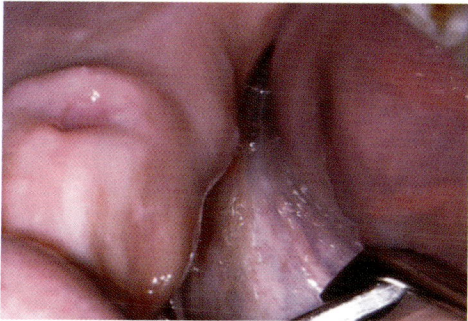

Fig. 1: Pre-op. Torus is noted lingual to the extended right mandibular first molar.

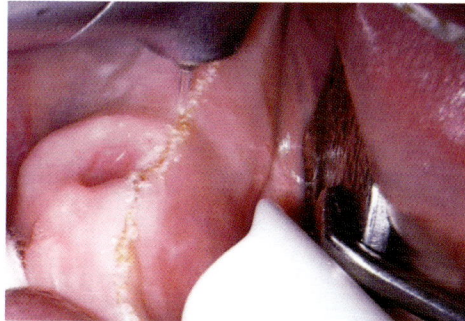

Fig. 2: After a mandibular block and a long buccal are given, a MT-4 tip is used to make an incision for flap at mesial and distal to the extracted tooth area. The setting is 2.50W, 7% Water, 11% Air, 50 Hz.

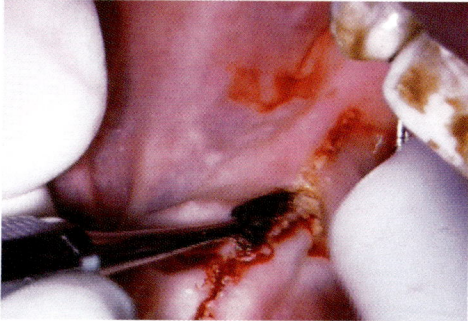

Fig. 3: A periosteal elevator is used to reveal the lingual torus.

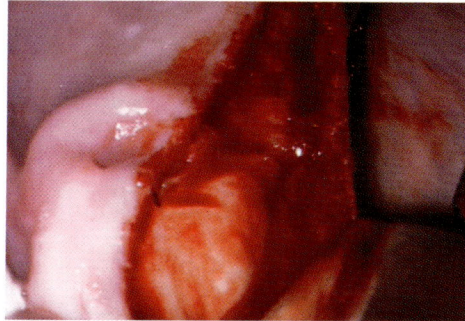

Fig. 4: The outline of the lingual torus is cleanly revealed.

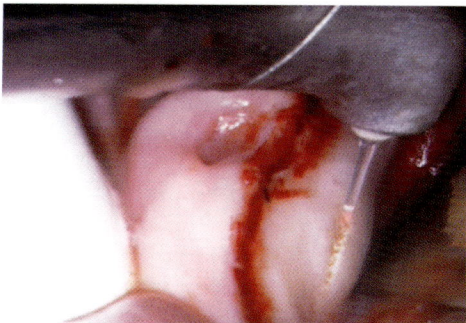

Fig. 5: A MG-6 tip is used to ablate bone from the occlusal area to outline the bone lesion. The setting is 6.00W, 60% Water, 65% Air, 20 Hz.

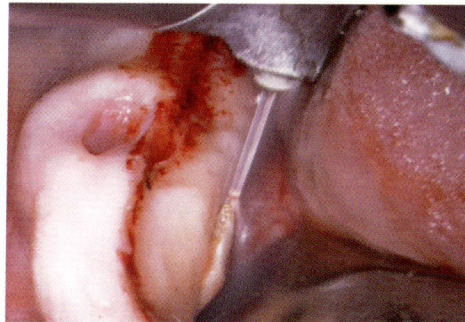

Fig. 6: Osteotomy continues to the apical area of the torus.

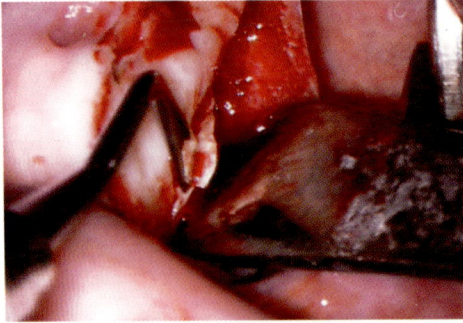

Fig. 7: An elevator is used to elevate out the torus that has been cut by the laser.

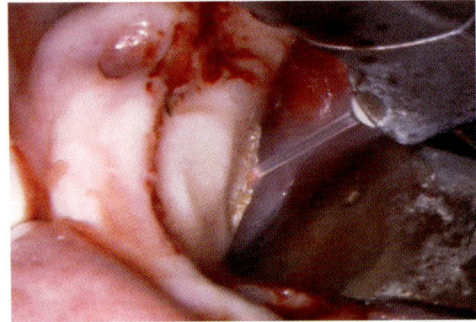

Fig. 8: Smoothing the surgical site with a setting of 4.50W, 60% Water, 65% Air, 40 Hz.

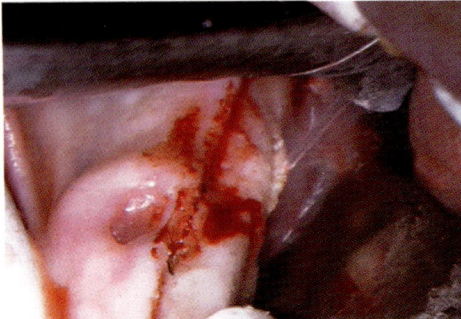

Fig. 9: A MC-3 tip is used to complete bone smoothing.

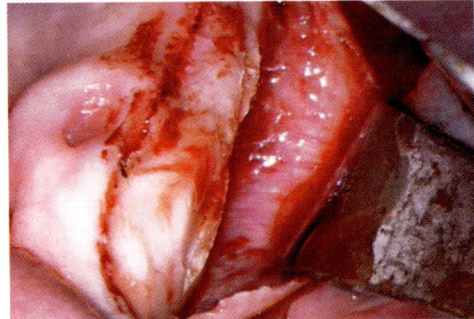

Fig. 10: Osteotomy of the lingual torus is complete.

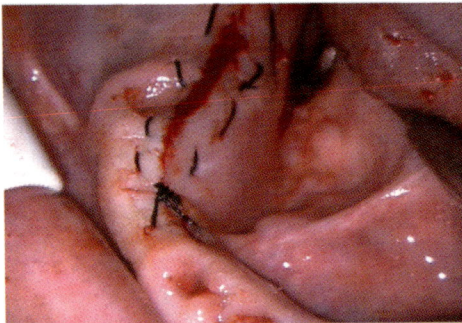

Fig. 11: A 3-0 black suture and a mattress technique are used to close the surgical site.

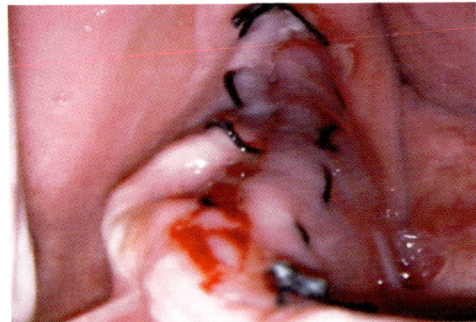

Fig. 12: Post-op at three days. No complication is noted.

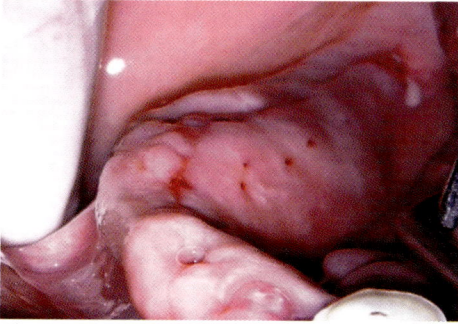

Fig. 13: Post-op at one week. The stitches are removed and good healing is noted.

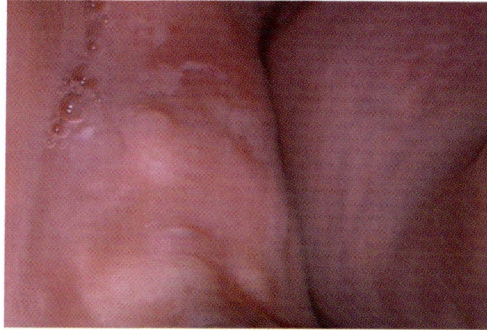

Fig. 14: Post-op at 12 weeks. Healing is complete.

Hemostasis

At the conclusion of any soft tissue surgical procedure, any bleeding may be halted quickly by using the laser at low power, air and water settings to induce hemostasis. Different fiber tips should be used at slightly different settings to achieve best results.

For fiber tip MG-6, the laser setting used is 1.25W, 0% Water, 11% Air, 30 Hz.

For fiber tip MC-6, the laser setting used is 1.25W, 0% Water, 11% Air, 30 Hz,

For fiber tip MC-12, the laser setting used is 1.50W, 0% Water, 11% Air, 30 Hz.

The MC-12 tip covers a very broad surface, as it has twice the diameter of the MG-6 or MC-6 tips, and is very effective in coagulating a laser frenectomy, a large fibroma removal, and any hyperplastic tissue removal.

In all instances, the technique used is a defocused mode (3-5mm), with a slow circular motion. The coagulated tissue should appear white and dry. The H mode is preferred over the S mode in performing the biologic band-aid. However, where the surgical site has excessive bleeding present, the S mode is more effective in coagulating the opened vessels. The tradeoff is there will be more charring present after prolonged use of the S mode setting.

Case 1: Hemostasis and Biologic Band-aid, after a Maxillary Labial Frenectomy performed by the MD

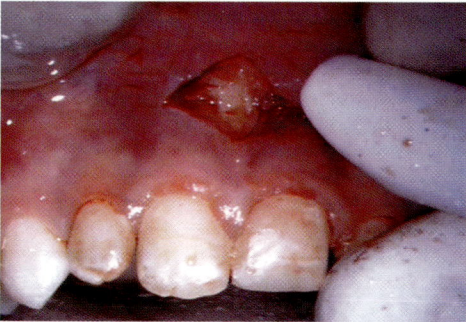

Fig. 1: Pre-op. Maxillary labial frenectomy is performed. Some bleeding is noted.

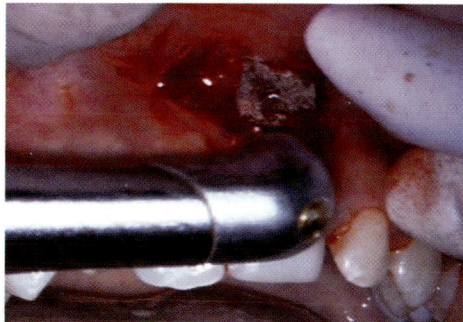

Fig. 2: A MG-6 tip is used to stop bleeding at the left side of the surgical site. The setting is 1.25W, 0% Water, 11% Air, 30 Hz.

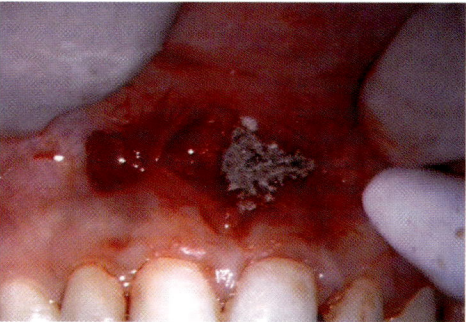

Fig. 3: Hemostasis is established at the left side of the surgical site.

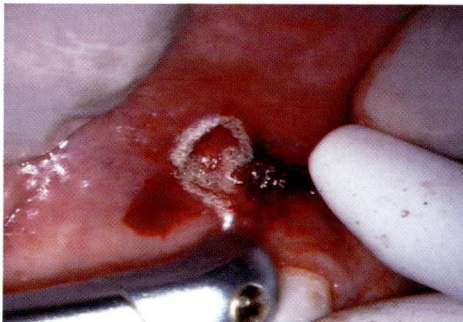

Fig. 4: A MC-12 tip is used to stop bleeding at the right side of the surgical site. The setting is 1.50W, 0% Water, 11% Air, 30 Hz. Half the time is needed to stop bleeding at the right half of the surgical site due to a larger diameter tip.

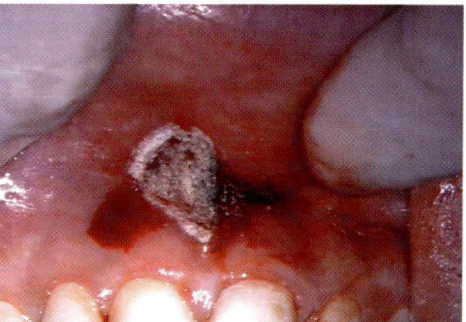

Fig. 5: Biologic band-aid is complete.

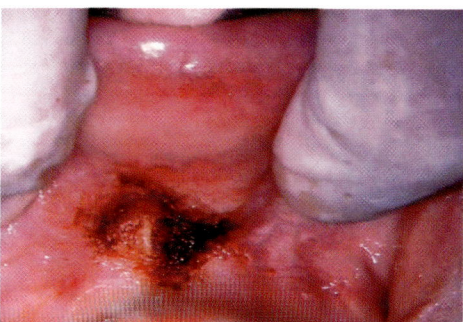

Fig. 6: Some bleeding still persists.

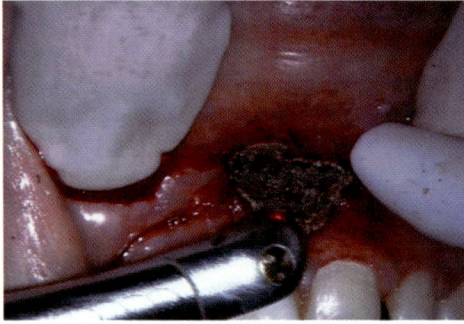

Fig. 7: More hemostasis is performed with the MC-12 tip. This time the setting is done with S mode at a more defocused mode (5-8mm).

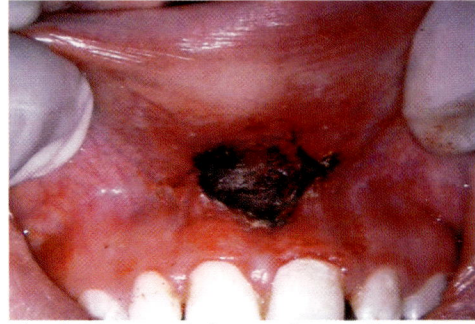

Fig. 8: Hemostasis is complete. A little charring of the tissue is noted.

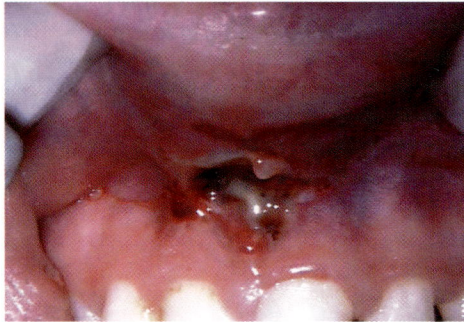

Fig. 9: Post-op at 5 days. No complications are observed.

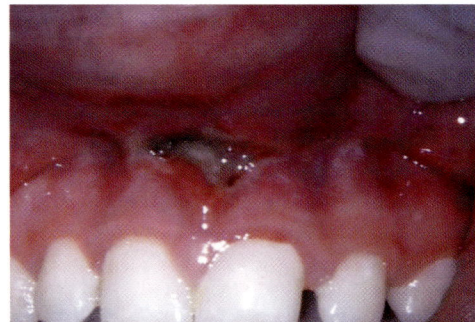

Fig. 10: Post-op at one week. Slower healing is observed when using H mode and pressure to perform hemostasis.

Gum Bleaching (De-Pigmentation of Gingiva)

Some patients may possess dark pigments in their gingiva. While the pigmentation is harmless, patients may desire to remove such pigmentation for esthetic reasons. The Er,Cr:YSGG laser system is very effective in performing this procedure of gum bleaching with no injection anesthesia needed.

Laser Parameters, Set 1: Ablation of Pigmented Gingiva

Waterlase MD laser system settings: MG-6 tip, 1.25-1.75W, 7-11% Water, 11% Air, 30 Hz

Other Er,Cr:YSGG laser system settings: G-6 tip, 1.00-1.50W, 7% Water, 11% Air

> Before using the laser, apply concentrated topical (Emla or Tac-gel) for at least 3 minutes. The tip is placed perpendicular to the gingiva and mucogingival surface where dark pigments are concentrated.
>
> Use the laser to ablate the pigmented gingiva and mucogingival tissues. This may take several rounds of surface ablation to disrupt the pigmented tissue. Use a sterile water soaked cotton swap to rub out the loose pigmented gingiva and mucogingival tissue.

Laser Parameters, Set 2: Hemostasis and Low Level Laser Therapy

Waterlase MD laser system settings: MG-6 tip, 1.25W, 0% Water, 11% Air, 30 Hz
Other Er,Cr:YSGG laser system settings: G-6 tip, 1.00W, 0% Water, 11% Air, defocused

> To finish, use the laser to apply low-level laser therapy to the open wound. No suturing is required.

Case 1: De-pigmentation of Gingival and Mucogingival Tissue of Tooth #7 Using a M2 with G-6 Tip

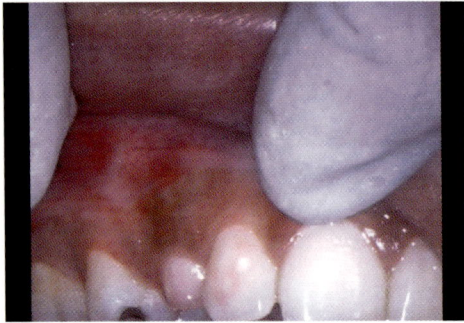

Fig. 1: Pre-op. Melanin pigments are prominent at the gingival and mucogingival areas of #6. Patient wants the de-pigmentation procedure to be performed.

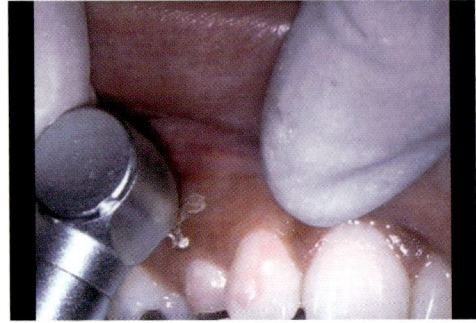

Fig. 2: A G-6 tip is used. The setting is 1.25W, 7% Water, 11% Air. The tip is defocused 1-2mm from the gingiva and mucogingival areas and is aimed to ablate and loosen up the surface tissue.

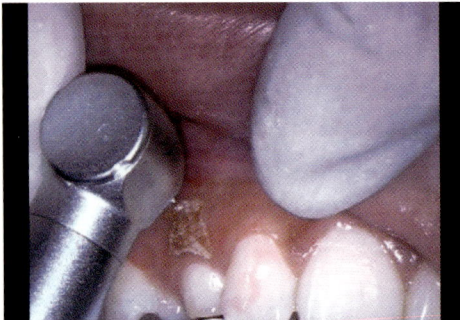

Fig. 3: The soft tissue ablation continues to cover the entire heavy pigmented area. Care should be taken to avoid exposing bone.

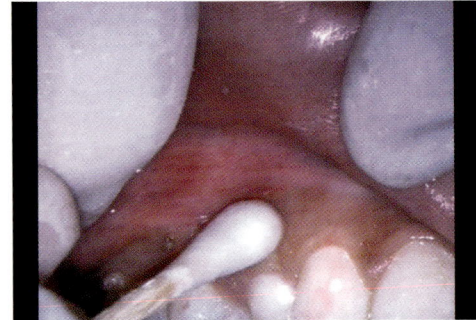

Fig. 4: A water soaked Q-tip is used to peel off the loose pigmented tissue.

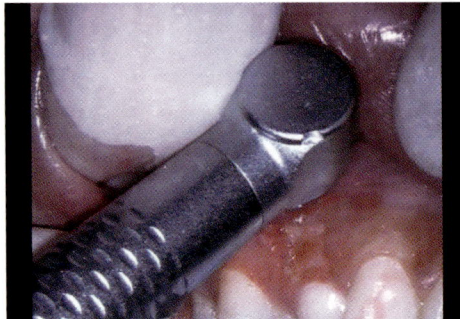

Fig. 5: A laser biologic band-aid is applied to the surgical site to complete the procedure. The setting is 1.00W, 0% Water, 11% Air, defocused to approximately 5mm.

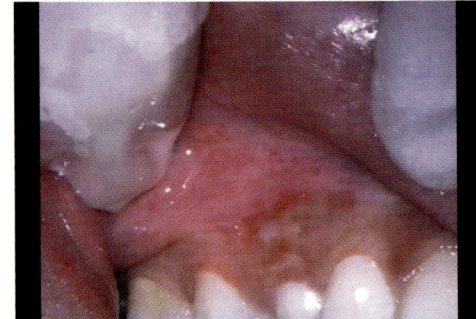

Fig. 6: Immediate post-op.

Er,Cr:YSGG Laser System Gingivectomy to Uncover Implant

No local anesthesia should be needed. Locate the healing cap by means of a plastic explorer probing the edentulous gingiva. Use some concentrated topical to treat the area.

Laser Parameters, Set 1: Ablation of Gingiva

Waterlase MD laser system settings: MG-6 tip, 1.25-2.00W, 7-11% Water, 11% Air, 30 Hz

Other Er,Cr:YSGG laser system settings: G-6 tip, 1.25-1.75W, 7% Water, 11% Air

A gingivectomy is performed to uncover the healing cap. The gingival tissue ablation takes place slowly and carefully until the outline of the healing cap is obtained. The ablation of the gingiva is conservative. As soon as enough access to remove the healing cap is established, the gingivectomy is completed.

Case 1: Gingivectomy to Uncover Endosseous Implant, MD Regular HP with MG-6 Tip

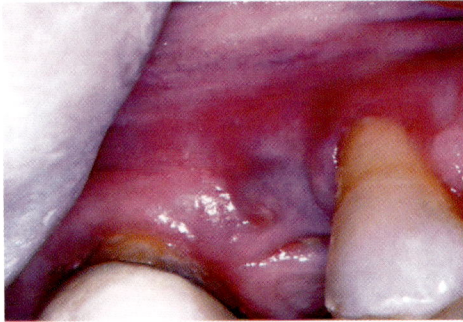

Fig. 1: Pre-op. An endosseous implant at right maxillary first molar area has healed well and is ready for restoration.

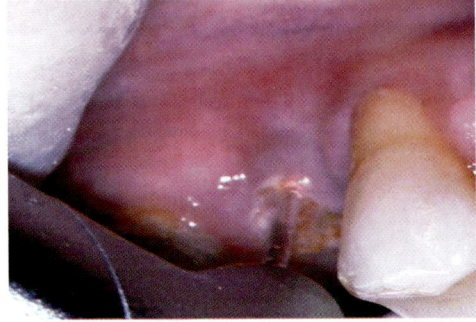

Fig. 2 A MG-6 tip is used to uncover the implant. The setting is 1.25W, 7% Water, 11% Air, 30 Hz.

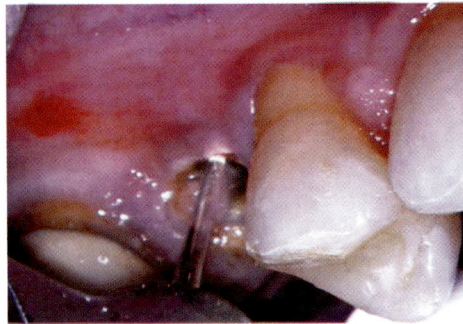

Fig. 3: The healing screw is revealed. The ablation does not go into bone. Minimum soft tissue is removed to enable removal of healing screw.

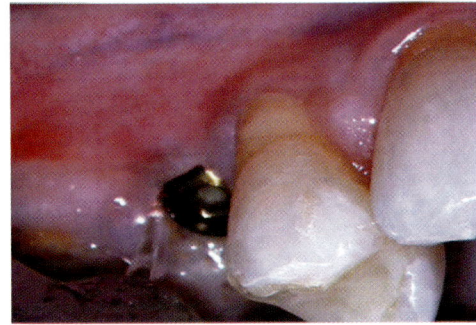

Fig. 4: The outline of the healing screw is revealed precisely.

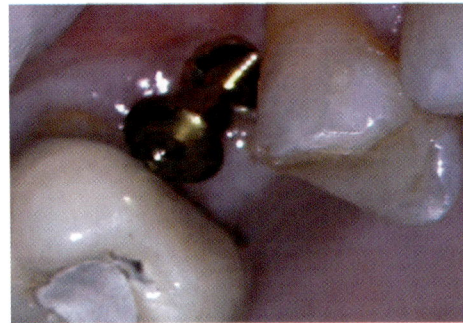

Fig. 5: The healing screw is removed.

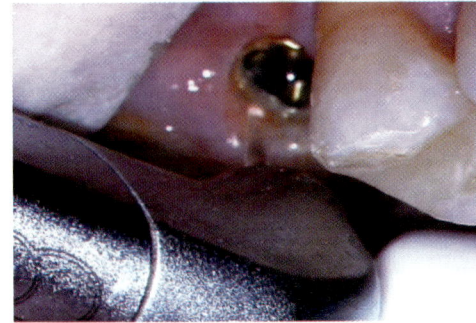

Fig. 6: Irregularities of soft tissue around the implant are smoothed by using 1.25W, 9% Water, 11% Air, 30 Hz, S mode.

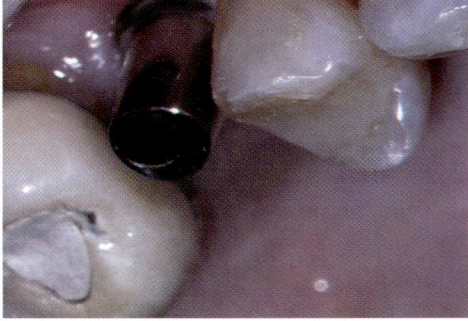

Fig. 7: Direct abutment is fitted to the implant.

Er,Cr:YSGG Laser System-Assisted Placement of Endosseous Implant

Laser Parameters, Set 1: Outline Surgical Site

Waterlase MD laser system settings: MG-6 tip, 0.75W, 0% Water, 11% Air, 30 Hz
Other Er,Cr:YSGG laser system settings: G-6 tip, 0.75W, 0% Water, 11% Air

Administer local anesthesia and use a template to guide the laser and mark the location of the implant osteotomy. The estimated diameter of the implant is outlined at the marked location.

Laser Parameters, Set 2: Ablation of Gingiva

Waterlase MD laser system settings: 1.50-2.50W, 7-11% Water, 11% Air, 30 Hz
Other Er,Cr:YSGG laser system settings: 1.25-1.75W, 11% Water, 20% Air

Continue the ablation of gingiva all the way to the bone level. If you are starting at the lowest power level and ablation is proceeding slowly, increase the power in 0.25Watt increments until a satisfactory speed is achieved.

Laser Parameters, Set 3: Osteotomy

Waterlase MD laser system settings: 4.00-6.00W, 60% Water, 80% Air, 20-25 Hz
Other Er,Cr:YSGG laser system settings: 4.50W, 60% Water, 65% Air

Using indelible ink, mark the laser fiber tip at a distance of 2mm shorter than the expected depth of cutting. The laser will be used to ablate the bone to the length of the implant. This serves as the "pivot drill" of the implant preparation.

Complete the osteotomy using conventional series implant preparation drills.

Laser Parameters, Set 4: Treat Implant Site for Decontamination

Waterlase MD laser system settings: 0.75W, 7% Water, 11% Air, 30 Hz
Other Er,Cr:YSGG laser system settings: 0.75W, 7% Water, 11% Air

After the drill preparation, laser energy is used to treat the implant site for decontamination. The tip should be moved in slow circular motion with a slow up-and-down motion to ensure that all faces of the implant site have received laser energy. This is followed in turn by the placement of the endosseous implant.

Laser Parameters, Set 5: Low Level Laser Therapy

Waterlase MD laser system settings: 1.00-1.50W, 7% Water, 11% Air, 30 Hz
Other Er,Cr:YSGG laser system settings: 0.75W, 7% Water, 11% Air

To finish, the laser is used to apply low-power laser energy to de-epithelialize a band of 4-5mm of the peri-implant gingiva.

Case 1: Laser-Assisted Osteotomy for Endosseous Implant Placement at #19

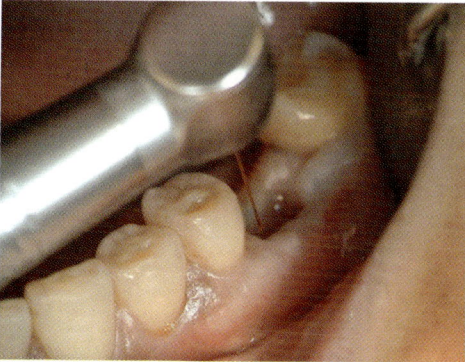

Fig. 1: Tooth #19 was extracted 10 days prior. An endosseous implant is planned to replace #19. Incision for a full thickness flap is made with a Z-4 tip. The setting is 1.00W, 7% Water, 11% Air.

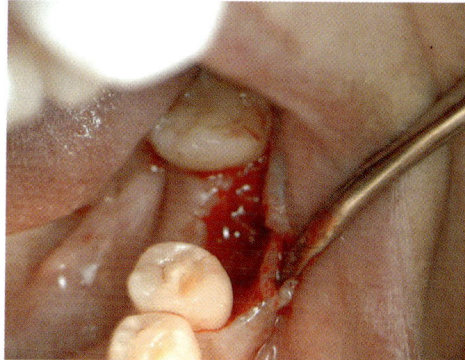

Fig. 2: Periodontal tissue is retracted to reveal the implant surgical site.

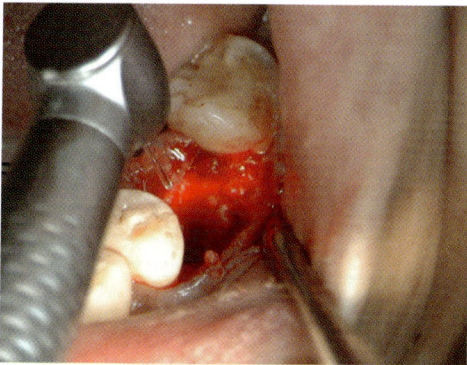

Fig. 3: A G-6 (9mm) or Z-6 (9mm) is used for the initial osteotomy that serves the purpose of a pivot drill. The implant length is established. The setting is 4.50W, 60% Water, 65% Air. A periodontal probe is used to periodically gage the depth of preparation.

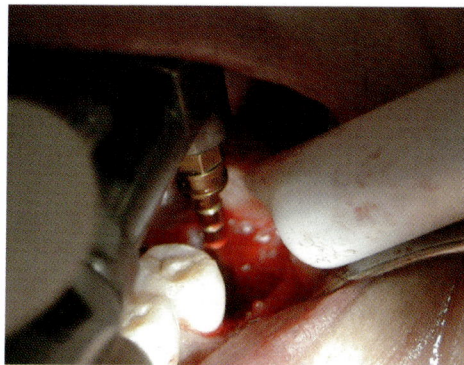

Fig. 4: Implant osteotomy is completed by using the manufacturer's sizing drills.

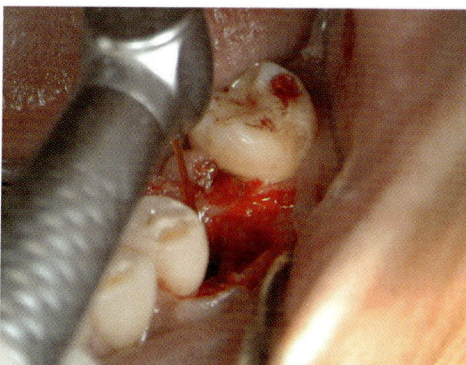

Fig. 5: Laser decontamination before the implant placement. The setting is 0.50W, 7% Water, 11% Air.

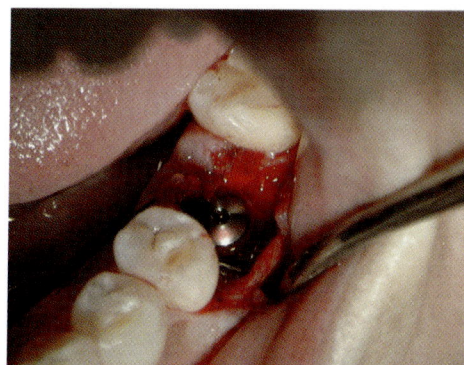

Fig. 6: After placement of the endosseous implant, the surgical site is ready to be closed.

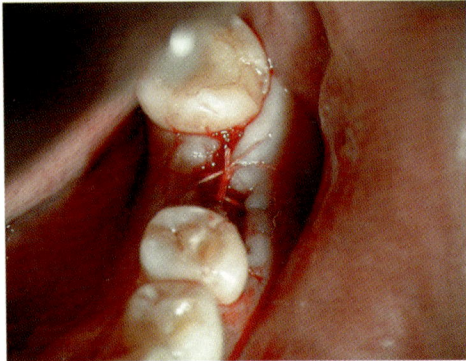

Fig. 7: A resorbable suture is placed and a laser biologic band-aid is applied. The setting is 1.00W, 0% Water, 11% Air.

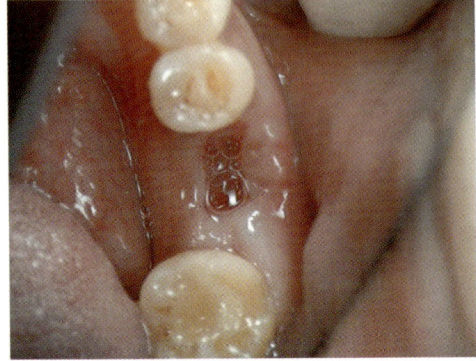

Fig. 8: One month post-op. The surgical site is healing well.

Case 2: Laser-Assisted Osteotomy for Endosseous Implant Placement at #31, Immediately After Extraction of Vertically Fractured #31

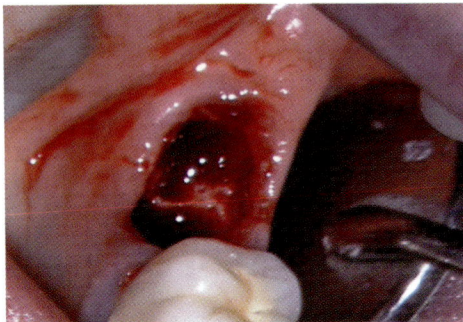

Fig. 1: Pre-op. #31, which had a vertical fracture, has been exposed. Immediate placement of an endosseous implant is planned.

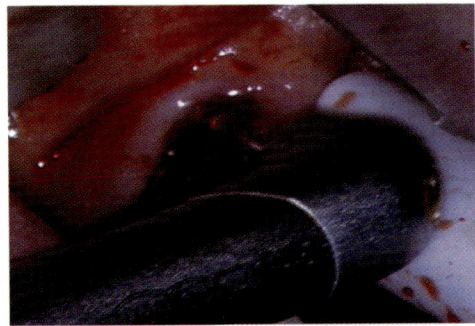

Fig. 2: Debridement of the fresh extraction site by the laser. The tip is MG-6 (9mm). The setting is 3.00W, 15% Water, 11% Air, 30 Hz.

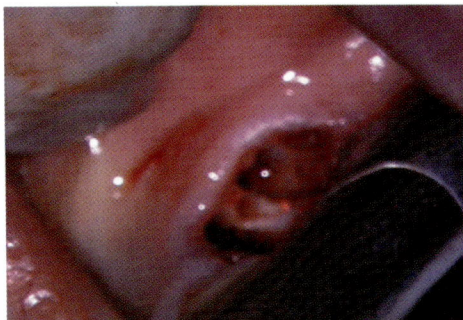

Fig. 3: Osteotomy of the endosseous implant starts with the laser at the furcation area. Care must be taken on the approximate diameter and the exact depth of the preparation. The setting is 4.25W, 60% Water, 80% Air, 20 Hz.

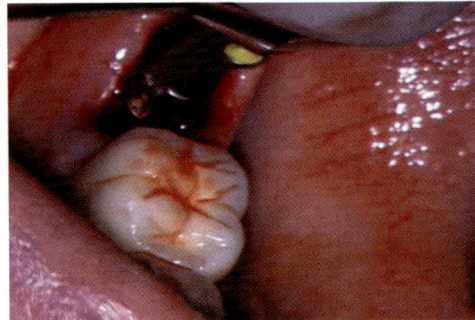

Fig. 4: Only one sizing drill is used to coagulate osteotomy and preparation for the implant.

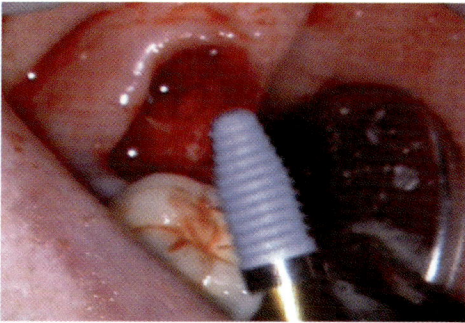

Fig. 5: A hydroxyapatite-coated endosseous implant is ready to be placed at #31.

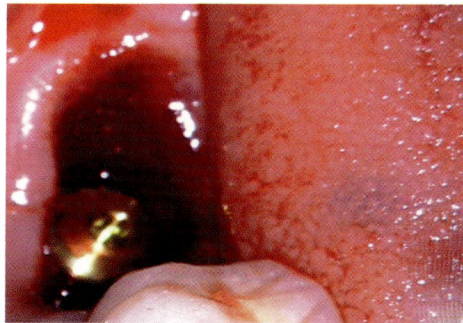

Fig. 6: Placement of the endosseous implant is complete.

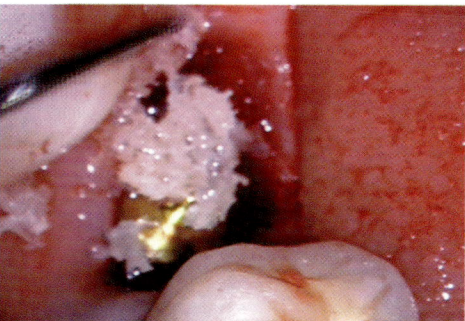

Fig. 7: Demineralized, freeze-dried bone graft is placed around the implant in the #31 extraction site.

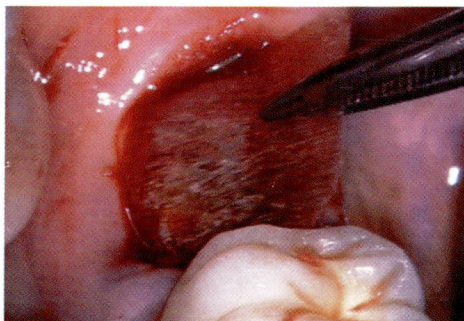

Fig. 8: A resorbable membrane is placed over the bone graft and implant.

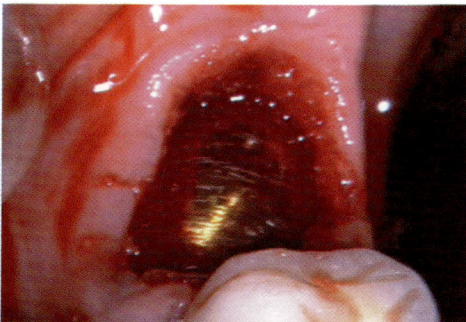

Fig. 9: The resorbable membrane is in place.

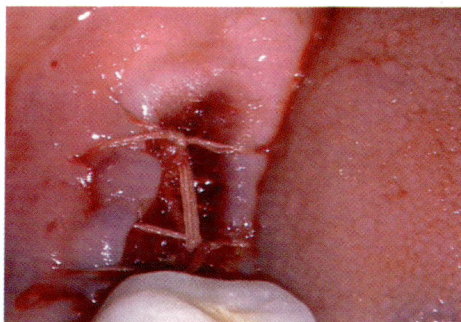

Fig. 10: Vicryl suture is placed.

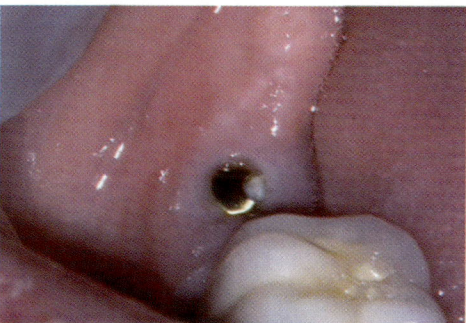

Fig. 11: Three-month post-op.

Er,Cr:YSGG Laser System-Assisted Placement of Implant in Very Narrow Ridge

Laser Parameters, Set 1: Outline Surgical Site

Waterlase MD laser system settings: MG-6 tip, 0.75W, 0% Water, 11% Air, 30 Hz
Other Er,Cr:YSGG laser system settings: G-6 tip, 0.75W, 0% Water, 11% Air

> Administer local anesthesia and use a template to guide the laser and mark the location of the implant osteotomy. The estimated diameter of the implant is outlined at the marked location.

Laser Parameters, Set 2: Ablation of Gingiva

Waterlase MD laser system settings: 1.50-2.50W, 7-11% Water, 11% Air, 30 Hz
Other Er,Cr:YSGG laser system settings: 1.25-1.75W, 11% Water, 20% Air

> Continue the ablation of gingiva all the way to the bone level to expose the diameter and site for the implant.

Laser Parameters, Set 3: Osteotomy

Waterlase MD laser system settings: 4.00-6.00W, 60% Water, 80% Air, 20-25 Hz
Other Er,Cr:YSGG laser system settings: 4.50W, 60% Water, 65% Air

> Using indelible ink, mark the laser fiber tip at a distance of 2mm shorter than the expected depth of cutting. The laser will be used to ablate the bone to the length of the implant. Laser osteotomy is used to finish the preparation like a pivot drill.

> Next, the laser osteotomy is continued by widening the implant site systematically to the rough diameter of the proposed implant. Ensure that the laser preparation is smaller in diameter than the actual implant. Unlike the previous laser implant procedure, laser osteotomy will be more extensive. The laser affords greater precision than a drill, and will avoid creating microfractures in the bone, which is critical in a narrow ridge.

> The final sizing of the implant site will still be performed by the implant drill preparation.

Laser Parameters, Set 4: Treat Implant Site for Decontamination

Waterlase MD laser system settings: 0.75W, 7% Water, 11% Air, 30 Hz
Other Er,Cr:YSGG laser system settings: 0.75W, 7% Water, 11% Air

> After the drill preparation, laser energy is used to treat the implant site for decontamination. The tip should be moved in a slow circular motion with a slow up-and-down motion to ensure that all faces of the implant site have received laser energy. This is followed in turn by the placement of the endosseous implant.

Laser Parameters, Set 5: Low Level Laser Therapy

Waterlase MD laser system settings: 1.00-1.50W, 7% Water, 11% Air, 30 Hz
Other Er,Cr:YSGG laser system settings: 0.75W, 7% Water, 11% Air

> To finish, the laser is used to apply low-power laser energy to de-epithelialize a band of 4-5mm of the peri-implant gingiva.

Case 1: Laser-assisted Placement of Two Endosseous Implants in Very Narrow Ridge, MD Regular HP with MG-6 Tip

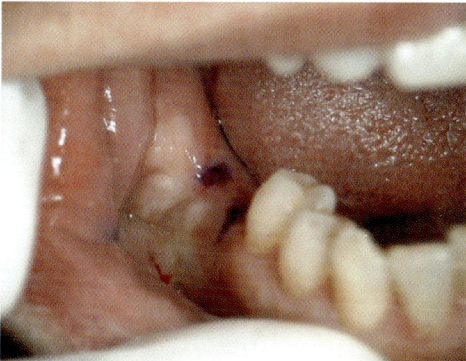

Fig. 1: Pre-op. Right mandibular first and second molar area is showing a relatively narrow ridge. Patient does not want to go through an extra procedure of bone grafting before the placement of implant. Smaller sized implants with laser-assisted osteotomy is planned to restore first and second molars. The indelible ink marks the two surgical sites.

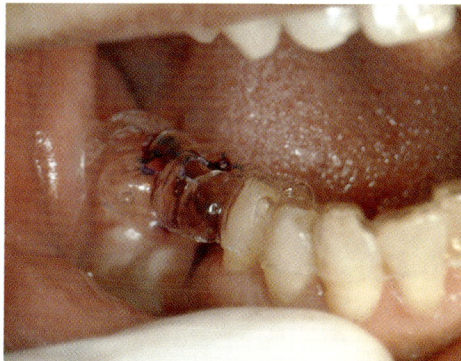

Fig. 2: A surgical template is in place to mark the two surgical sites.

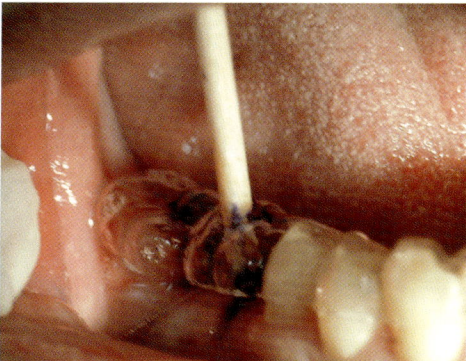

Fig. 3: Indelible ink is used to mark the surgical sites.

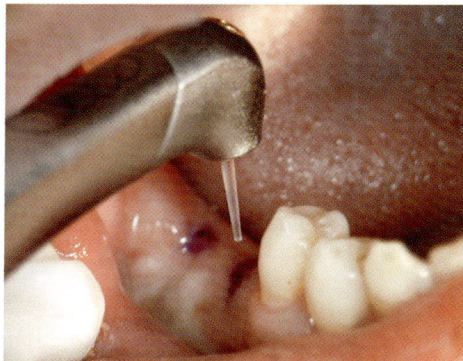

Fig. 4: A MG-6 (9mm) tip is used to perform gingivectomy at the implant sites. The setting is 1.75W, 7% Water, 11% Air, 30 Hz.

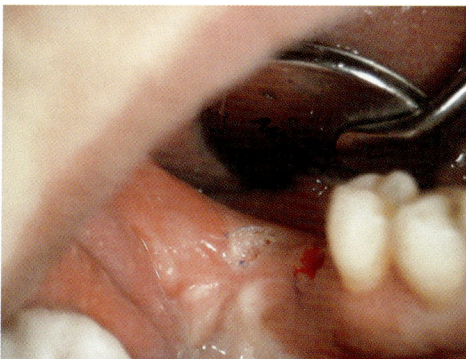

Fig. 5: No flap is made. Gingivectomy is complete for the first molar and the outline for the second molar is made.

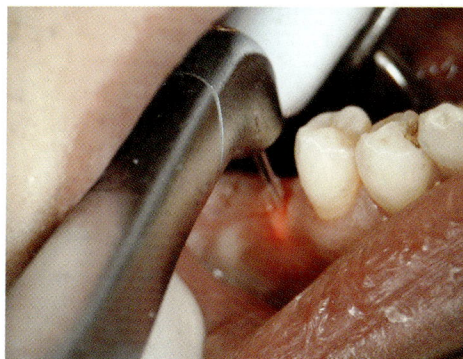

Fig. 6: Osteotomy at the first molar is prepared with the laser. The setting is 4.50W, 60% Water, 65% Air, 20 Hz.

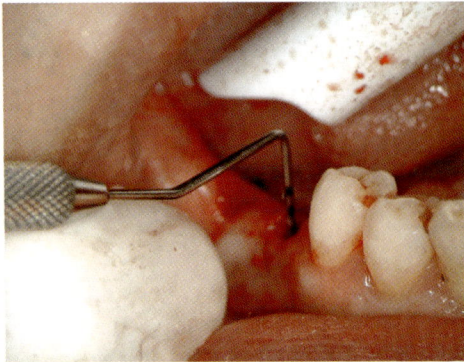

Fig. 7: A periodontal probe is used periodically to check both the depth and diameter of preparation.

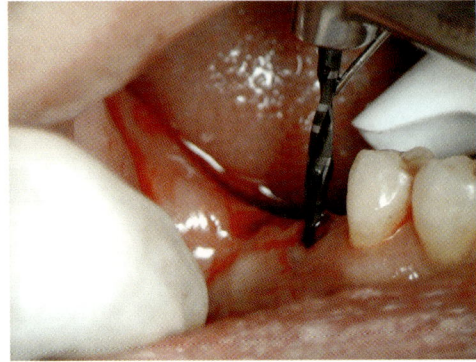

Fig. 8: Osteotomy is completed by using the last sizing drill of the implant series.

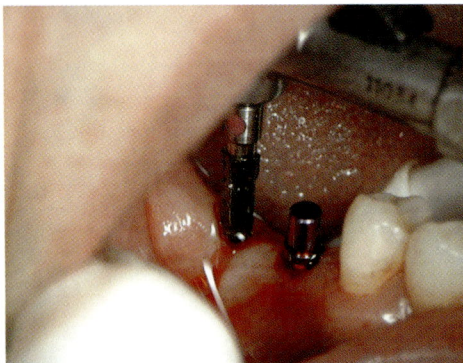

Fig. 9: The last sizing drill is used in the second molar site. The direction of preparation is referenced by the trial module in place at the first molar site.

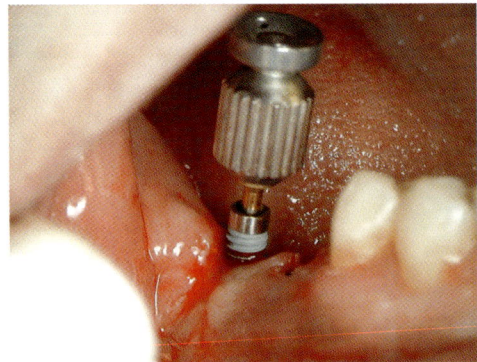

Fig. 10: Placement of an endosseous implant at the second molar site.

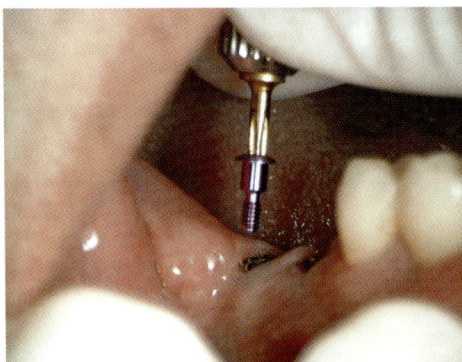

Fig. 11: Placement of healing screw.

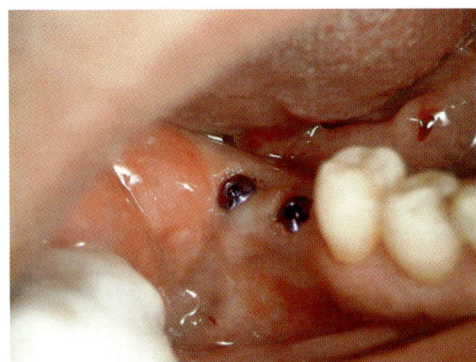

Fig. 12: Implant placement is complete for both the first and second molar.

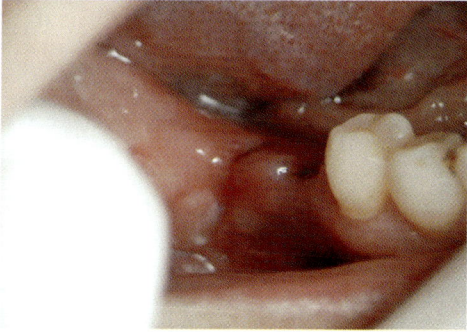

Fig. 13: One week post-op. The site is healing well and no complications are noted.

MD Gold Handpiece

The newest accessory for the Waterlase MD laser system is the MD Gold™ Handpiece. The system also consists of two new laser fiber tips, the MZ-5 and MGG-6 tips. Almost all other tips can be used with the MD Gold Handpiece, except for the MG-6 tip, which has been replaced by the MGG-6 tip. The applications for soft and hard tissue are the same as the standard Waterlase MD laser system.

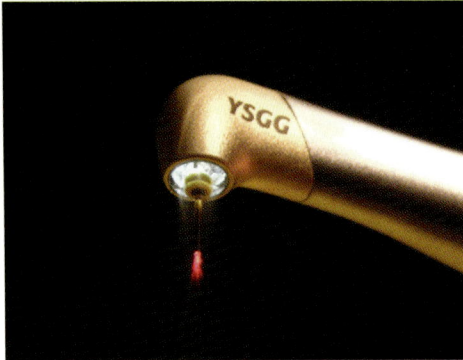

Fig. 1: The MD Gold Handpiece

The design of the mirror of the MD Gold Handpiece allows laser energy to be applied in a higher power density, and Biolase has shown through published test results that the depth of penetration with a MD Gold Handpiece is significantly deeper than with the standard MD handpiece system.

In using the MD Gold Handpiece and tips, the clinician will find ablation in both hard and soft tissue to be significantly faster. In principle, a similar setting as used in the standard system can be used as an initial setting. However, where the speed of cutting is too fast for minimally invasive dentistry, or the power density is too high, resulting in patient discomfort, the power should be adjusted to a lower intensity. From my experience, it is good practice to lower the power 0.25W at a time, until you have achieved a satisfactory response in terms of ablation speed or patient comfort. This reduced power can go as far as 0.75W below the starting setting.

The MZ-tips can be used in either contact or non-contact modes. These laser fiber tips are all cylindrical in shape and, per Biolase's description, the laser energy exiting the tip is evenly distributed. The tips also transport energy well and are capable of delivering a higher power density to the target tissue.

In contact mode, the MZ-tip is placed touching the enamel lightly. This will result in very focused laser energy from the laser tip to the target surface. This energy will eventually melt the surface of the MZ-tip and simultaneously create a photo acoustic effect on tissue, resulting in rapid ablation of enamel. Most of the laser energy is used in cutting the enamel and not much of this laser energy is reflected back into the mirror of the MD

Gold Handpiece. A consequence is that the MZ-tip is a one-use item; the tip will be damaged after one use, although the handpiece mirror should remain undamaged. In my opinion, after several months clinical testing, it seems that the speed of ablation using the MZ-5 tip in contact mode may approach the speed of high-speed drilling.

In non-contact mode, the MZ-tip is placed 1-2mm from the target tissue and the technique is similar to using standard MD handpieces. Because of the increased distance to the tissue, the power density is not as high as in the contact mode, though in my opinion, the speed of cutting is still faster than with the standard MD handpiece. When not in contact, the tips may be used more than once, although it is critical that you use a hand-held microscope to check the surface of the MZ tips before and after procedures. If you observe any modifications or changes to the surface of the tip, discard the tip, even if the tip has never been used. Continual use of damaged tips may damage the MD Gold Handpiece mirror and even the fiber trunk.

There is much to be explored with the MD Gold Handpiece system. Currently, most clinicians favor using the MZ-5 tip. The following are a potpourri of clinical cases using a variety of tips, including the MZ-5.

Class I Cavity Preparation with the MD Gold Handpiece

Laser Parameters, Set 1: Pre-Conditioning

MZ-5 tip, 2.00W, 60% Water, 80% Air, 30 Hz

Utilize the Turtle Technique, the same procedure as described in Section 1 for Class I cavity preparations. Spend 60 seconds going back and forth over the fissure, keeping the defocused distance as constant as possible. Allow the patient to close his/her mouth momentarily and then repeat.

Laser Parameters, Sets 2-5: Enamel Ablation

MZ-5 tip, 3.00-4.50W, 60% Water, 80% Air, 15 Hz

Utilize the Turtle Technique, the same procedure as outlined in Section 1 for Class I cavity preparations, laser parameters sets 2-5.

Laser Parameters, Set 6: Complete Prep

MZ-5 tip, 2.00W, 60% Water, 80% Air, 15 Hz

Complete the preparation using the same technique for Class I cavity preparations.

Case 1:

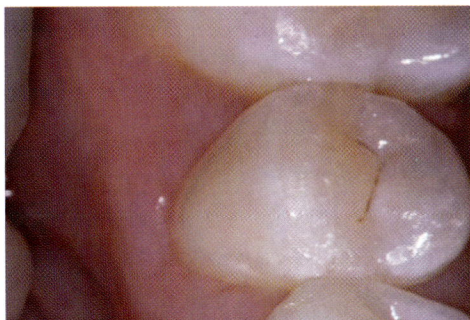

Fig. 1: Pre-op. An occlusal caries is noted in the mandibular second premolar.

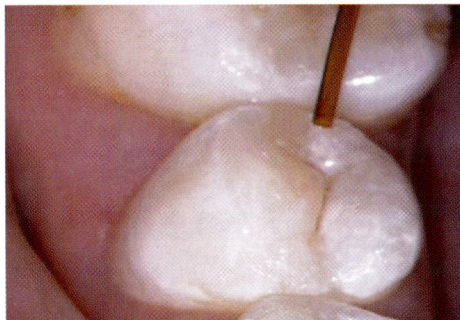

Fig. 2: Pre-conditioning is done with the laser using a MZ-5 tip focused and aiming at the occlusal lesion. The setting is 2.00W, 60% Water, 80% Air, 30 Hz. Time spent is 60 seconds. Have patient close the mouth momentarily. This is followed by another 60 seconds of pre-conditioning.

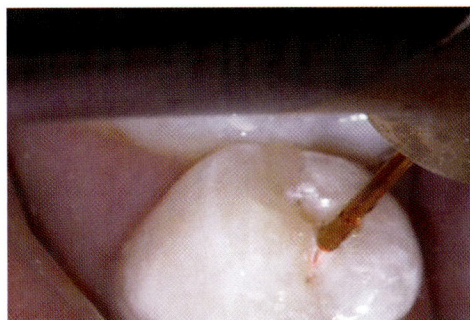

Fig. 3: The MZ-5 tip is angled, aiming at the buccal border of the cavity. The buccal edge is extended by the laser. The setting is 3.50W, 60% Water, 80% Air, 15 Hz.

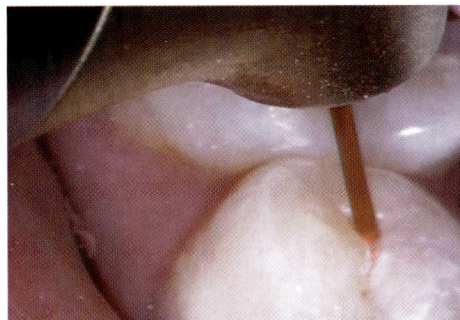

Fig. 4: The MZ-5 tip is angled and aiming at the lingual border of the cavity. The lingual edge is extended by the laser.

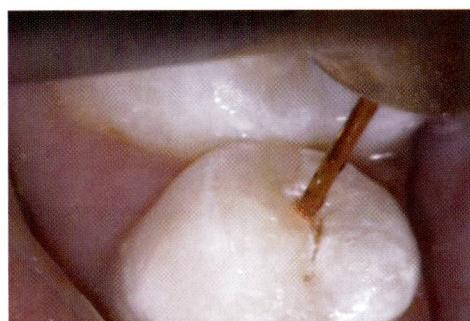

Fig. 5: The MZ-5 tip is perpendicular, aiming at the pulp floor. The laser is used to deepen the cavity.

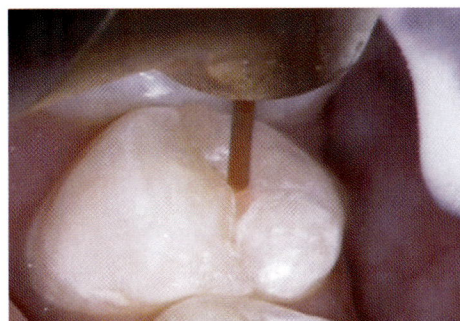

Fig. 6: With sides of tubules now exposed, the laser is used to remove caries and finish the preparation more efficiently.

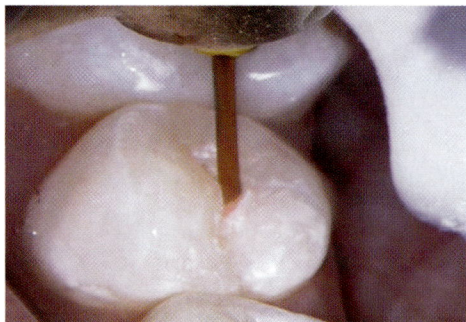

Fig. 7: To complete preparation, the setting is changed to 2.00W, 60% Water, 80% Air, 30 Hz, before placement of composite.

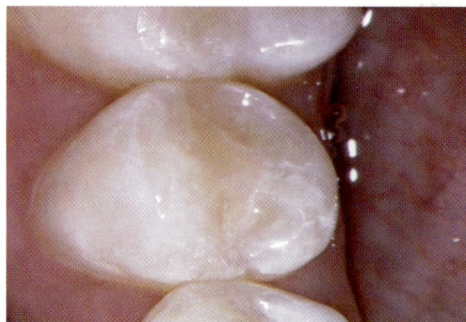

Fig. 8: Post-op. Composite restoration is complete in the occlusal surface.

Case 2:

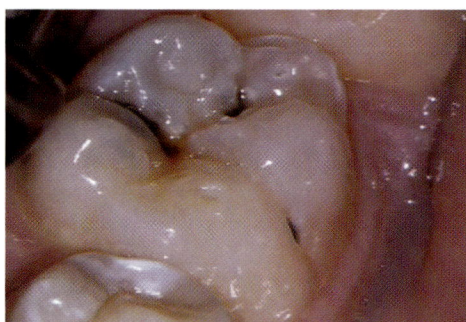

Fig. 1: Pre-op. Caries is present at the buccal pit and the occlusal surfaces of the mandibular left first molar.

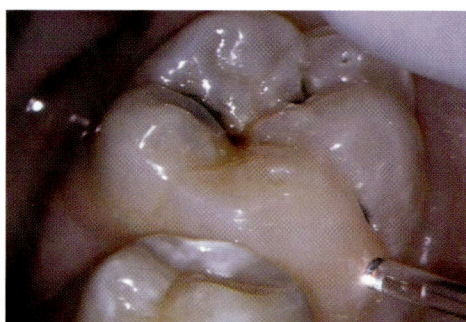

Fig. 2: A MC-12 tip is used to pre-condition the tooth. The setting is 0.50W, 0% Water, 0% Air, 50 Hz. The tip is defocused 1mm and is moved along the shape of the pulp. Total pre-conditioning time is 2 minutes.

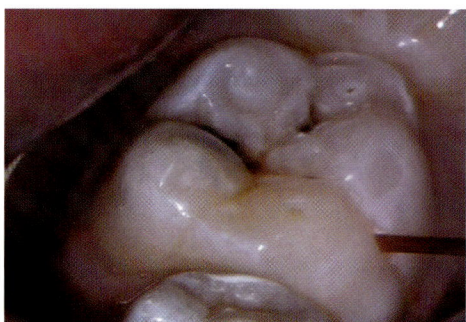

Fig. 3: A MZ-5 tip is used to prepare the cavity at the buccal pit. The setting is 4.50W, 60% Water, 80% Air, 15 Hz.

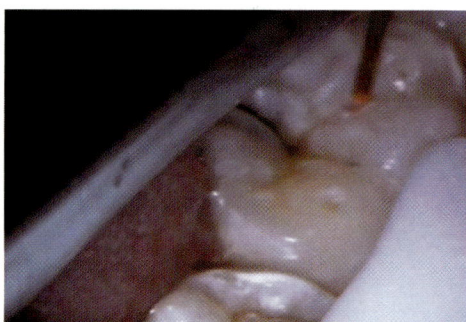

Fig. 4: Efficient ablation can be done with the tip being angled to the decay.

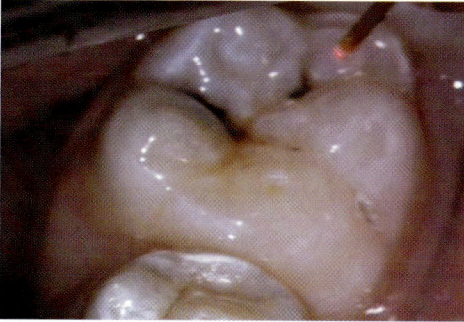

Fig. 5: The preparation on the occlusal surface is minimally invasive in the form of dots and grooves. The design is determined by the extent of the caries.

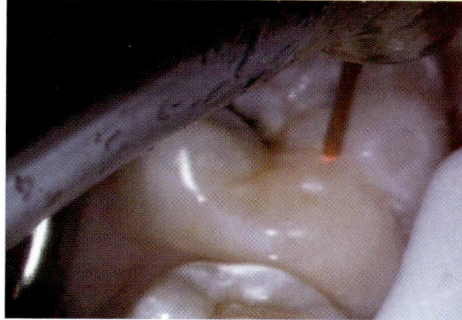

Fig. 6: Ablation of the cavity continues to buccal fossa.

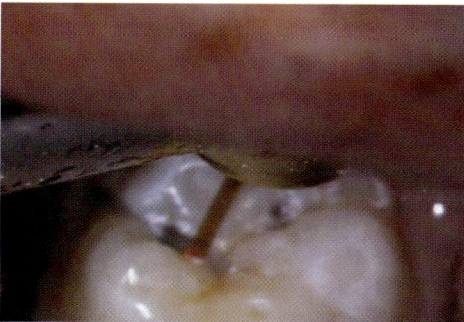

Fig. 7: Laser ablation of caries at the central fossa.

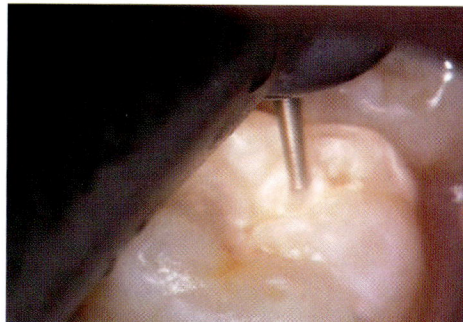

Fig. 8: Modified technique is used by a sharp #1 round bur from an electric high-speed handpiece. All sclerotic dentin is removed.

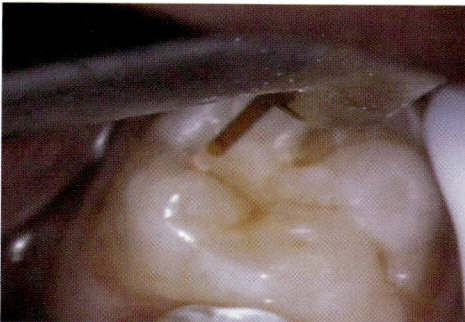

Fig. 9: The laser is used to finish the cavity preparation. The setting is 2.00W, 60% Water, 80% Air, 30 Hz.

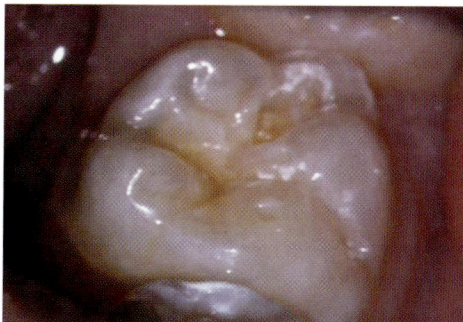

Fig. 10: Cavity preparation is complete.

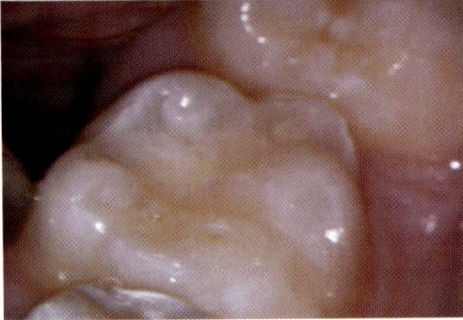

Fig. 11: Post-op. Composite restoration is placed.

Class II Cavity Preparation with the MD Gold Handpiece

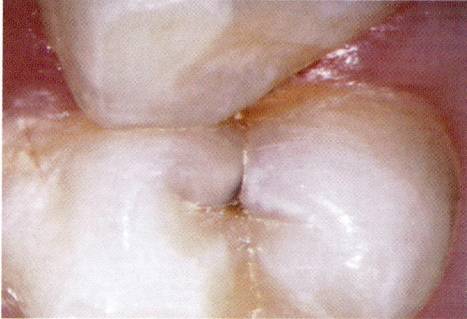

Fig. 1: Pre-op. An occlusal-distal lesion is shown on the maxillary left first premolar.

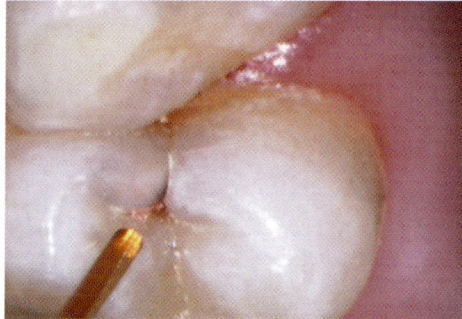

Fig. 2: Pre-conditioning is done by a MZ-5 tip aimed at the occlusal surface of the lesion. The setting is 2.00W, 60% Water, 80% Air, 30 Hz. After 60 seconds of pre-conditioning the patient is instructed to close the mouth momentarily. This is followed by another 60 seconds of low-level laser therapy.

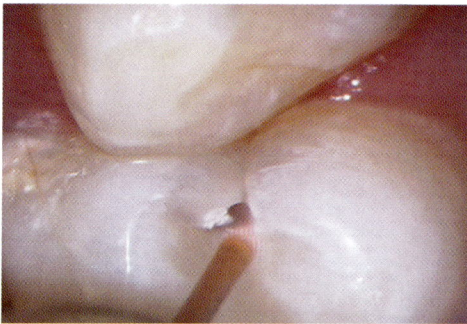

Fig. 3: Noticeable ablation starts with the tip aimed at the border of the cavity. The setting is 3.50W, 60% Water, 80% Air, 15 Hz.

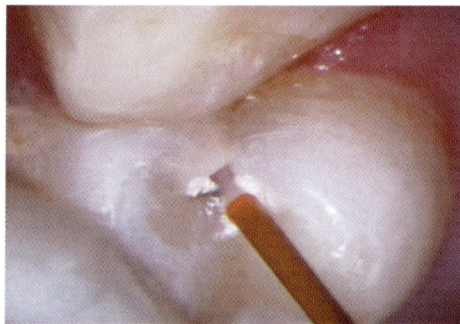

Fig. 4: The tip is aimed at the other border of the cavity. Extension of the edge of the buccal side is established. The same setting as in Fig. 3 is used.

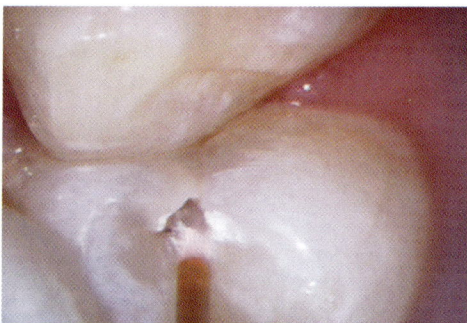

Fig. 5: The cavity is deepened by the tip aimed at the pulpal floor.

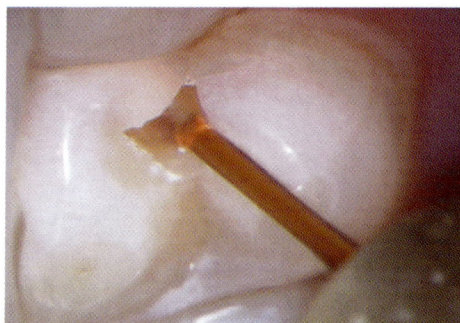

Fig. 6: With sides of tubules exposed, more efficient ablation takes place.

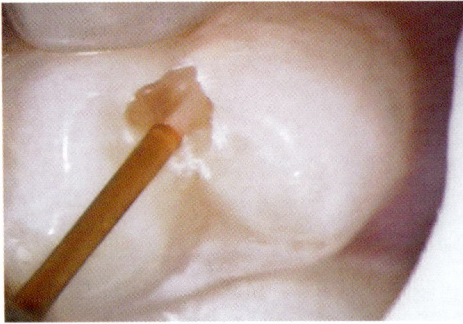

Fig. 7: Caries is removed by the laser at the lingual surface.

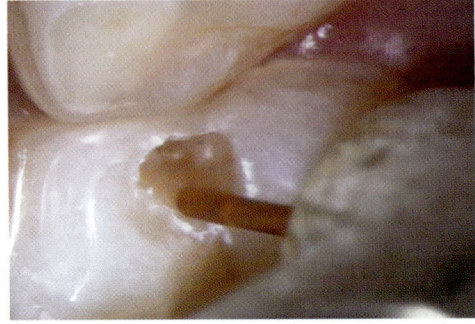

Fig. 8: More caries removal is being conducted by the laser at the pulpal floor.

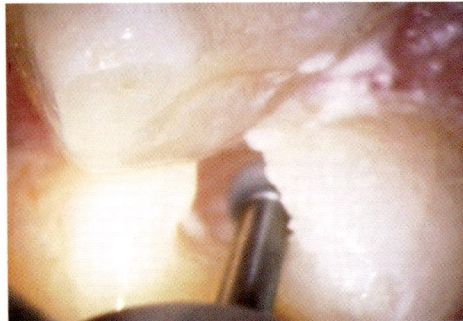

Fig. 9: A slow-speed round bur (from an electric handpiece) is used to extend the preparation to the interproximal area, breaking the thin enamel wall. After caries removal has been completed, the laser is used to finish the cavity preparation. The setting is 2.00W, 60% Water, 80% Air, 30 Hz.

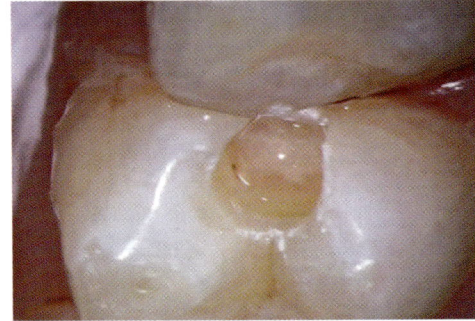

Fig. 10: The cavity preparation is complete.

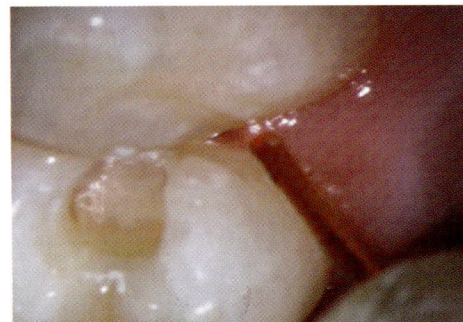

Fig. 11: The interproximal gingival sulcus is pre-conditioned with the laser before the matrix is placed for the restoration procedure. The setting is 0.25W, 20% Water, 20% Air, 30 Hz.

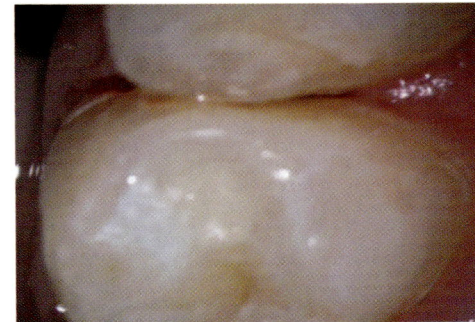

Fig. 12: Post-op. Composite restoration is complete.

Class III Cavity Preparation with the MD Gold Handpiece

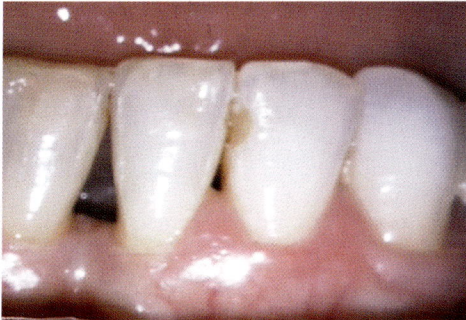

Fig.1: Pre-op. Recurrent decay is present at the mesial surface of the mandibular left lateral incisor.

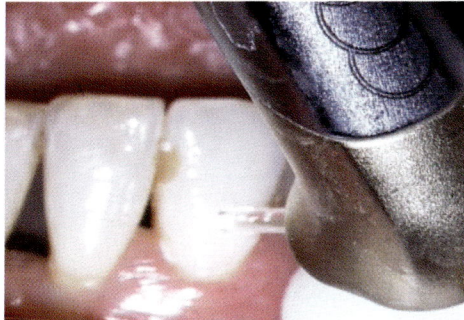

Fig. 2: Pre-conditioning of tooth is done using a MC-12 tip. The setting is 0.50W, 0% Water, 0% Air, 50 Hz, at the cervical area.

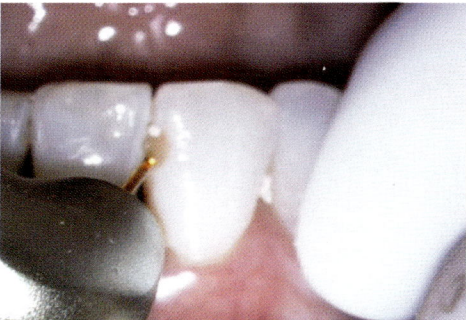

Fig. 3: The old composite is removed by using a MZ-5 tip. The setting is 3.50W, 60% Water, 80% Air, 15 Hz.

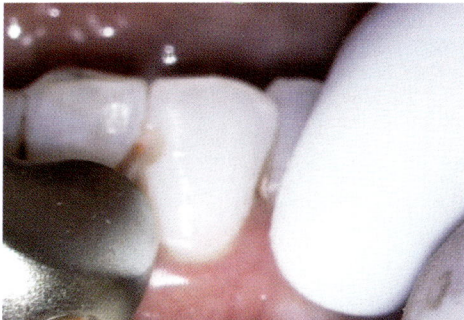

Fig. 4: After caries check with a slow-speed round bur, the laser is used to remove smear and debris. The setting is 2.00W, 60% Water, 80% Air, 30 Hz.

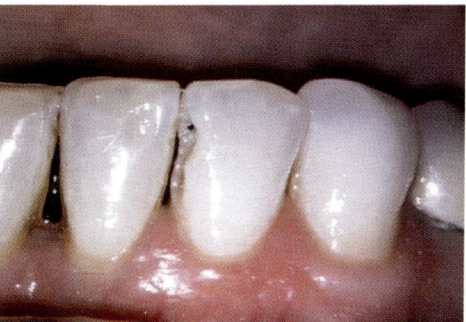

Fig. 5: Class III preparation is complete.

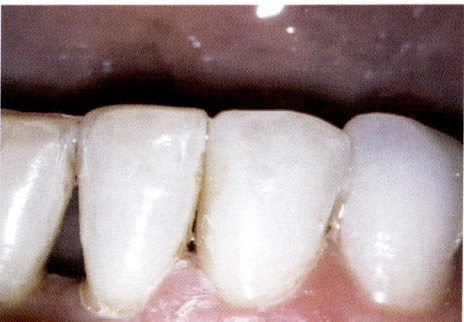

Fig. 6: Post-op, composite restoration is placed at the mesial surface of the mandibular left lateral incisor.

Class IV Cavity Preparation with the MD Gold Handpiece

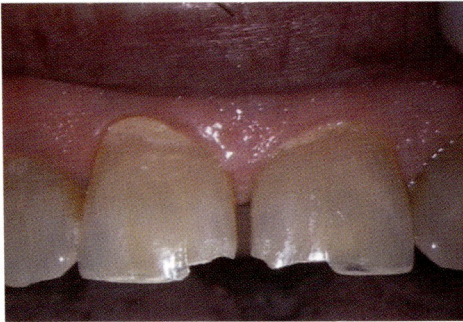

Fig. 1: Pre-op. Class IV lesions are present in both maxillary central incisors.

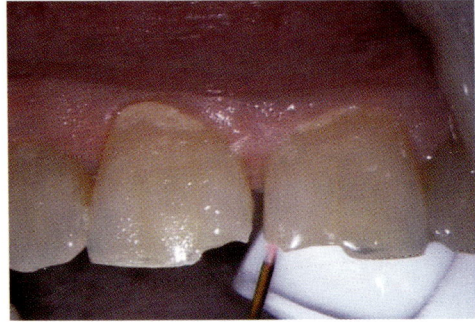

Fig. 2: A MZ-5 tip is used and is defocused at 1-2mm. The setting is 1.25W, 60% Water, 80% Air, 30 Hz.

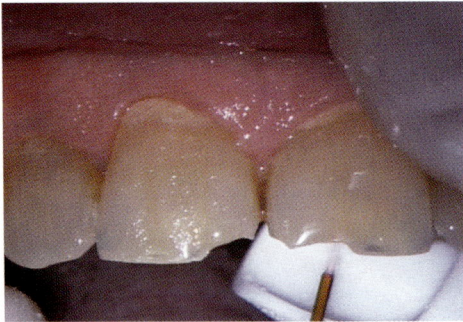

Fig. 3: The power is raised to 1.50W and the preparation involves the entire incisal surface. from mesial to distal of the left central incisor.

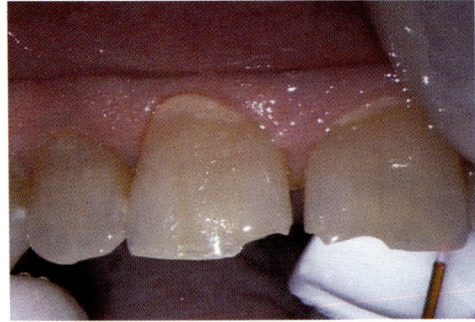

Fig. 4: The power setting is raised to 1.75W to complete the preparation.

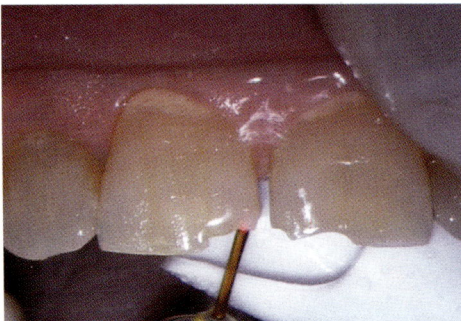

Fig. 5: The preparation of the right central incisor starts with a setting of 1.25W, 60% Water, 80% Air, 30 Hz.

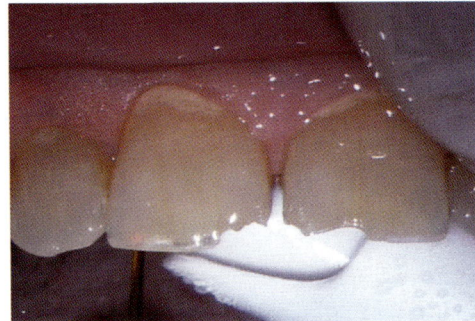

Fig. 6: The preparation continues with the power raised to 1.50W and involving the entire incisal surface.

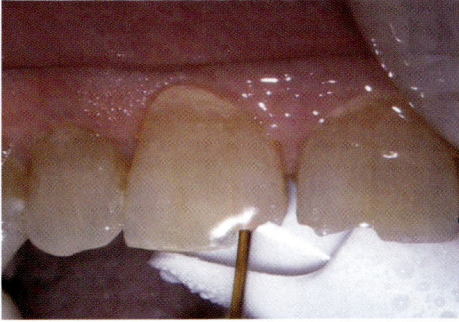

Fig. 7: The power setting is raised to 1.75W to finish the preparation.

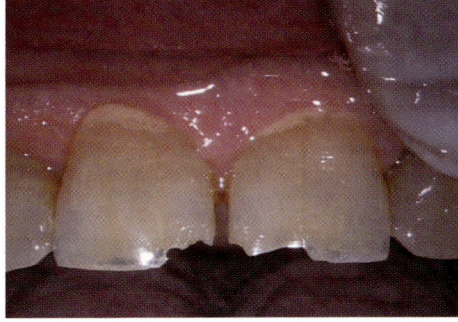

Fig. 8: Immediate post-op after preparation.

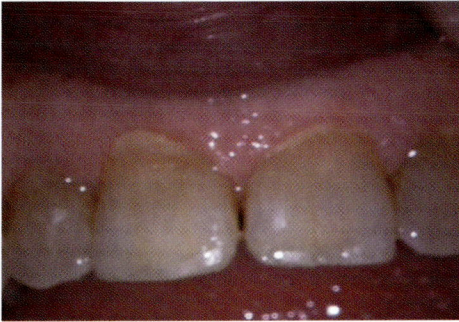

Fig. 9: Post-op. Composite restorations are complete for both maxillary central incisors.

Class V Cavity Preparation with the MD Gold Handpiece

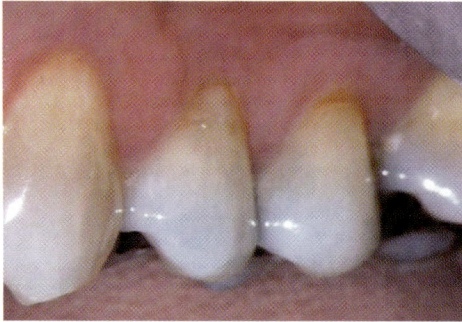

Fig. 1: Pre-op. A Class V cavity is present at the buccal of the maxillary left first premolar.

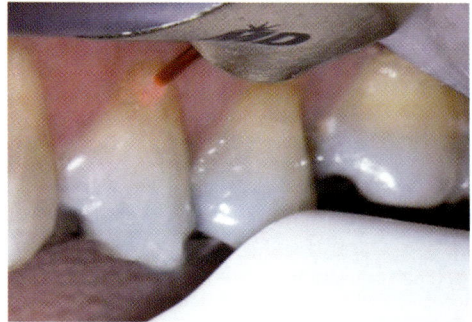

Fig. 2: A MZ-5 tip is used, defocused at 1mm from the lesion. The setting is 1.25W, 60% Water, 80% Air, 30 Hz.

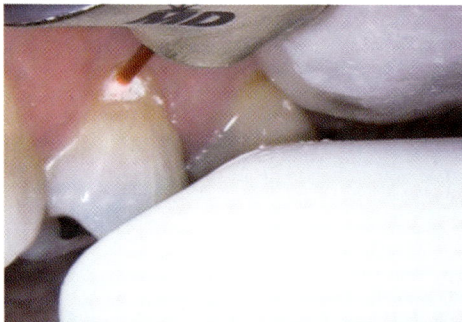

Fig. 3: The power is increased 0.25W after 30 seconds, until efficient ablation of lesion is noted. The highest power setting is 1.75W, 60% Water, 80% Air, 30 Hz.

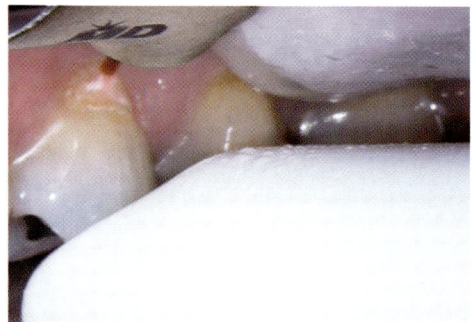

Fig. 4: The setting is changed to 1.50W, 60% Water, 80% Air, 30 Hz to finish prep.

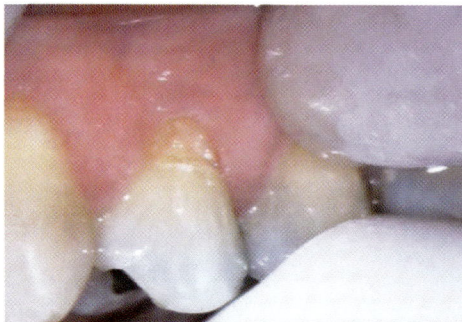

Fig. 5: Post-op. Class V cavity preparation is complete.

Pediatric Class I Cavity Preparation with the MD Gold Handpiece

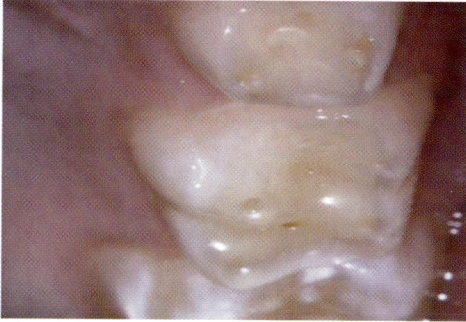

Fig. 1: Pre-op. An occlusal caries is present at the occlusal surface of the distal fossa of the maxillary left deciduous second molar.

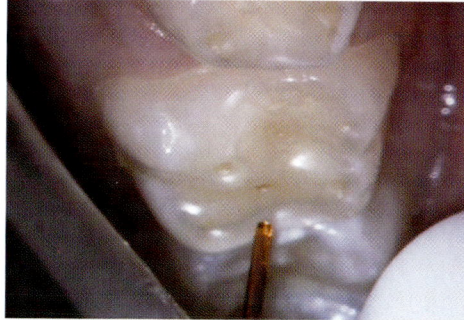

Fig. 2: A MZ-5 tip is used and defocused at 1mm from the distal fossa. Pre-conditioning starts with a setting of 2.00W, 60% Water, 80% Air, 30 Hz.

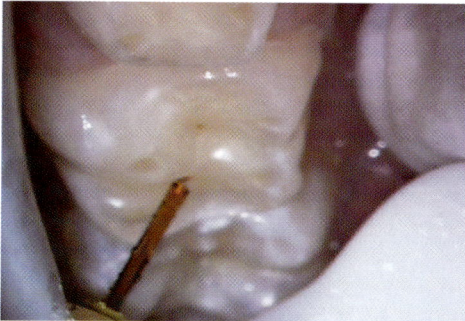

Fig. 3: The tip is angled to get more efficient ablation. The setting is 4.50W, 60% Water, 80% Air, 30 Hz.

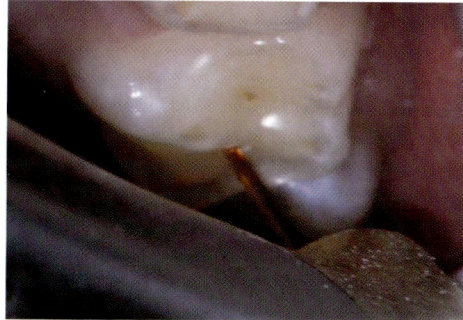

Fig. 4: The tip is angled and aimed at the border of the opposite side of the cavity to extend the preparation.

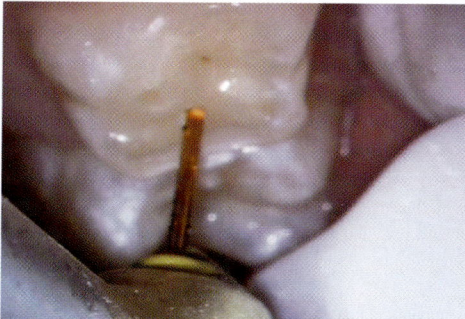

Fig. 5: The pulpal floor is deepened and caries removal continues.

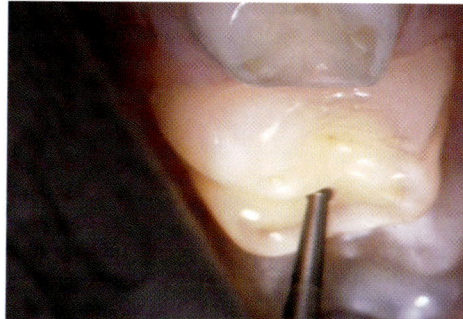

Fig. 6: An electric slow-speed round bur is used for caries check.

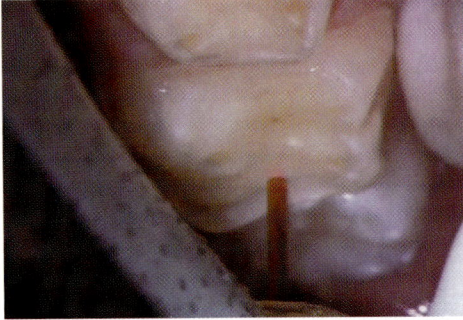

Fig. 7: Laser is used to finish the cavity preparation. The setting is 2.00W, 60% Water, 80% Air, 30 Hz.

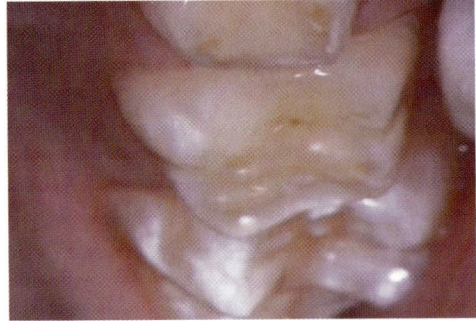

Fig. 8: Post-op. Composite restoration is placed.

Pediatric Class II Cavity Preparation with the MD Gold Handpiece

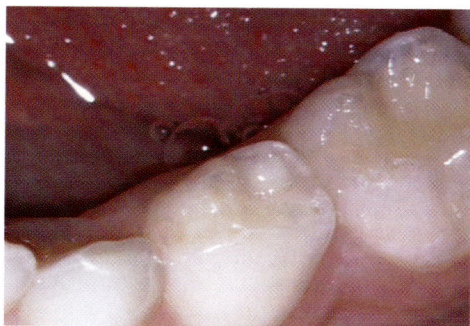

Fig. 1: Pre-op. Mandibular left first deciduous molar has a DO lesion.

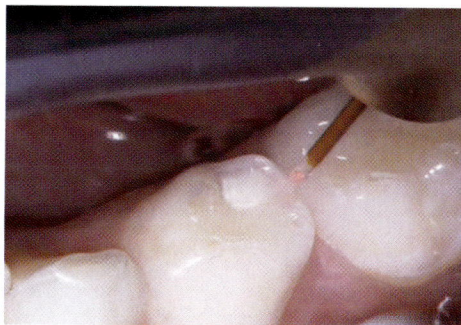

Fig. 2: A MZ-5 tip in a MD Gold Handpiece is used. The tip is aimed at the distal ridge. The setting is 2.00W, 60% Water, 80% Air, 30 Hz.

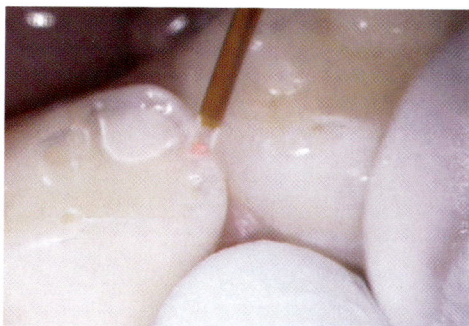

Fig. 3: After pre-conditioning, the tip is angled and the power setting is raised to 3.00W, 60% Water, 80% Air, 15 Hz, for enamel ablation. A slot-prep is started with laser energy.

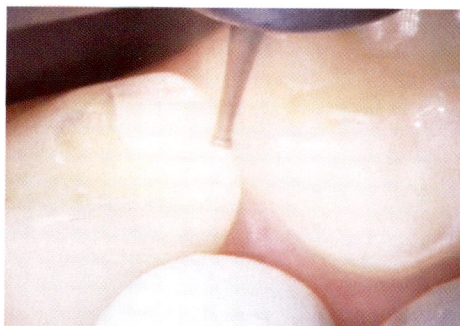

Fig. 4: A high-speed ¼ round bur from an electric handpiece is used to quickly outline the slot prep.

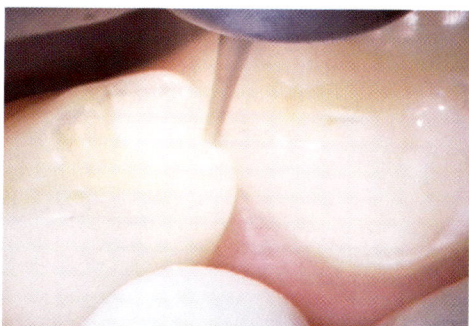

Fig. 5: A slow-speed round bur is used to remove and check caries.

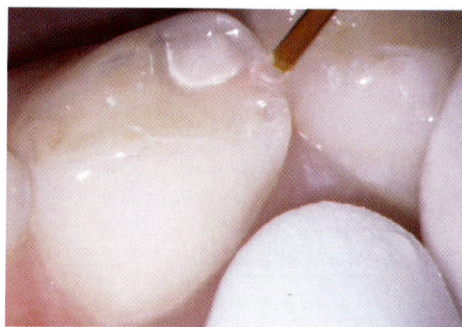

Fig. 6: The DO preparation is finished with laser energy. The setting is 2.00W, 60% Water, 80% Air, 30 Hz.

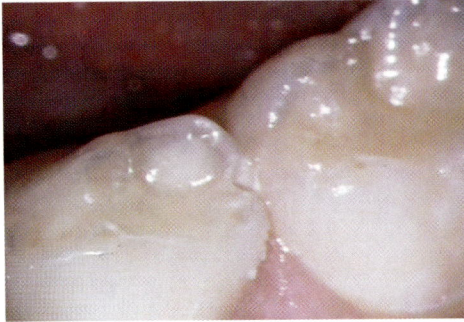

Fig. 7: The DO slot preparation is complete.

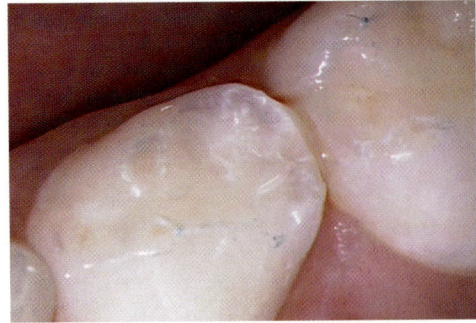

Fig. 8: Post-op, after composite restoration is placed.

Biopsy with the MD Gold Handpiece

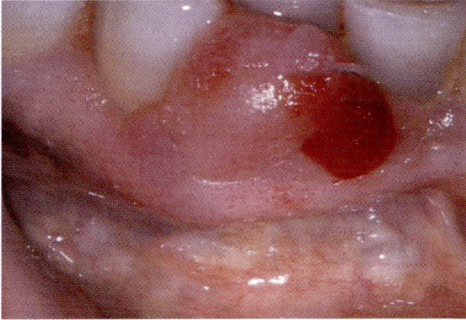

Fig. 1: Pre-op. A large epulis is present at the facial area of the mandibular right lateral incisor.

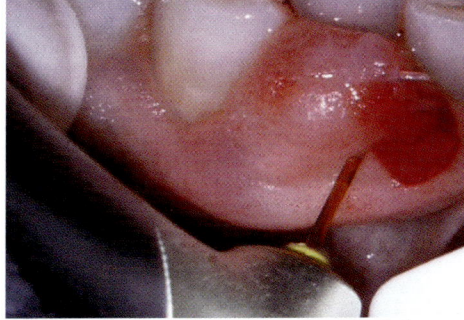

Fig. 2: After a right mandibular block is administered, the MD Gold MZ-5 tip is placed to aim at the outline of the lesion to make an incision cut. The setting is 2.25W, 7% Water, 11% Air, 30 Hz.

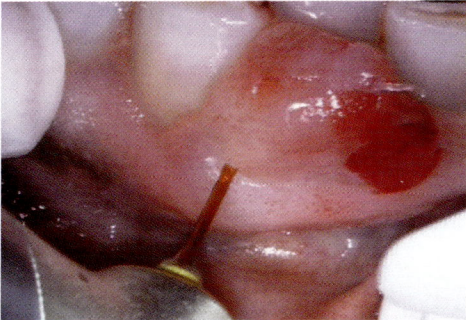

Fig. 3: The incision cut continues to the outline of the lesion.

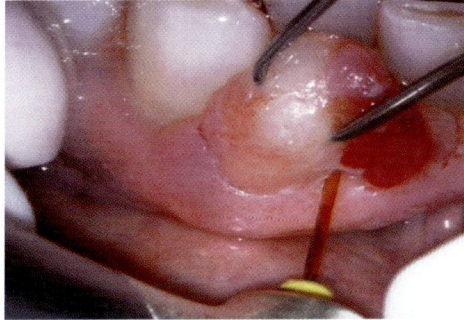

Fig. 4: The lesion is held with pain tissue forceps.The excision of the lesion begins. The same setting as the incision is used.

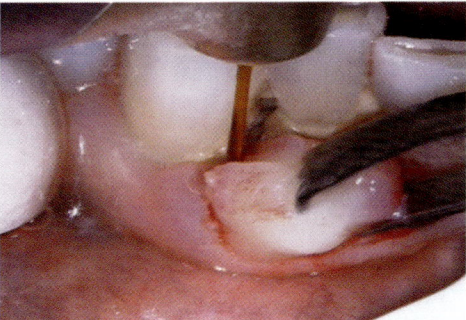

Fig. 5: The excision of the lesion is continued.

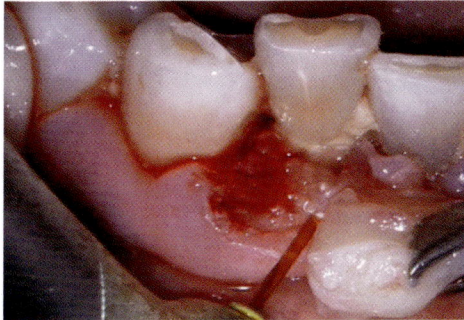

Fig. 6: The lesion is pulled away from the mucogingivia as laser energy continues to excise the lesion.

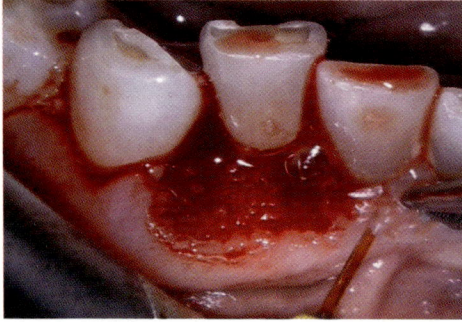

Fig. 7: The lesion is almost completely excised.

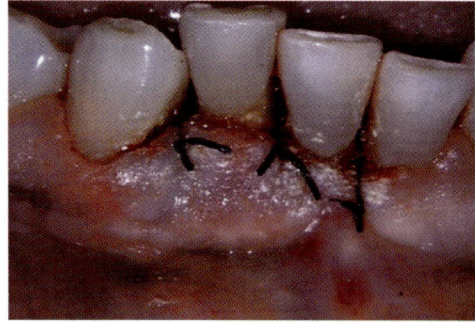

Fig. 8: Three interrupted 3-0 black silk sutures are placed to close the lesion. Laser biologic band-aid is complete.

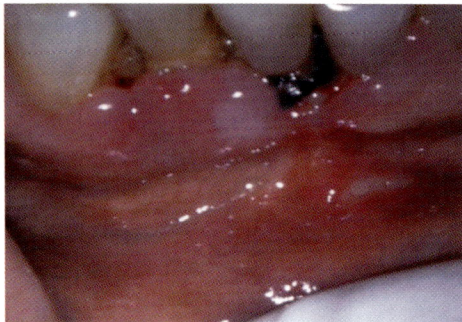

Fig. 9: 24 hours post-op. Healing is rapid.

Frenectomy with the MD Gold Handpiece

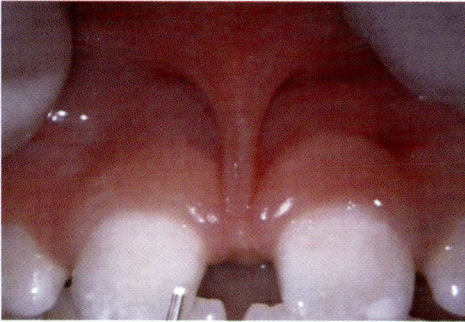

Fig. 1: Pre-operative. Labial frenum of the maxilla causes a large diastema between the maxillary central incisors.

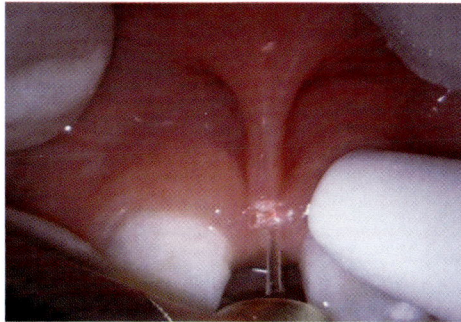

Fig. 2: A MGG-6 tip is placed parallel to the long axis of the central incisor aiming at the maxillary frenum. The laser is used to perform the frenectomy. The setting is 2.50W, 7% Water, 11% Air, 30 Hz, S mode.

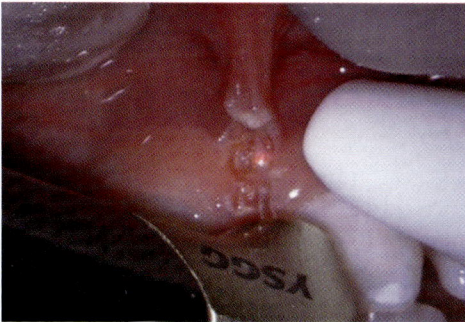

Fig. 3: The muscular relief reaches the mucogingival level.

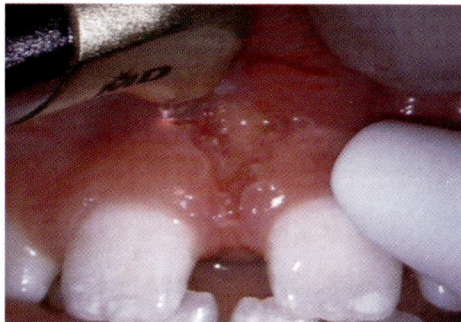

Fig. 4: The tip changes direction and is now perpendicular to the long axis of the central incisor. A horizontal relief is made at the mucogingival line.

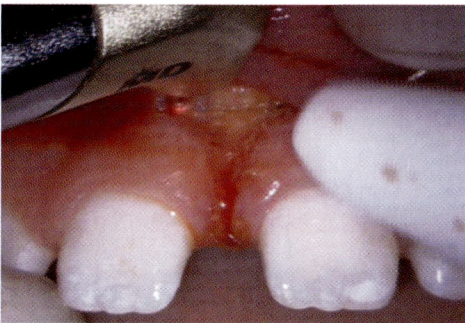

Fig. 5: The horizontal scarring procedure reaches the bone.

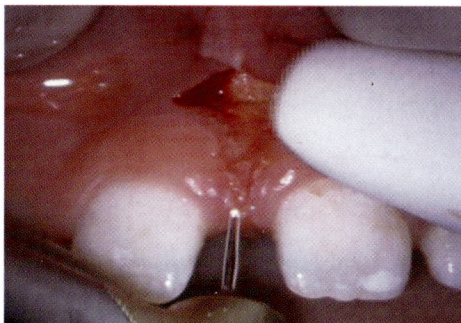

Fig. 6: The fibrous muscular impingement is ablated all the way to the palatal area.

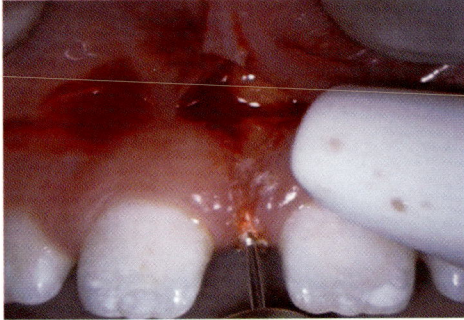

Fig. 7: Care is to be taken not to violate the nasopalatine area.

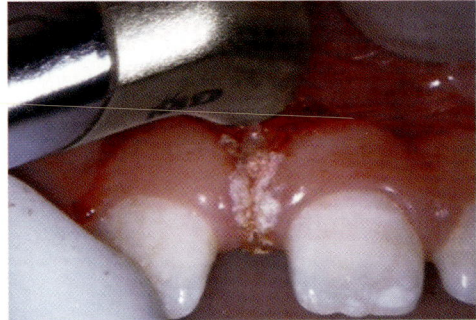

Fig. 8: A biologic band-aid is applied to the vertical relief area. The setting is 1.25W, 0% Water, 11% Air, 30 Hz.

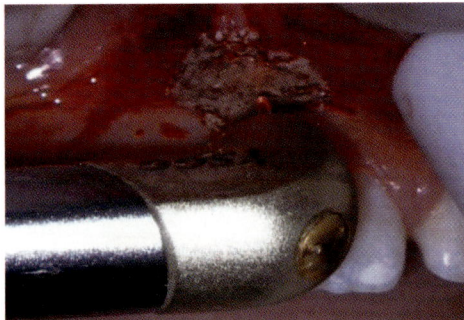

Fig. 9: A biologic band-aid is applied to the rest of the surgical site.

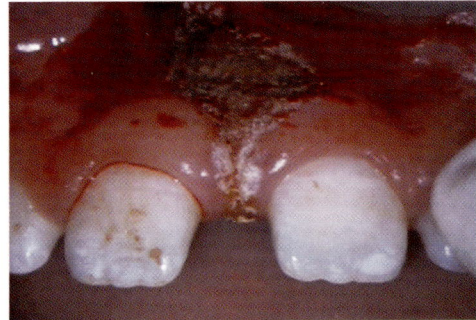

Fig. 10: Immediate post-op.

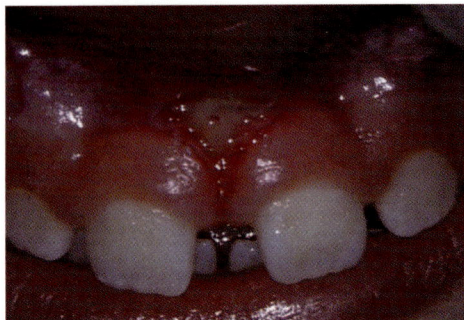

Fig. 11: One week post-op, showing no complications.

Laser Removal of a Fractured Crown with the MD Gold Handpiece

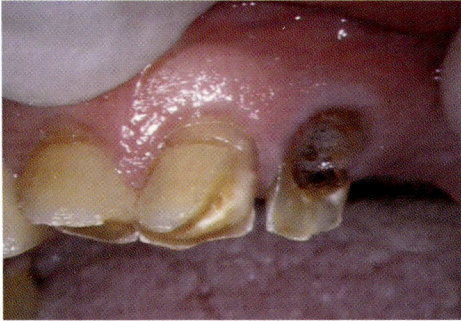

Fig. 1: Pre-op. A medically compromised patient who is on blood thinner medication is presented with a fractured crown at the maxillary left lateral incisor. Palliative treatment is planned to remove the loose crown without injection.

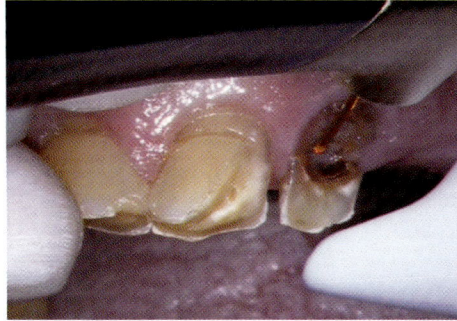

Fig. 2: The laser is used to carefully section the loose crown from the root. A MZ-5 tip is used. The setting is 2.00W, 60% Water, 80% Air, 30 Hz.

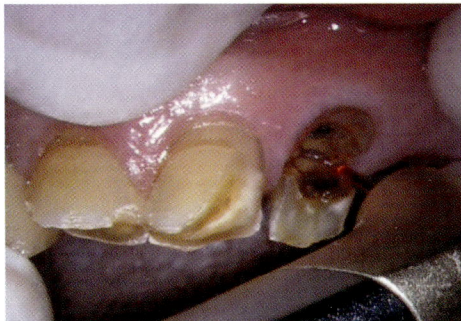

Fig. 3: The laser sectioning the crown moves from the mesial to the distal area.

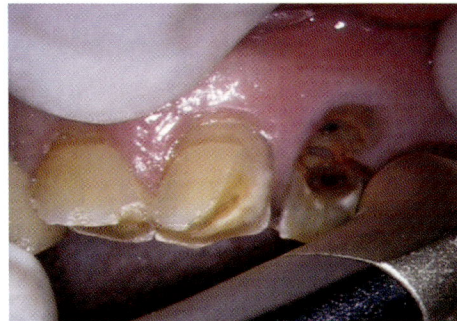

Fig. 4: The sectioning of the crown continues until the crown becomes detached from the root.

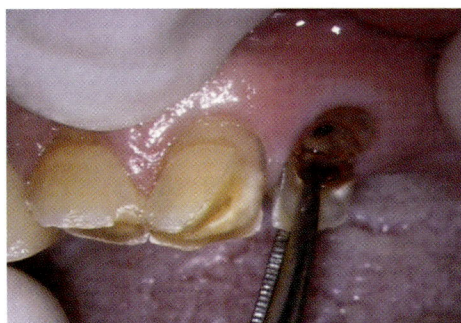

Fig. 5: Removal of the fractured crown is done with a hemostat.

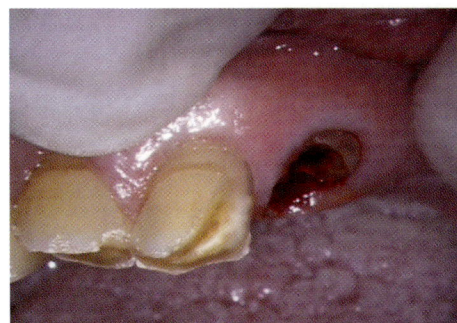

Fig. 6: Some bleeding occurs at the lingual area.

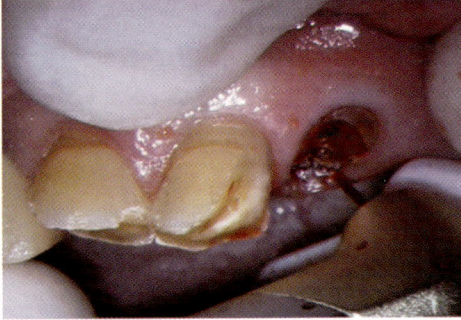

Fig. 7: The laser is used to stop bleeding. The setting is 1.00W, 0% Water, 11% Air, 30 Hz. This is followed by 0.75W, 0% Water, 11% Air, 30 Hz, S mode.

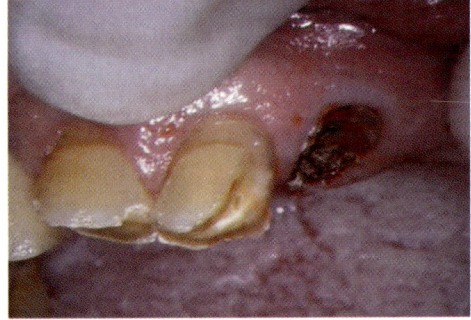

Fig. 8: Completed prep.

Root Canal Therapy with the MD Gold Handpiece

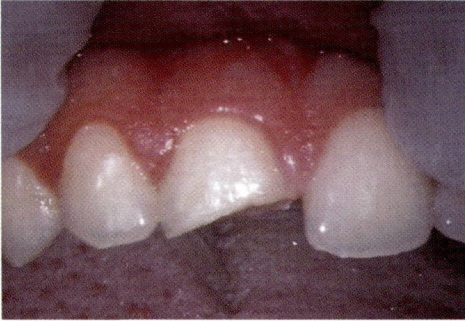

Fig. 1: Pre-op. The maxillary right central incisor is diagnosed to have an irreversible pulpitis due to a traumatic accident that resulted in a fracture of the crown. A root canal therapy is treatment planned.

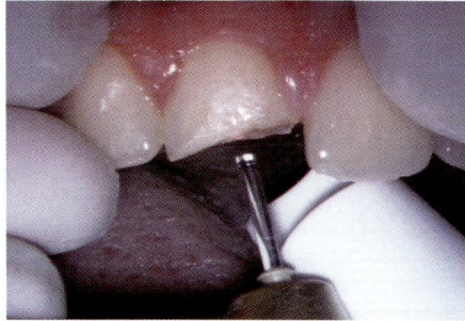

Fig. 2: A MC-12 in the MD Gold Handpiece is used to aim directly at the pulp. The setting is 0.50W, 0% Water, 0% Air, 50 Hz.

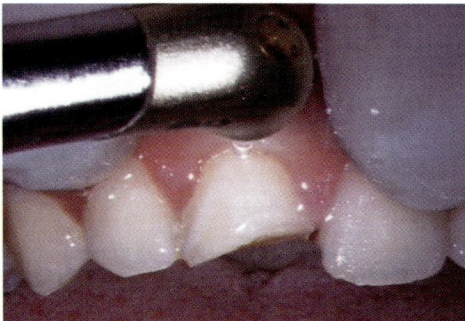

Fig. 3: The MC-12 tip is aimed at the cervical-sulcular area to pre-condition the tooth and periodontal area.

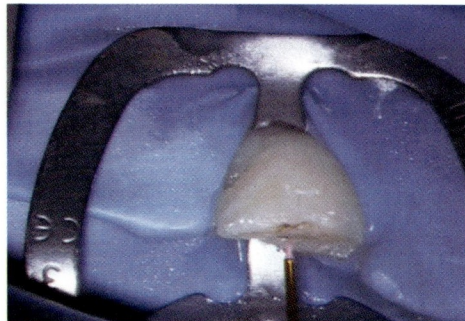

Fig. 4: A rubber dam clamp and rubber dam are placed. A MZ-5 tip is used to ablate and begin access opening into the pulp. The setting is 3.50W, 60% Water, 80% Air, 15 Hz.

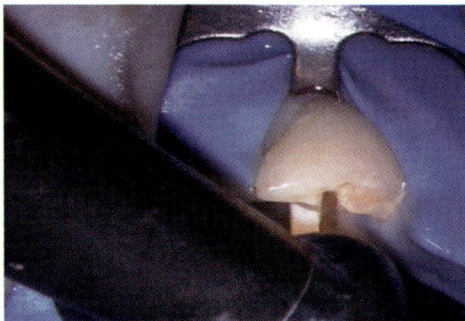

Fig. 5: A #2 high-speed round bur is used to accelerate access opening into the root canal.

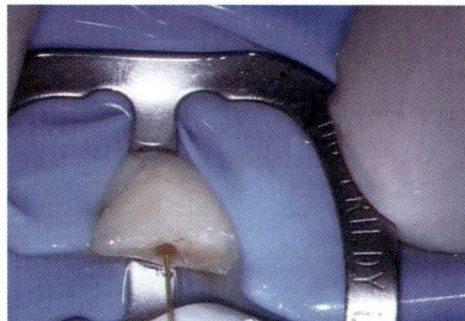

Fig. 6: Direct nerve analgesia is performed with a MZ-2 tip, which slowly move into ½ to 1/3 of the estimated working length. The setting is 0.25-0.75W, 20% Water, 20% Air, 30 Hz.

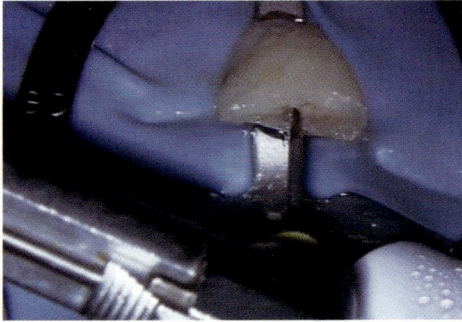

Fig. 7: After the working length is measured by a #15 K-file and an apex locator, a series of Gates Glidden is used to enlarge the opening of the root canal.

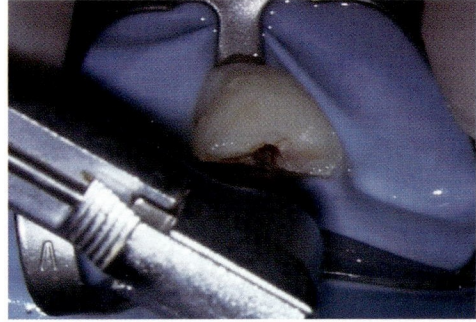

Fig. 8: This is followed by a short series of crown-down nickel-titanium rotary instrumentation to enlarge the root canal to 250µm.

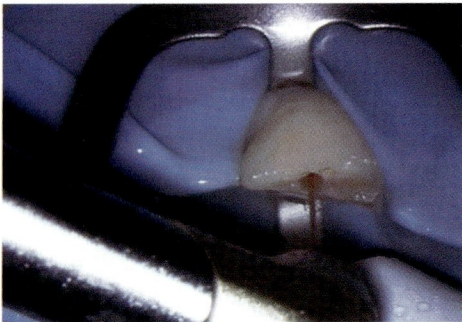

Fig. 9: The MZ-2 is used to clean debride and enlarge the root canal. The setting is 1.50W, 24% Water, 34% Air, 30 Hz.

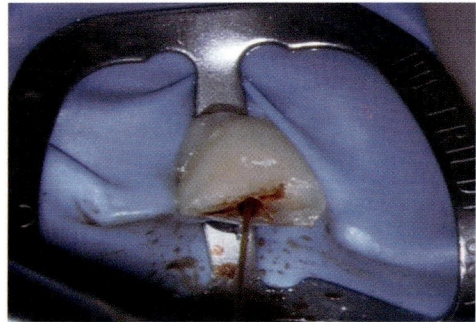

Fig.10: A MZ-3 tip is used to continue cleaning, debridement and enlarging the root canal. The setting is 1.50W, 24% Water, 34% Air, 30 Hz.

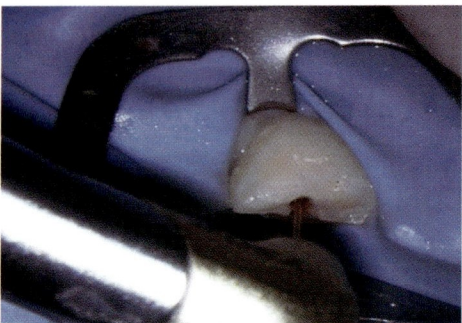

Fig. 11: A MZ-4 tip is used to complete cleaning, debridement and enlarging the root canal. The setting is 1.50W, 24% Water, 34% Air, 30 Hz.

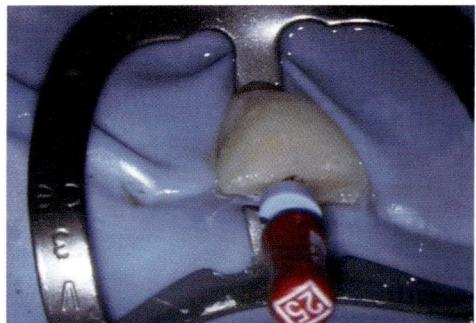

Fig. 12: A #25 K-file is used to check the patency.

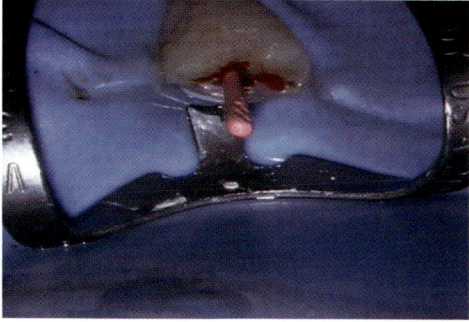

Fig. 13: A master gutta-percha point is tried in.

Torus Removal with the MD Gold Handpiece

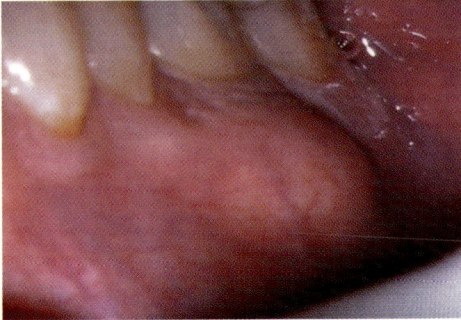

Fig. 1: Pre-op. Bone tori are present at the buccal of mandibular left first and second molars. Patient complains about pain and bleeding from the area during eating. Surgical intervention is indicated.

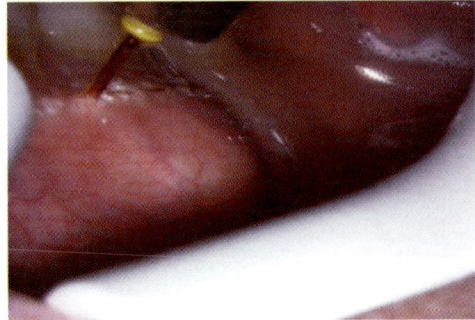

Fig. 2: After profound local anesthesia, the laser is used to make the incision at the mucogingival area for a flap. A MZ-5 tip is used. The setting is 2.25W, 9% Water, 11% Air, 30 Hz.

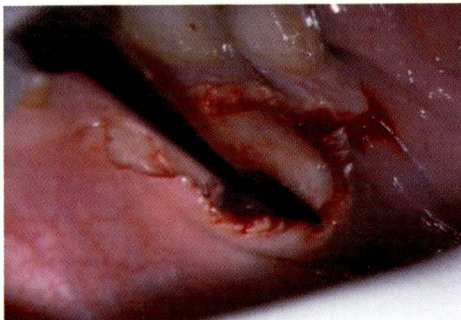

Fig. 3: Mucogingival tissue is retracted to expose the buccal torus.

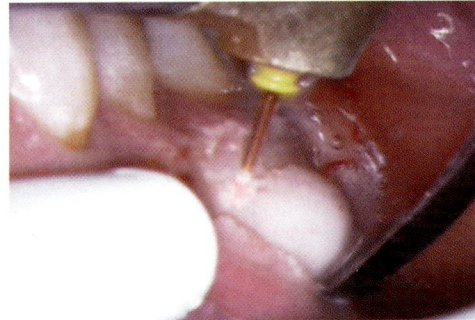

Fig. 4: The MZ-5 tip is used to section the torus from the occlusal aspect. The setting is 6.00W, 75% Water, 90% Air, 20 Hz.

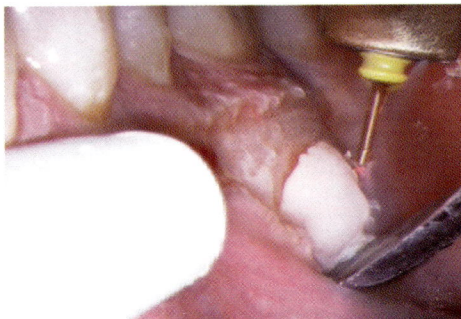

Fig. 5: Vertical cuts are made to fragmentize the torus.

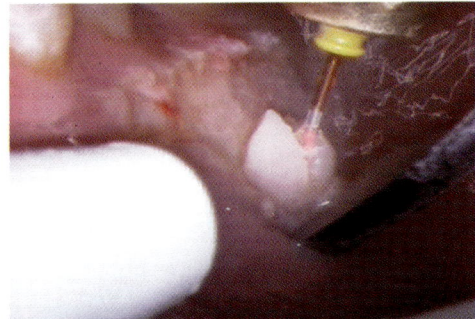

Fig. 6: The torus is removed in fragments.

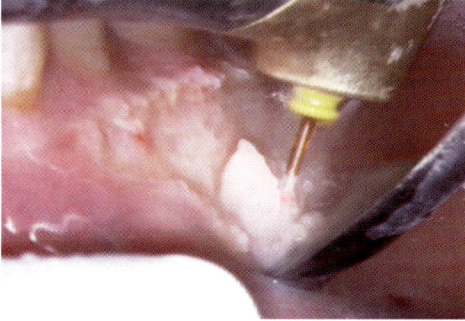

Fig. 7: The torus removal continues until all fragments are removed.

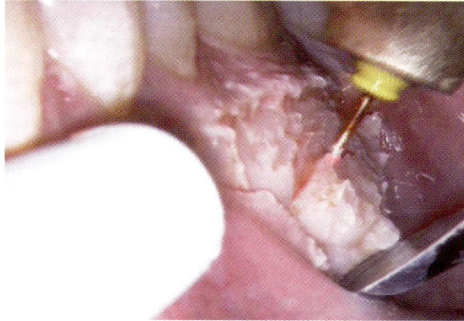

Fig. 8: A rough bone surface is produced from the gross reduction of the torus.

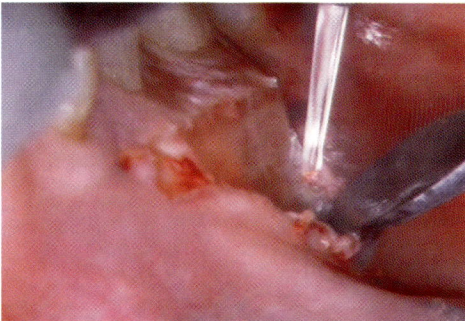

Fig. 9: A MC-3 tip is used to smooth the bone. The setting is 2.00-4.00W, 60% Water, 80% Air, 30 Hz.

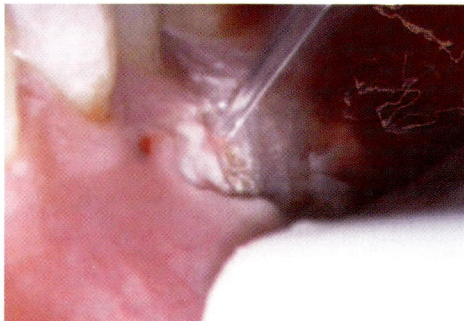

Fig. 10: The smoothing of the bone surface is completed with the setting of 2.00W, 60% Water, 80% Air, 40 Hz.

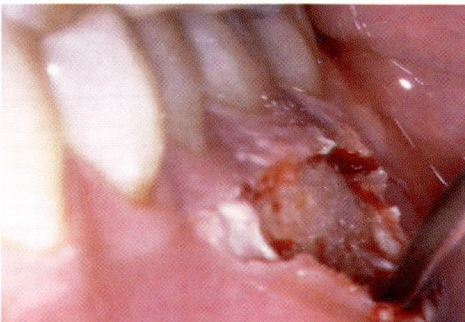

Fig. 11: Bone surface is smoothed before closure.

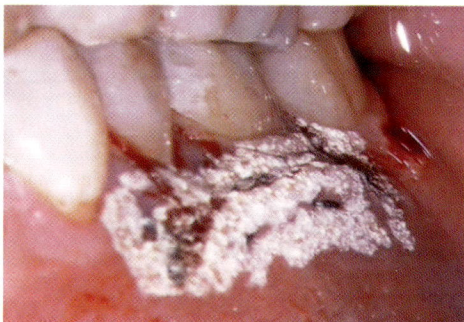

Fig. 12: After suture is placed, a biologic band-aid is performed. A MC-12 tip is used at 1.75W, 0% Water, 11% Air.

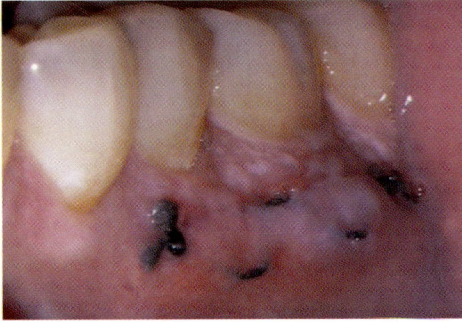

Fig. 13: One week post-op. No complications.

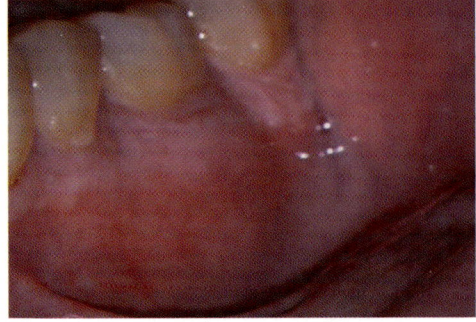

Fig. 14: Two months post-op. No more bleeding, and no pain during eating.

Apicoectomy with the MD Gold Handpiece

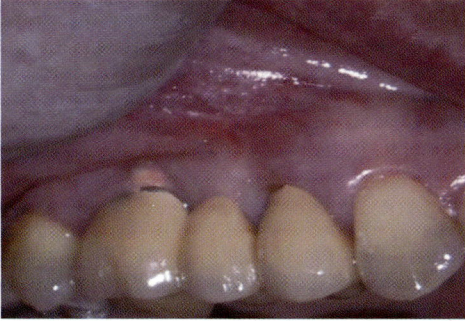

Fig. 1: Pre-op. Reinfection of a root canal is treated on the maxillary right first premolar. A fistula is noted at the apical area.

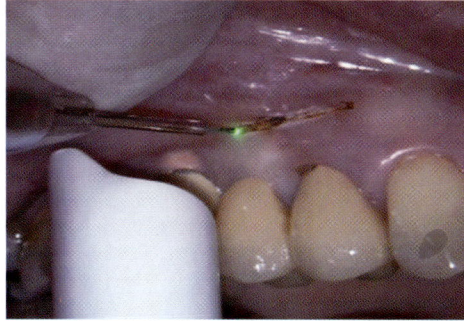

Fig. 2: After profound injection anesthesia is administered, a 940nm diode laser is used to make the incision for a flap at the mucogingival area.

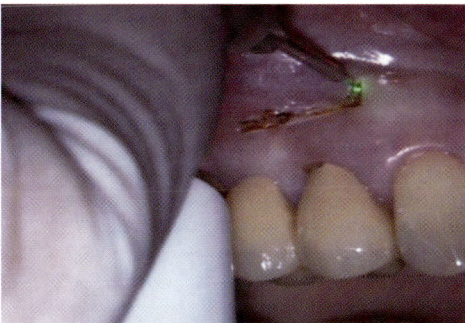

Fig. 3: A trapezoid flap design is used, extending the flap from mesial of the first premolar to the distal of the second premolar.

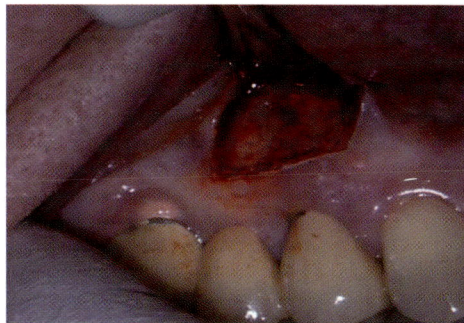

Fig. 4: After the retraction of the flap, the lesion in the apical area of the first premolar is revealed.

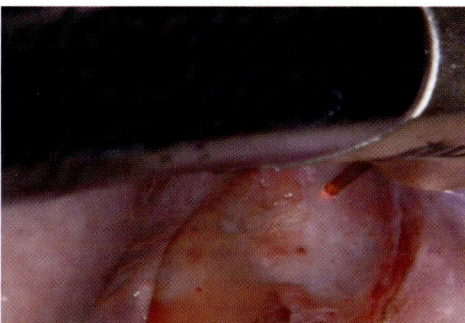

Fig. 5: The Waterlase MD Gold Handpiece is used to ablate bone to reveal the infected root end of the first premolar. The setting is 4.00W, 60% Water, 80% Air, 20 Hz.

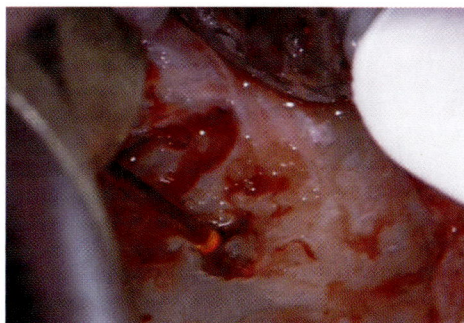

Fig. 6: The laser is used to remove granulation tissue around the root end area. The setting is 2.00W, 7% Water, 11% Air, 30 Hz.

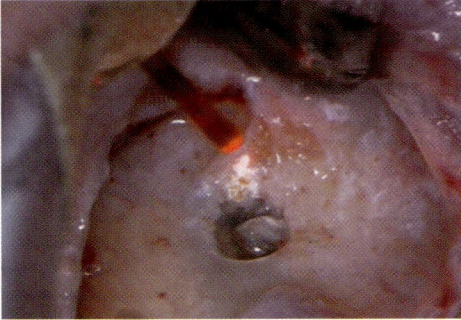

Fig. 7: Granulation in the alveolus bone area is also removed.

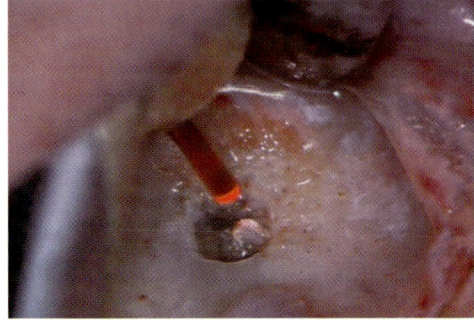

Fig. 8: About 3mm of the root end is sectioned. The setting is 3.00W, 60% Water, 80% Air, 30 Hz.

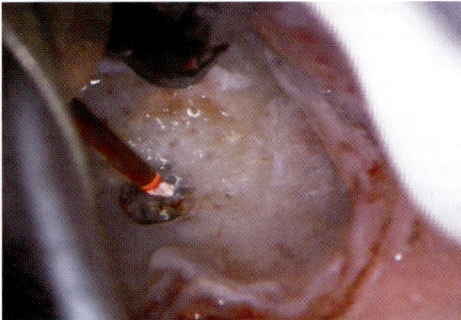

Fig. 9: More granulation tissue is removed from the area behind the root end.

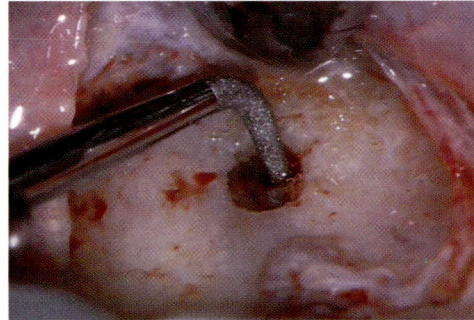

Fig. 10: A surgical endodontic cavitron tip is used to remove gutta percha from the root end.

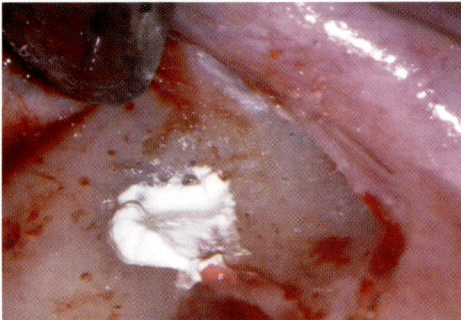

Fig. 11: MTA is placed as a retrofill material.

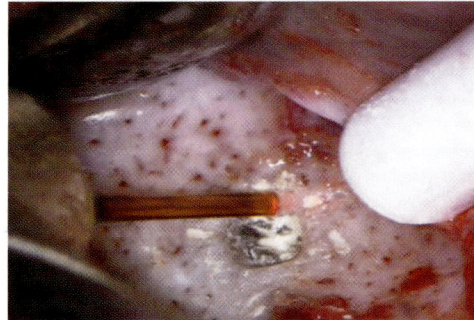

Fig. 12: Before closure, the laser is used to finish debridement. The setting is 2.00W, 60% Water, 80% Air, 30 Hz.

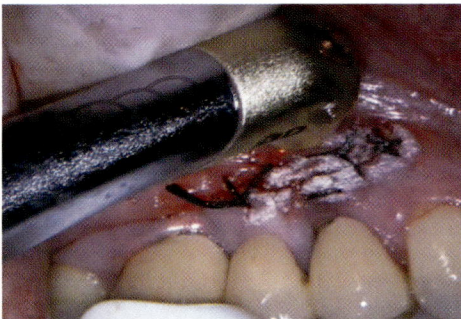

Fig. 13: After suture placement, a laser biologic band-aid is applied. The setting is 1.00W, 0% Water, 11% Air, 30 Hz.

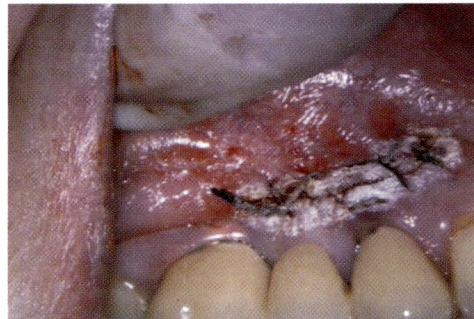

Fig. 14: Post-op.